Nursing Theories

Nursing Theories

BT Basavanthappa MN, PhD

Principal, Govt. College of Nursing,
Fort, Bangalore
PhD Guide (Recognized by INC and Indian Universities)
Examiner for UG, PG and Doctoral Courses in Nursing
Ex-Programme In-charge, IGNOU BSc, Nursing Course

Life Member
Trained Nurses Association of India, New Delhi
Govt. Nurses Association of Karnataka, Bangalore
Academy of Nursing Studies, Hyderabad
United Writers Association of India, Chennai
Nursing Research Society of India, New Delhi

President
RGUHS Nursing Teachers Association, Karnataka

Winner
Bharat Excellence Award and Gold Medal
Vikas Ratan Gold Award
UWA Lifetime Achievement Award

Author
Ten Books on Nursing

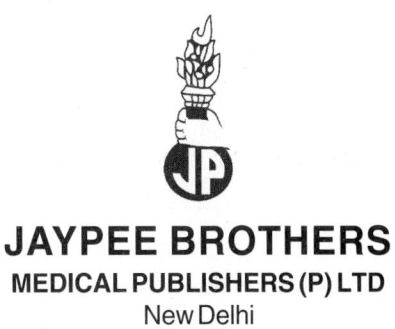

JAYPEE BROTHERS
MEDICAL PUBLISHERS (P) LTD
New Delhi

Published by
Jitendar P Vij
Jaypee Brothers Medical Publishers (P) Ltd
B-3 EMCA House, 23/23B Ansari Road, Daryaganj
New Delhi 110 002, India
Phones: +91-11-23272143, +91-11-23272703, +91-11-23282021, +91-11-23245672,
Rel: 32558559, Fax: +91-11-23276490, +91-11-23245683
e-mail: jaypee@jaypeebrothers.com
Visit our website: www.jaypeebrothers.com

Branches

- 2/B, Akruti Society, Jodhpur Gam Road Satellite
  Ahmedabad 380 015, Phones: +91-079-26926233, Rel: +91-079-32988717,
  Fax: +91-079-26927094, e-mail: jpamdvd@rediffmail.com

- 202 Batavia Chambers, 8 Kumara Krupa Road
  Kumara Park East, **Bangalore** 560 001, Phones: +91-80-22285971, +91-80-22382956,
  Rel: +91-80-32714073, Fax: +91-80-22281761, e-mail: jaypeemedpubbgl@eth.net

- 282 IIIrd Floor, Khaleel Shirazi Estate, Fountain Plaza
  Pantheon Road, **Chennai** 600 008, Phones: +91-44-28193265, +91-44-28194897,
  Rel: +91-44-32972089, Fax: +91-44-28193231, e-mail: jpchen@eth.net

- 4-2-1067/1-3, 1st Floor, Balaji Building, Ramkote Cross Road
  Hyderabad 500 095, Phones: +91-40-66610020, +91-40-24758498, Rel:+91-40-32940929,
  Fax:+91-40-24758499, e-mail: jpmedpub@rediffmail.com

- No. 41/3098, B & B1, Kuruvi Building, St. Vincent Road
  Kochi 682 018, Kerala, Phones: 0484-4036109, +91-0484-2395739, +91-0484-2395740
  e-mail: jpkochi@rediffmail.com

- 1-A Indian Mirror Street, Wellington Square
  Kolkata 700 013, Phones: +91-33-22451926, +91-33-22276404, +91-33-22276415,
  Rel: +91-33-32901926, Fax: +91-33-22456075, e-mail: jpbcal@dataone.in

- 106 Amit Industrial Estate, 61 Dr SS Rao Road
  Near MGM Hospital, Parel, **Mumbai** 400 012, Phones: +91-22-24124863,
  +91-22-24104532, Rel: +91-22-32926896, Fax: +91-22-24160828,
  e-mail: jpmedpub@bom7.vsnl.net.in

- "KAMALPUSHPA" 38, Reshimbag, Opp. Mohota Science College, Umred Road, **Nagpur** 440 009
  (MS), Phones: Rel: 3245220, Fax: 0712-2704275, e-mail: jaypeenagpur@dataone.in

Nursing Theories

© 2007, BT Basavanthappa

All rights reserved. No part of this publication should be reproduced, stored in a retrieval system, or transmitted in any form or by any means: electronic, mechanical, photocopying, recording, or otherwise, without the prior written permission of the author and the publisher.

> This book has been published in good faith that the material provided by author is original. Every effort is made to ensure accuracy of material, but the publisher, printer and author will not be held responsible for any inadvertent error(s). In case of any dispute, all legal matters are to be settled under Delhi jurisdiction only.

First Edition: **2007**
ISBN 81-8061-963-X
Typeset at   JPBMP typesetting unit
Printed at   Sanat Printers, Kundli.

Dedicated

to

My Ever Loving Parents

and

My Dear Students of

Noble Nursing Profession

Preface

It gives me an immense pleasure and satisfaction to introduce and present this book *Nursing Theories* to our honorable Nursing community. I have been very much pleased with utilization of my earlier nine books; namely, Community Heath Nursing, Medical Surgical Nursing, Pediatric/Child Health Nursing, Midwifery and Reproductive Nursing, Fundamentals of Nursing, Nursing Education, Nursing Administration and Nursing Research.

In the past nursing was based on principles borrowed from the physical and social sciences and other disciplines. Today, however, there is a body of knowledge that is uniquely nursing, while this was not always same, amount of investigation and analysis of nursing care has expanded rapidly in recent years. Nursing is no longer based on task orientation, situation or trial and error but it increasingly relies on researcher as a basis for practice; now we have several theoretical models of nursing which have been developed by our own nursing theorists.

This book is a synthesis and extension of what we believe that theoretical models now serve a newer and more important role within nursing. Nursing theories and model have come to be understood on the embodiment of nursing philosophies, presenting nursing beliefs understanding and purposes it has been believed that theoretical models are excellent and tangible sources of the perspective of nursing across time. Certainly some of the models serve as sources for extensive programmes of research, as curriculum organizers and as templates for practice. It has been suggested that the nursing perspectives may be used to guide knowledge development within nursing. Since it fulfils one of the criteria of the profession that there is special body of knowledge which continuously enlarges the body of knowledge uses and improves its techniques of education and service by the use of scientific method to fulfil the purpose. I have tried my level best to select some of the important contributions of nurse theorists and put it in an understandable language so that every one will be aware and acquainted with knowledge of nursing theories, which help them in nursing practice, nursing education and nursing research.

When Nursing develops its own theory, validates research knowledge in the practice setting and relies on this knowledge to direct nursing practice, it will be recognized as an independent autonomous profession.

I hope this book will continue to serve not only nursing student of all levels for whom it is intended but also nursing teachers and practitioners. Theory improves nursing practice by describing, explaining, predicting and controlling phenomena of interest to nurses. Theory allows professional autonomy by guiding the practice, education and research functions of the profession. The study of theory helps develop analytical skills, challenges, thinking and clarifying values and assumptions.

I am aware of manifold reasons, error might be crept in and shall feel oblige, if such errors are brought to my notice. I sincerely welcome constructive criticism from readers, that would help me to enrich myself and suggestions will be incorporated in the next edition.

BT Basavanthappa

Acknowledgements

I owe a great deal of thanks to many who encouraged and supported me with their time and encouragement throughout.

- Shri G Basavannappa, Formerly, Minister and presently, MLA of Karnataka for having initiated and supported me to take up this "Noble Nursing Profession" as my career.

- Dr (Mrs) Manjula K Vasundhra, Formerly, Professor and HOD of Community Medicine, Bangalore Medical College, who continuously encouraged me to write texts in the field of Nursing since nursing is a major force in Medical and Health Services.

- My Father Shri Thukkappa, who continues his grace for the progress of my career and all-round development of my personality for the welfare of the community.

- My Mother Smt Hanumanthamma, who continue to be a bright spot in the lives of all who knew her and whose grace gave me strength to progress of my life.

- My Wife Smt Lalitha, who gives meaning to my life in so many ways. She is the one whose encouragement keeps me motivated, whose support gives me strength and whose gentleness gives me comfort.

- My lovely children BB Mahesh and BB Gaanashree, for all the joy they provided me and all the hope that they instill me and who bare with patient throughout my works of the nursing texts. They keep me young at heart.

- Finally, my warmest appreciation goes to M/s Jaypee Brothers Medical Publishers (P) Ltd, New Delhi, for sharing my vision for this book and giving me the chance to turn vision into reality.

Contents

1. Introduction to Theory 1
2. Nightingale's Environment Model 40
3. Abdellah's Typology of 21 Problems 52
4. Henderson's Unique Function of Nurses 61
5. Orem's Self-care Theory 72
6. Hall's Core, Care and Cure Models 86
7. Watson's Philosophy and Science on Caring 96
8. Peplau's Interpersonal Relations Theory 109
9. Orlando's Nursing Process Theory 121
10. Wiedenbach's Helping Art of Clinical Nursing 130
11. King's Theory of Goal Attainment 147
12. Paterson and Zderad Theory of Humanistic Nursing 169
13. Erikson, Tomlin, Mary Ann's Theory of Modelling and Role Modelling 179
14. Boykin and Schoenhofer Theory of Nursing as Caring 186
15. Johnson's Behavioural System Model 190
16. Roy's Adaptation Model 205
17. Neuman's Systems Model 225
18. Levine's Four Conservation Principles 242
19. Leininger's Cultural Care Theory 257
20. Rogers' Science of Unitary Human Beings 273
21. Newman's Theory of Health 286
22. Fitzpatrick's Rhythm Model 298

23. Travelbee's Human-to-Human Relationships 304
24. Benner's Excellence and Power in Clinical Nursing Practice 313
25. Mercer's Theory in Maternal Role Attainment 327
26. Adam's Conceptual Model on Nursing 337
27. Parse's Man-Living-Health Theory 348
28. Joan Riehl's Symbolic Interactionism 366
29. Barnard's Parent-child Interaction Model 375
30. Pender's Health Promotion Model 384
31. Other Theories 389
    Index *401*

Chapter 1

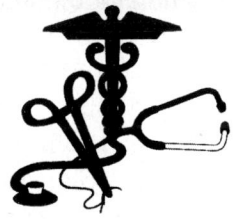

Introduction to Theory

The term "theory" is used in many ways. For example, Nursing teachers and students use the term "theory" to refer to the content covered in classroom, as opposed to the actual practice of performing nursing activities. Sometimes the term "theory" is used to refer to someone's hunches or ideas as in "My theory is that if I postpone cleaning my room, long enough, my mother will clean it for me", or "My theory is not to tell lie or not to bluff any body", etc. Whatever the usages the term, "theory" almost always connoted an abstraction or generalization.

DEFINITIONS OF THEORY

Scientists generally use the term "theory" in a precise way, i.e. theory has always been defined in a number of ways as given below.

- "A theory is a statement that purports to account for or characterize some phenomenon" and that "it pulls out the salient parts of a phenomenon so that one can separate the critical and necessary factors for relationships, from the accidental and unessential factors or relationships" (Barnum 1990).

- "Theory is a systematic abstraction of reality that serves some purpose (Chinn and Kramer 1991). They describe each part of the definition, i.e. **systematic** implies a specific organizational pattern, **abstraction** means that theory is a representation of reality and **purposes** include description, explanation, and prediction of phenomena and control of some reality."

- "Theory enables to explain a maximum number of observable relationships, by setting limits on "What question to ask and what methods to use to pursue answers to the questions" (Meleis 1985).

- "A theory is a set of interrelated constructs (concepts adapted for a scientific purpose), definitions, and prepositions that present a systematic view of phenomena by specifying relations among variables, with the purpose of explaining and predicting the phenomena" (Kerlinger 1986). This definition takes a basic view of science, that development of a general explanation about natural phenomena via theories.

- Theory is a set of interrelated concepts, definitions and propositions that present a systematic way of viewing facts/events by specifying relations among variables, with the purpose of explaining and predicting the fact or event (Kerlinger 1973).

The key ideas of this definition are, interrelation of concepts, propositions specifying relations among the variables and stated purposes of explaining or predicting facts or events. This definition states that a theory suggests a direction in how to view facts and events. For example, Nightingale proposed a beneficial relationship between fresh air and health.

- Theory is a "Creative and rigorous structuring of ideas that project a tentative, purposeful and systematic view of phenomena (Chinn and Kramer 1991).

This definition adds additional element, i.e. focus on the tentative nature of theory. It says that theories cannot be equated with scientific laws. Laws are the basis of natural science. Nursing is a human science. The rigour and objectivity of the laboratory are both inappropriate and impossible to duplicate.

- A theory can be defined as an organizing statement about abstract concepts that gives them meaning in relation to the real world. Theories describe, explain or predict relationships among abstract concepts. Abstract concepts are mental images of reality; they may be highly abstract and non-observable, such as intelligence, or relatively concrete and directly measurable, such as caring behaviour. Theories are linked to the real world through definitions that specify how concepts will be known, experienced, observed and measured. Theories guide decision making by providing the supporting conceptualisation for the study such as "significance of the problem, background, and problem definition or statement of the problem (Phillips, 1986). Thus, theory is an abstract generalization that presents a systematic explanation about the relationships among phenomena. Theories embody principles for explaining, predicting and controlling phenomena. So theory construction and testing are intimately related to the advancement of scientific knowledge, and it may even be claimed that theory is the ultimate goal of science. Theoretical and conceptual systems represent the highest and most advanced efforts of humans to understand the complexities of the world in which they live.

The ideal of theory carries varying conceptualisations within and outside the discipline of nursing. Belief about the nature of theory arise in part from the various fields of inquiry from which nursing knowledge is developed. Some nursing theorists come from traditions in which the ideal theory is logically linked sets of confirmed hypothesis. Others view theory as loosely connected hypothetic conjectures. Still others think of theory as philosophically based sets of belief and values about human nature and action. As a result, the nursing literature contains for theory, but this diversity serves to stimulate further understanding and development of theory. The following definitions in the nursing literature emphasize important dimensions of theory.

- "Theory is a logically interconnected set of confirmed hypotheses" (McKay 1969).

This definition implies a specific form of expression based on rules of logic. It also requires that hypotheses are tested and confirmed by using methods of research to qualify as a theory.

- "Theory is a conceptual system of framework invented to some purpose" (Dickoff and James, 1963). In this definition, the purpose for which a theory is created is emphasized. The term **invented** implies a creative purpose.
- "Theory is an imaginative grouping of knowledge, ideas, and experience that are represented symbolically and seek to illuminate a given phenomenon" (Watson, 1985). Here creativity again emphasized, but the purpose for which theory is created shifts away from a specific purpose to the aim of enhancing understanding of a given phenomenon.
- "Theory is a conceptual and pragmatic principle forming a general frame of reference for a field of inquiry" (Ellis, 1968). This definition implies that theory provides a philosophic view that guides inquiry in a discipline and also that theory serves a pragmatic or practical purpose for the discipline.

From the above definition, all theory comprises a creative and rigourous structuring of ideas. The ideas are structured as concepts that are represented by word symbols. For theory to project a systematic view of phenomena, the concepts contained within the theory must be conveyed within the relationship statement and defined within the context of the theory. The theorists created a language and structure that impart the theory for some reason. The purpose may take many forms. Theory is tentative and thus is grounded in assumptions, value choices and the creative and imaginative judgement of the theorist. Therefore, "theory is a creative, rigorous structuring of ideas that projects a tentative, purposeful and systemic view of phenomena. Theories are general explanations which scholars use to explain, predict, control and understand commonly occurring events. Theory is defined as a "set of propositions used to describe, explain, predict and control of events" in which

- Set: a group of circumstances, situations, and so on, joined and treated as a whole. For example, negative number is treated as set in mathematics.
- Propositions, statements about how two or more concepts are related, e.g. heart rate increase as anxiety increases.
- Concept. Abstract classification of data, e.g. 'temperature' increases.
- Describe: to tell about in detail.
- Explain: to offer reason for
- Predict: to foretell
- Control: to exercise a regulating influence over.
- Phenomenon: an occurrence or incident; event.

PURPOSES OF THEORY

The overall purpose of theory is to make scientific finding meaningful and generalizable. Theories allow scientists to knit together observations and facts into an orderly system. They are efficient, mechanises for drawing together and summarizing accumulated facts from separate and isolated investigations. The linkage of findings into a coherent structure makes the body of accumulated knowledge more accessible, and thus more useful both to practitioners who seek to implement findings and to researchers who seek to extend the knowledge base, in addition to summarizing, theories serve to explain scientific findings. Theory guides the scientists understanding of not only the 'what' of natural phenomena but also the 'why' of that occurrence. The power of theories to explain, lies in their specification of which variables are related to one another and what the nature of that relationship is. Finally theories help stimulate research and the extension of knowledge by providing both direction and impetus. On the basis of theory scientists draw inferences (formulate hypothesis) about what will occur in specific situations. These hypotheses are then subject to empirical testing in research studies. Theories thus serve as a spring board for scientific advances.

Theories provide a method of classifying and organizing data in a logical and meaningful manner. It is important to remember that theory is an explanation that has not yet been disapproved. For example, Einstein's theory of relativity, which states that matter and energy are equivalent and form the basis for nuclear energy and that space and time are relative rather than absolute concepts (It is good working definition of theory).

According to the above definitions, there are four functions of theory—i.e. description, explanation, prediction and control—represents a different phase of theory development. The perfect theory would do all four things well. However, no perfect theories exist in any discipline. Because science is evolving and because humans are fallible, that is liable to make mistakes. Theories are always changing at any given point of time. In a given area of study, theories in all stages of development can be found. This is certainly true in Nursing.

As a science, Nursing is in its infancy. Professional nurses are aware of this and conscious of the need for both nursing theory development and theory-based practice. As nursing comes of age, not only as a practice discipline but also as a scholarly discipline, there will be increasing interest in delineating the theory base for nursing. Some believe that theory development is the most crucial task facing nursing (Chinn and Jacobs 1978).

There are three reasons for this interest in theory as given below:

1. Firstly, one criterion for profession is a distinct body of knowledge upon which practice is based. There has been interest in identifying a body of nursing knowledge that is essential to professional nursing practice. Theory development contributes to knowledge building and is seen as a means of establishing nursing as a profession.

2. Secondly, commitment to practice based on sound, reliable knowledge is intrinsically valuable to nursing. That is to say, knowledge is desirable by its very nature. The growth and enrichment of theory in and of itself is an important goal for nursing, as a scholarly discipline to pursue.

3. And thirdly, theory is useful. Nursing practice settings are complex and the amount of data available to nurses is virtually endless. Nurses must analyse a tremendous amount of information about each patient and decide what to do. If a theory helps practising nurses categorize

and understand what is going on in nursing practice, if it helps them predict patient's responses to nursing care, and if it is helpful in clinical decision making it is useful as a guide to practice.

THE NATURE OF THEORY

Concepts are the basic ingredients of a theory. Examples of nursing concepts are health, interaction, and adaptation. Theories also consist of a set of statements or propositions, each of which indicates a relationship. Relationships are denoted by such phrases as "is associated with," "varies directly with," or "is contingent upon." In theories the propositions must form a logical interrelated deductive system.

This means that the theory must provide a mechanism for logically arriving at new statements from the original propositions.

A simple illustration is classical learning theory, also referred to as the theory of reinforcement. According to this theory, behaviour that is reinforced (i.e. that is rewarded) will tend to be repeated and therefore, learned. This theory consists of broad concepts (reinforcement and learning) and a proposition stating the relationship between those concepts. Furthermore, the proposition readily lends itself to deductive hypothesis generation. For example, if the theory of reinforcement is valid, then we could deduce that hyperactive children who are praised or rewarded when they are engaged in quiet play will exhibit less acting-out behaviours than similar children who are not praised. Or we could deduce that elderly nursing home residents who are praised or given a reward for self-grooming activities will be more likely than others to care for their appearance and personal hygiene. Both of these predictions, as well as many others based on the theory of reinforcement, could then be tested in a research investigation.

Two additional nature of theories should be emphasized. The first concerns their origin. Theories are not discovered by scientists; they are created and invented by them. The building of a theory depends not only on the observable facts in out environment but also on the scientist's ingenuity in pulling those facts together and making sense of them. Thus, theory construction is a creative and intellectual enterprise that can be engaged in by anyone with sufficient imagination. But imagination alone is not an adequate qualification; theories must be congruent with the realities of the world around us and with existing knowledge.

The second concerns to the tentative nature of theories. It cannot be stressed too strongly that a theory can never be proven or confirmed. A theory represents a scientist's best efforts to describe and explain phenomena; today's successful theory may be relegated to tomorrow's intellectual garbage dump. This may happen if new evidence or observations disprove or discredit a theory that previously had some support. It is also possible that a new theoretical system can integrate new observations with the observations that the old theory made and result in a more parsimonious explanation of some phenomena. Furthermore, the theories that are not congruent with a culture's values and philosophical orientation may be discredited. This link between theory and values may surprise those who think that science is completely objective. It should be remembered, however, that theories are deliberately invented by human; they can, thus, never be freed totally from the human perspective, which is amenable to change over time. For example, numerous theories, such as psychoanalytic theory, that had widespread support for decades have come to be challenged by changes in society's views about the roles of women. In sum, no theory, no matter what its subject matter, can ever be considered final and verified. There always remains the possibility that a theory will be modified or discarded.

CHARACTERISTICS OF A THEORY

Torres (1990) presented the following characteristics of a theory.

1. *Theories can interrelated concepts in such a way as to create a different way of looking at a particular phenomenon.*

   Theories are constructed from concepts, which are mental images representing reality. Theory must identify more than one concept and then the relationship between these concepts must be clear. These concepts need to be explicitly defined so that one can picture the events and experiences that the theory is designed to describe, explain or predict. For example, needs-oriented theorist must identify the concepts of "Self-care deficit and nursing." The concept of self-care deficit may be described as a client who experiences an inability to perform health promotion activities. Nursing may be defined in terms of actions that can be taken to assist the client to perform health promotions activities. Theories guide practice by directing the nurse to look for needs or deficits that the client may be experiencing.

2. *Theories must be logical in nature.*

   Logic is an orderly reasoning. Interrelationship of concepts must be sequential and consistently used within the theory. There should not be any contradictions between the definitions, of concepts, their relationships within the theory and the goals of the theory. These relationships and goals should flow directly from the theoretical assumptions. For example, if "man-universe" is defined to be continuous interaction, this concept must be consistent with all parts of the theory, from the assumptions to the practice methodology.

3. *Theories should be relatively simple yet generalizable.*

   A theory may be defined as "tight" or "parsimonious," if it is stated in most simple terms possible but at the same time describes, explains, or predicts wide range of possible experiences in nursing practice. A theory of communication can be explained simply and generalized to all person-to-person interaction would be considered parsimonious.

4. *Theories can be the bases for hypotheses that can be tested or for theory to be expanded.*
   - **Quantitative** research tests hypotheses in clinical practice and uses statistical analysis to arrive at findings. These findings represent the testing of the precision of the theory in describing, explaining or predicting reality.
   - **Qualitative** research expands theory by using different research methodology that focuses on the lived experiences of persons. These findings represent determining. Identifying and exploring themes in the reality lived by the persons who participate in the studies.

5. *Theories contribute to and assist in increasing the general body of knowledge within the discipline through the research implemented to validate them.*

   Theories that can be tested, whether by quantitative or qualitative research methods, contribute to the general body of knowledge of discipline of nursing. Validation of the theories enhances the ability of the nurse to describe, predict or control of nursing practice.

6. *Theories can be used by practitioners to guide and improve their practice.*

   One of the most significant characteristics of a theory is its usefulness to the practitioner. Theories guide practice by describing, explaining, or predicting events in clinical practice.

7. *Theories must be consistent with other validated theories, laws, and principles but will leave open unanswered questions that need to be investigated.*

   Logic of theories and their assumptions must be based on underlying laws, previously validated knowledge, and humanitarian values that are generally accepted as good and right, however, tentative nature of theory continues to raise questions that challenge aspects or knowledge that have not yet been challenged.

Analysis and Evaluation of Theory

There is a variety of methods for analysing and evaluating nursing theories. Analysis gather, refers to examining the content of the theory, whereas evaluation refers to a critique or judgement about the theory.

Chinn and Kramer (1991) suggested that one should consider the following four criteria for analysis and evaluation of theory.

- Clarity (semantic and structural)
- Simplicity
- Generality
- Empirical applicability and
- Consequences (derivable)

   i. *Clarity*: Semantic and structural clarity and consistency are important. To assess these, one should identify the major concepts and subconcepts and identify definitions for them. Words should be invented only if necessary and they should be carefully defined. Sometimes, words have multiple and competing meanings within and across discipline. Therefore words should be borrowed cautiously and defined carefully. Diagrams and examples may provide more clarity and should be consistent. The logical development should be clear and assumption should be consistent with theory's goals.

   ii. *Simplicity*: In nursing, practitioners needs simple theory to guide practice. That a theory should be maximally comprehensive and concrete, and it should do so with the fewest concepts and the simplest relations of concepts and simply counting the number of concepts is not sufficient, but most useful theory provides the greatest sense of understanding.

   iii. *Generality*: To determine generality of theory, the scope of concepts and goals within the theory are examined. The more limited the concepts and goals the less general the theory.

   iv. *Empirical precision/applicability*: Empirical precision is linked to the testability and ultimate use of a theory and refers to the extent that the defined concepts are grounded in observable reality. In theory there should be match between theoretical claims and the empirical evidence. Theories should be clearly recognized as tentative and hypothetical. If the theory cannot generate hypothesis, it is not useful to anyone and does not add to the body of knowledge. So, testability of the theory can be sacrificed in favour of scope, complexity and clinical usefulness. If research, theory, and practice are meaningfully related, then theory in nursing should lend itself to research testing, and research testing should guide nursing practice.

v. *Derivable consequences*: Nursing theory ought to guide research and practice, new ideas, and differentiate the focus of nursing from other professions. Theories should reveal what knowledge nurses must and should spend time pursuing. It is essential for nursing theory to develop and guide practice. The nursing profession should make use of existing theory to predict certain outcomes and control events in such a way that desired outcomes are achieved.

Fawcett (1989) differentiates between analysis and evaluation. She developed this framework of analysis and evaluation of conceptual models but it can readily be applied to theories.

- For analysis, she proposes a consideration of the historical evolution of the theory the approach to model development, content and source of concern.
- For evaluation, she proposes evaluation of explicitness of the assumption, degree of competitiveness of content, logical congruences, ability of the model to test and generate hypothesis, how much the model contributes to nursing knowledge development and social conditions.

Barnum (1990) proposes evaluative criteria for internal criticism (internal construction) and external criticism (the theory and its relationship to people, nursing and health).

- The criteria for internal criticism are clarity, consistency, adequacy, logical development and levels of theory development.
- The criteria for external criticism are reality convergence, utility.

Meleis (1991) suggests a model that defines evaluation as encompassing description, analysis, critique, and testing.

THEORY OF STRUCTURE AND DEVELOPMENT

A theory is a set of concepts, definitions, and propositions that project a systematic view of phenomena by designing specific interrelationships among concepts for purposes of describing, exploring, explaining and predicting. The purpose of scientific theory is to describe, explore and predict a part of the empirical world. The same purpose can be ascribed to nursing theory.

To identify nursing theory in its various stages of development, it is necessary to understand the components parts of theory and the steps through which theory is developed.

- A *concept* is a complex mental formulation of object, property of event that is derived from individual perceptual experience. It is an idea, a mental image, or generalization formed and developed in the mind. Concepts may be abstract or concrete. Abstract concepts are completely independent of time or place, for example,

temperature. A concrete concept is specific to time and place, for example body temperature.
- *Definitions* are the statements of the meaning of the word, phrase of term. Theoretical definitions convey the general meaning of the concept in a manner that fits the theory and operational definitions specify "the activities of operations" necessary to measure a construct or a variable. Constructs are complex concepts.
- *Propositions* are theorems or statements derived from axioms. Axioms are a basic set of statements each independent of the others (they say different things) from which all statements of the theory may be logically derived. The proposition often used interchangeably with hypothesis to mean any idea or hunch that is prescribed in the form of a scientific statement, thus describe a relation between two or more concepts.
- A *phenomenon* is any occurrence or fact that is directly perceptible by senses. It is in reality on what exists in the real world.

Theory development is a process that primarily involves induction, deduction and retroduction.
- *Induction* is a form of reasoning that moves from the specific to the general. In inductive logic, a series of particulars is combined into a larger who or set of things. In inductive research, particular events are observed and analysed as a basis for formulating general theoretical statements, often called grounded theory.' This is a research is theory approach.
- *Deduction* is a form of logical reasoning that progresses from general to specific. This process involves a sequence of theoretical statements derived from few general statements or axioms. Two or more relational statements are used to draw a conclusion. Abstract theoretical relationships are used to draw a conclusion. Abstract theoretical relationships are used to derive specific empirical hypothesis. This is a theory to research approach.
- *Retroduction* combines induction and deduction.
- Research is application of systematic methods to obtain reliable and valid knowledge and to test impirical reality. Research may generate theory with an inductive approach or test it a deductive approach.

STEPS OF THEORY DEVELOPMENT

According to Dickoff, James and Weidenbach (1968) theory building is practice and is refined through research, and then is returned to practice. After elaboration on their work as well as on the work of Jacox (1974) the steps of theory development can be seen as follows:

Criticism or Fault Finding

Criticism is the result of concern. One does not bother to criticize something about which one is indifferent. A criticism serves to articulate a belief that something is amiss and brings to awareness one or more salient features of the situation. Frequently the process is aborted at this initial step, and movement to a more constructive reaction is never achieved.

Statement of the Problem

A desire to improve the situation results in a delineation of the problem with a refinement of the criticism to the point of being articulate about the defect in the situation. Delineation of the problem involves following steps.

Concept Identification

A concept is a term that has been given an operational meaning. Key ideas, thoughts, and words in a problem become concepts that require further exploration and delineation to create a precise meaning. Concepts are individual, idiosyncratic impression with distinguishing attributes that can be related within a framework. Thus attributes of concepts can be divided into categories such as values, number, form, dominance, size and colour. Jacox described concepts on the abstract representation of reality that indicate the subject matter of theory. Constructs are more complex entities constructed of concepts that are directly or indirectly observable.

Concepts are traditionally defined as a class of stimuli having common characteristics but in reality they are impressions individual and idiosyncratic, that cause factors to be related in a framework—a framework into which the person expresses experience, interpretations and emotional component, so that the very stimuli are distorted, e.g. anaemia patient.

Concept can be conjunctive, disjunctive, or relative in nature. In **conjunctive** concepts, several similar values are jointly present, e.g. Anaemias have pale and other signs and symptoms similar as hen face, fatigue, cold, weakness, etc.

Disjunctive are those in which one or more attributes do not match, e.g. anaemic patient also have other than similar signs and symptoms. Relational concepts clearly define the relationship between two attributes such as distance and direction, e.g. cause and effect. In nursing one might sum these up as conjunctive or comparative concepts, disjunctive or contrasting concepts, need relational or cause and effect concepts.

Proposition or Principle Formulation

A statement of generalization called as proposition or principle relates two or more concepts or facts, there by serving to reduce the complexity of the problem. The statement of relationship between two or more concepts becomes a rule for generalizations and is called a principle. For example, if the patient haemorrhages and the blood volume decreases, the heart rate will increase. The relationship between the concepts of haemorrhage, blood volume and heart rate is combined into one if, then principle is formulated.

Theory Construction

The product of linking, propositions or principles deductively in theory, a conceptual framework designed to show interrelationships. Theory construction, then, is the systematic hierarchical arrangement of propositions. Rules of generalisation provide one type of guide for prediction of outcome and thus serve as guide to action. Theory is existing on four levels, i.e.
- Factor-isolating
- Factor-relating
- Situation-relating
- Situation-producing (Prescriptive theory)

Each of these levels of theory presupposes lower-level supporting theories. Prescriptive theory has the essential ingredients of justifiable goal, a prescription of activity to achieve that goal, and a number of component parts which are defined as follows:

a. Agency: the performer of the action.
b. Patience: the recipient of the action.
c. Framework: the context of the situation.
d. Terminus: the end point of the activity.
e. Procedure: the protocol for the activity.
f. Dynamics: the type and amount of energy utilized.

By the systematic organization of proposition about these attributes, prescriptive theory may be constructed utilizing the process of induction and deduction. To clarify the role of theory in nursing practice further. Jacox (1974) stated that theory in one field may be utilized as a model in another field if the elements of the theory behave in the same way in both fields. Kaplan (1964) identified an empirical theoretical continuum to theory that any given theory can be located at some point on the continuum where it will have some reference of reality. Theory may be clarified with the use of models.

Validation of Theory

Once developed, theory can serve as a guide for:
- Collection of facts.
- Search for new knowledge.
- Explanation of the nature of the phenomena being studied.
- Further action.

The professional nurse can put theory to the same use. She/he can and should develop and use theory to collect facts, seek new knowledge, explain phenomena and direct nursing action. With such use of theory, the nurse functions at a professional level as opposed to becoming the heir to routines born of habit; however, theory can be taken one more step. By testing theory in practice, theory can be validated and then be considered to be doctrine or essential truth. Validation of theory is the endpoint of theory and the beginning of scientific fact that can be utilized in nursing practice.

To sum up the steps in development of theory are as follows:
1. Articulation of criticism.
2. Statement of the problem through.
   - Identification of the concepts involved.
   - Formation of propositions or principles from two or more concepts.
3. Construction of theory by relating concepts and propositions in hierarchical order.
4. Testing theory in practice to validate it and produce a fact which can be incorporated into nursing practice as evidence of scientific basic or nursing action.

Testing Theory

Researchers test theory by formulating hypothesis deductively from the theory and testing the hypothesis in research construction of theory, on he other and, begins after observation. The researcher uses inductive reasoning to order the observation into categories and concepts, and attempts to relate one concept to the other in a statement—the empirical generalization. From the empirical generalization the researches deduces hypotheses for further testing. As the evidence for relationships between concept grows, the researcher may use creative abilities to purpose a general explanation for the interrelationships among the concepts and propositions. Thus a theory formulated that summarizes the interrelationships and predicts the relationships that will be found in the future observations. Theory construction involves observation, forming categories, conceptualisation, and both inductive and deductive reasoning.

Jacox (1981) summarizes the efforts to develop a theory:
1. Specifying, defining, and classifying the concepts used to describe the phenomena of the field.
2. Developing statements or propositions that propose how two or more concepts are related.
3. Specifying how all of the propositions are related to each other in a systematic way.

In the first step, the emphasis on concepts, in the second step, the emphasis on the propositions and in the third step, the propositions are related to one another.

Dickoff and James (1968) suggest that theory is a mental invention for some purposes to describe, explain, predict, or prescribe. Theories may be constructed (As stated earlier) in their view at four different levels.
1. *Situation-producing theory* prescribes the activities necessary to reach defined goals.
2. *Situation-relating theory* explains the interrelationships among concepts or propositions. Once such explanations have been formulated, predictive statements or hypothesis may be deduced. The hypothesis may produce causation or correlation.
3. *Factor-relating theory*. It relates the named concepts to one another. This is also the same level as the construction of empirical generalization-statement that proposes the relationship between two concepts.
4. *Naming theory* (factor-isolating theory) is the lowest level of theory construction but also the most basic. This kind of naming and describing theory is basic because the higher level depends on its development for their own emergence. Naming theory puts observation into named categories and includes both the name of the phenomenon and its description. Nursing diagnosis are an example of naming theory.

Each level of theory construction presupposes that the lower level have been developed. Not all the theorists would induce description and naming on a theory unless a relationship between the names is shown. However, such as **Diers** have found the approach useful for proposing on research in nursing practice.

THEORY AND NURSING RESEARCH

Nurses traditionally have based their practice on intuition, experience or the "way I was taught." These methods lead to role and stereotypical practice. Practice based on theories however allows for hypothesis about practice, which make it possible to derive a rationale for nursing actions. Testable theories provide a knowledge for the science of nursing. As the science of nursing develops, nurses will be able to (i) more accurately understand and explains past events and (ii) provide a basis for predicting and controlling future events. In addition, practice-based on science will suggest the image of nursing as a professional discipline.

When evaluating published nursing research, reader will see terms such as theoretical framework and conceptual framework used in some, but not all, of these studies. Several basic definitions should help to understand terms related to the use of theory in research studies as follow:
- *A concept* is an idea or a complex mental formulation of a specific phenomenon. For example, if you think of the word "table", what comes to your mind? Is it a piece of wooden furniture that is round and has

four legs? Or is it square like a card table? Or is your table a food chart? Or is it a table of contents for a book you are using in your nursing courses? Most likely, each person who is asked to think about the concept of "table" will have a different idea or mental formulation of what this abstract phenomenon called "table" looks like. Concepts range from being relatively concrete and more directly observable and measurable (such as height and weight) to being relatively abstract (such as wellness and self-esteem).

- *A construct* is a highly abstract and complex concept—such as intelligence—that is deliberately invented (constructed) by researchers for scientific purposes. A construct cannot be directly measured but must be indirectly measured by nothing the presence of indicators of concept. For example, the more concrete concept of weight (in pounds) can be directly determined by reading the numbers on a scale. The more abstract and complex construct of intelligence cannot be as directly measured but must be interred from such indicators of intelligence as verbal skills and mathematical reasoning on a standardized intelligence test.
- *A model* is a symbolic representation of reality used to demonstrate the interrelationships among a set of concepts or phenomena that cannot be directly observed but that do represent reality. Examples of models include verbal models, which are worded statements; schematic models, which may be diagrams, drawings, graphs, or pictures; and quantitative models, which are mathematical symbols. Models may function to provide a sense of understanding as to how "theoretic relationships develop and are useful to illustrate various forms of theoretic relationships." Models may be presented as part of a theory or can be constructed to show links between related theories. In nursing, a model is most often characterized as a conceptual models, a term that is used interchangeably with the term conceptual framework."

Conceptual models of nursing include Dorothy Orem's Self-Care Model, Sister Callista Roy's Adaptation Model, Betty Neuman's Systems Model, Martha Roger's Model: Science of Unitary Persons, and Imogene King's System Framework (Fitzpartick and Whall, 1996). Each of these nursing theorists "developed conceptual models that helped direct theory development." Concepts are the major components or building blocks of theories. A **theory** is a set of logically interrelated statements that is "a creative and rigorous structuring of ideas that project a tentative, purposeful, and systematic view of phenomena." Note that a theory consists of ideas—theory is not reality—and that these ideas are created and structured by the theorist. It is important to note the tentative nature of theory and that theory cannot be proved: theory is "grounded in assumptions, value choices, and the creative imaginative judgement of the theorist."

The basic function of theory is to describe, explain, and predict phenomena. A specific type of theory—prescriptive theory—is intended to control or change phenomena by identifying a goal and specifying the specific procedures to attain the goal. A theory contains propositions. A **propositions** a statement of a relationship between two or more concept in the theory. The proposition is stated in such a way that a testable hypotheses can be derived from the abstract statements of the theory. A **hypothesis** is a statement of the predicted relationship between two or more variables in a research study.

Thus, concepts are the components of theory. A theory consists of propositions, which are the testable part of a theory from which research hypotheses can be derived.

Theory helps to provide knowledge to improve nursing practice by describing, explaining, predicting, and controlling the specific phenomena related to nursing. Nurses power is increased through theoretical knowledge because systematically developed methods are more likely to be successful. In addition, nurses will know why they are doing what they are doing if challenged. Theory provides professional autonomy by guiding the practice, education, and research functions of the profession.

Classification of Theory

Theory can be classified according to the range and specificity of the phenomena dealt with in the theory. The subject matter for a theory can range from being very broad and all-inclusive to being very narrow and limited.

- *Broad-range theories* (also called grand theories) are "systematic constructions of the nature of nursing, the mission of nursing, and the goals of nursing care." Broad-range theories in nursing deal with the scope, philosophy, and general characteristics of nursing. For example, a conceptualisation of nursing's goal for high-level wellness for all individuals in society would be classified as nursing as broad-range theory. Although not all conceptual models can be classified as nursing theories, the following are examples of conceptual models that are classified as grand theories in nursing: Dorothea E. Orem's Self-Care Deficit Theory of Nursing; Martha E. Roger's Unitary Human Beings; Imogene King's Systems Framework and Theory of Goal Attainment; and Betty Neuman's Systems Model.
- *Middle-range theories* (also termed midrange theories) have a narrower focus than broad-range theories. "Middle-range theories are more precise than grand theories and focus on developing theoretical statements to answer question about nursing." Both middle-range and broad-range theories deal with a wide range of phenomena. However, unlike broad-range theories, middle-range theories do not deal with the entire range of phenomena of concern within a discipline. "When a theory is at the grand-theory level, many applications of that theory can be made in practice at the middle-range level by specifying such factors as the age of the patient, the situation, the health condition, the location, or the action of the nurse."

Chinn and Kramer (1995) describe an example of middle-range theory: "A theory of pain alleviation represents a midrange theory for nursing; it is broader than a theory of neural conduction of pain stimuli but narrower than the goal of achieving high-level wellness." A theory of pain alleviation would be classified as a middle-range theory in that the phenomenon of pain is only one of the many phenomenon of concern within the discipline of nursing. Other phenomena include quality of life, incontinence, and uncertainty in illness. Examples of middle-range nursing theories include Nola Pender's Health Promotion Model; Madeline Leininger's Culture Care: Diversity and Universality Theory; and Ida Jean Orlando's Nursing Process Theory.

- *Narrow-range theories* (also called microtheories) deal with a limited range of discrete phenomena of concern to a discipline. They are the most specific and least complex of the types of theories, and their theoretical formulations are not extended to link with the total range of phenomena of concern within a discipline. A discrete theory of neural conduction of pain stimuli (as cited above) is an example of narrow-range theory.
- *The conceptual models* of a discipline are broad conceptual structures or frameworks that provide a total perspective of the phenomena that are specific to that discipline. There is considerable agreement that nursing's metaparadigm (a specific type of paradigm) consists of the phenomena that are specific to the discipline of nursing. These central domain concepts are person, environment, health, and nursing. Nursing models can then be described as broad conceptual structures that provide a perspective of the total phenomena of nursing (details of conceptual model see page 20 towards).

What this means in terms of nursing practice is that the way nurses think about people and about nursing has a direct impact on how people are approached, what questions are asked, how information is learned and processed, and what nursing activities are included in nursing care.

The propositions or relationship statements of theories are consistent with the model or the framework from which they are derived. Theories, also consisting of sets of concepts, are less broad than models and propose more specific outcomes: "When the nurse approaches people from the perspective of a certain nursing model and asks questions, processes information, and carries out activities in a certain way according to that model, a specific outcome is proposed based on the application of the theory of that model."

The research proposal for example, "Compliance With Universal Precautions in Pediatric Settings," provides an example of a theory that has been derived from a model. The research study was developed within King's systems framework or model and its resultant theory of goal attainment. King developed her theory of goal attainment from her own systems framework. Two other theories that have been derived from King's systems framework are Frey's theory of social support and health and Sieloff's theory of departmental power.

In summarizing relationship of nursing theory to nursing models, the following definitions are offered. "The conceptual models of a discipline provide different perspectives or frames of reference for the phenomena identified by the metaparadigm of that discipline." The different perspectives identified by the nursing paradigm are person, environment, health and nursing. Nursing theory can be defined as:

An articulated and communicated conceptualisation of invented or discovered reality pertaining to nursing for the purpose of describing, explaining, predicting, or prescribing nursing care. Nursing theory is developed to answer central domain questions.

Although we have chosen to cite these particular definitions of nursing models and nursing theory, it must be noted that distinctions between to two are a debated issue and one on which not all authors agree.

PURPOSE OF THEORY IN A NURSING RESEARCH

Theory gives purpose and direction to a research study throughout the entire research process. Theory guides the research from the initial statement of the research problem through the analysis of the study data and provides a framework within which to analyze and interpret the results of the study. Analysing the study results within the framework of the theory not only guides the research in organizing and giving meaning to the phenomena, but may also increase the applicability and generalizability of the study findings.

The following hypothetical and very simplified–example should help clarify the function of theory in a research study. The purpose of this hypothetical study is to describe the characteristics of 100 hypertensive male adults who do or do not adhere to their medication regimen. If the study is not designed within a theory, the report of the results, although interesting, has limited applicability and generalizability to other than the 100 hypertensive male adults receiving medications who participated in the study.

If, however, the research were formulated within the framework of a theory, such as Orem's theory of self-care, the applicability and genralizability of the findings could then be broadened. Consider the following example of the same study formulated within Orem's self-care theory. In describing her theory of self-care Orem (1995) offered this definition of self-care.

The practice of activities that maturing and mature persons initiate and perform, within time frames, on their own behalf in the interest of maintaining life, healthful functioning, continuing personal development, and well-being.

In hypothetical study, formulated within Orem's self-care theory, the researcher was specifically looking for the relationship between adherence to medication regimens and self-care agency among the participants of the study. Self-care agency is defined by Orem's as "the complex acquired ability of mature and maturing persons to know and meet their continuing requirements for deliberate, purposive action to regulate their own human functioning and development." In analysing the study results within the framework provided by self-care theory, the research could now observe that study participants with enough self-care agency to adhere to their medication regimen could be viewed as having positive outcomes of good self-care: the ability to meet their own requirements for care that promotes health and well-being.

Thus, the knowledge gained from the study could now move from merely describing the 100 subjects of the study, as in the first design, to the broader area of describing hypertensive adult male's health and health care. Guided by the explanatory function of the theory, the research could now understand why the phenomena are occurring; the predictive feature could permit the ability to forecast what is most likely to occur in adult male hypertensive patients in the future. Providing we could assume that there is a prescriptive feature of self-care theory, caregivers could now be directed to assess systematically the self-care agency of medicated hypertensive adult males. They could then prescribe the enhancement of individual self-care agency, thereby potentially increasing adherence to the regimen and the attainment of positive outcomes of good self-care.

Research Frameworks

All research studies have a framework of background knowledge that provides the foundation for the study. This framework serves to organize the study by placing it in the context of existing related knowledge, as well as providing a context within which to interpret the results of the study. If a study is based on a conceptual model, the framework for the study is most often referred to as a *conceptual framework*; if a study is based on a specific theory or theories, the framework is most often referred to as a *theoretical framework*. The terms conceptual framework and theoretical framework are often used interchangeably.

Although all research studies have framework—that is, have conceptual underpinnings—not all researchers explicitly identify and describe their research framework, especially, when the research is not based on a specific theory or conceptual model. In a study based on a single concept or more than one concept, each major concept should be identified, defined, and discussed by the researcher.

Not all research studies linked to the theory development process. Chinn and Kramer (1995) describe two types of research, isolated research and theory-linked research, that "reflect certain basic standards that have been established in order to obtain results that are considered reliable and valid or accurately representative of empiric reality."

Isolated research is research that is not linked to the theory development process. Out hypothetical study of hypertensive adult male's adherence to their medication regimen, when designed without a theoretical or conceptual framework, is an example of isolated research. The study focused on a specific problem and offered little potential for applying the results beyond the findings of the study. However, isolated research does have certain merits, according to Chinn and Kramer (1995): "The results of isolated research can provide new insights that prompt the researcher, or someone reading the report of the research, to speculate about larger implications of the research for the discipline, which in turn can lead to developing theory that has broader meaning for the discipline."

Theory-linked research, on the other hand, "is designed with reference or linkage to theory." Theory-linked research is designed to develop theory or to test theory, and "it is this quality that sets the stage for the study to contribute to the larger knowledge of the discipline." Theory-linked research is linked to the theory development process in one of two ways: the research is either theory-generating (designed to develop theory) or theory-testing (designed to test how accurately the theory depicts phenomena and their relationships).

Theory-generating research is most often associated with the qualitative research approach. In a theory-generating qualitative study, the theory is "built up" from the data. The researcher does not begin with a theory or theories to test or verify; instead, "consistent with the inductive model of thinking, a theory may emerge during the data collection and analysis phase of the research or be used relatively late in the research process as a basis for comparison, with other theories."

Theory-testing research is most often associated with the quantitative research approach, in which deductive reasoning is used to test the theory. "In quantitative studies one uses theory deductively and places it toward the beginning of the plan for a study. In quantitative research the objective is to test or verify theory, rather that to develop it." The researcher tests a theory or theories by testing a hypothesis or research questions derived from the theory. Our hypothetical example using Orem's self-care theory was theory-testing research. The theory-guided the research, and the researcher could test how accurately the theory depicted the phenomena and their relationships.

Theory and research are reciprocal in their relationship, that is, theory guides research and research tests (validates) the theory. "If you begin with a theory, research derived from the theory is used to clarify and extend the theory. If you begin with research, theory that is formed from the findings can be subsequently used to direct research."

Chinn and Kramer (1995) provide the following observation regarding the role of both theory-linked and isolated research in the development of nursing knowledge: "From a research point of view, both can be of excellent quality. Both types of research can ultimately contribute to knowledge, although isolated research is much more limited in the contribution it can make to a discipline."

Selection of Theory in Research

Nurse researchers who use theories to guide their studies select theories that are unique to nursing as well as those borrowed from other disciplines. Selecting the most appropriate theory (or theories) depends on several considerations. Researchers must select a theory that has concepts and propositions that fit with the proposed study and one in which there are no contradictions between the theory and the variables selected for study. The theory should be one that provides a "best fit" with the proposed study and that can be useful in describing the relationship(s) between study variables.

It has already mentioned some of the nursing theories (conceptual frameworks) used by researchers. Examples of those from other disciplines include Selye's Stress Theory. Festinger's Cognitive Dissonance theory, Lazarus and Folkman's Coping Theory, Kohlberg's Moral Reasoning Theory, and Bandura's Social Learning Theory.

Statement of the Purpose of the Study

After formulating the research problem and deciding on the research approach and the role of theory in the study, researchers then state the purpose of the study. For both quantitative and qualitative research, the purpose of the study is a single sentence or a short paragraph that summarizes the essence of the study.

The statement of the research study's purpose can be written in three ways (i) as a declarative statement, (ii) as a question, or (iii) as a hypothesis. The form depends on the way the research question is asked and the extent of the researcher's knowledge about the problem. The statement of the purpose should include information about what the researcher intends to do to collect data (such as observe, describe, or measure some variable), information about the setting of the study (where the researcher plans the collect the data), and information about who the study subjects/participants will be.

The Purpose as a Declarative Statement

In previously formulated research question designed to describe the relationship between the type of teaching and success in breast-feeding by primiparas, the purpose of the study written as a declarative statement could read: "The purpose of this study is to describe the effect of structured individualized versus structured group instruction on successful breast feeding by primiparas in their home setting." Note that the statement includes information about what the researcher intends to (to describe), the setting of the study (home setting), and the subjects of the study (primiparas).

The Purpose as a Question

Using the same research question, the purpose of the study written as a question could read: "The purpose of this study is to answer the question: Is there a significant relationship between a specific method of teaching about breast-feeding and successful breast-feeding by primiparas in their home setting?" Specific methods of teaching might include structured individual teaching, structured group teaching, and unstructured (incidental) teaching. The primiparas in the study could be interviewed regarding their perceptions of their own success with breast-feeding and their satisfaction with the method of teaching to prepare them for breast-feeding.

The Purpose as a Hypothesis

Using the same research question, the purpose of the study, written as a hypothesis, could read: "The purpose of the study is to test the following hypothesis: Primiparas who receive individualized instruction about breast-feeding will have a significantly more successful breast-feeding experience in their home setting than primiparas who receive group instruction about breast-feeding."

CONCEPTUAL MODEL

The basic unit in the language of theoretical thinking is the concept:
- Concept is something conceived in the mind—a thought or notion.
- Concepts are words that represent reality and enhance our ability to communicate about it.
- Concept may be empirical or abstract, depending on their ability to observe in the real world.
  – Empirical concepts can be observed or experienced through the senses, e.g. stethoscope. In this there is an object.
  – Abstract concepts are those that cannot be observed through senses, e.g. hope, infinity. In these there is no object.

In nursing theories, which are developed by nurse scientists, usually four major concepts are emphasized which includes person, health environment, and nursing. These concepts formulate the metaparadigm of nursing which identifies the core content of a discipline. These concepts are presented as an abstraction here:

- *Person* may represent one individual, a family, a community, or all mankind. The person is the recipient of nursing care.
- *Health* represents a state of well-being mutually decided on by the client and the nurse.
- *Environment* may represent the immediate surroundings, the community or the universe and all it contains.
- *Nursing* is the science and art of the discipline.

Thus, concepts are the elements used to generate theories.

Concept is an image or symbolic representation of an abstract idea. It is an abstraction based on observation of certain behaviours or characteristics (e.g., stress, pain). It is formed by generalizing from particular characteristics. To illustrate, *health* is a concept formed by generalizing from particular behaviours. For example, being mobile, being free from infections and communicating appropriately. Other concepts include pain, intelligence, weight, grieving, self-concept, and achievement.

Concept is a complex mental formulation of experience. By experience we mean perceptions of the world—objects, other people, visual images, colour, movement, sounds, behaviour, interactions, the totality of what is perceived. Concepts are major components of theory and convey the abstract ideas within the theory.

Concept facilitates the delineation of ideas so that systematic inquiry can proceed. Some concepts are directly observable such as pen or rain and others are indirectly observable such as anxiety in intelligence. It is better to know the concepts because they are the basis for refining ideas and developing theory. So it is important to select those concepts that clearly reflect the subject matter being pursued.

Concepts, no matter what their level of abstraction, must be, defined as unambiguously as possible, so that they can be easily communicated to others. Even the word **'can'** is open to various interpretations. For example, a container, being able to or a commode.

A conceptual definition conveys the general meaning of the concept, as does a dictionary definition. It reflects the theory used in the study of that concept. The following are the example of conceptual definitions.

- *Recovery*: "The process of healing that takes place after an injury."
- *Adaptation*: "The degree to which an individual adjusts, psychologically, socially and physiologically to long-term illness."
- *Postoperative pain*: "Discomfort, an individual experiences after surgical procedure."
- *Coping effort*: Amount of physical and\or emotional energy an event or situation required to adjust to or handle the situation.

Operationalization is the process of translating concepts into observable, measurable phenomena. Operational definition refers to the measurements used to observe or measure a variable, delineates to procedures or operations required to measure the concept. In other words, operationalization adds another dimension to the conceptual definition by delineating the procedures or operational terms. For example, pulse and counting the number of beats or pulsations for a minute. Other concepts are more difficult to define operationally, such as coping, leaving it up to the investigator to locate and select an instrument that best measures the concepts as defined. The following are examples of operational definitions.

- *Dyspnea*: "The sensation of difficult breathing" is measured by the Visual Analogue Dyspnea Scale (VADS).
- *Hopelessness*: "The perceptual experience of anticipation of undesirable situation or (consequences that are largely beyond one's control) was measured by hopelessness scale" (Abraham, Neundorfer & Currie, 1992).
- *Body attitude*: "Individuals' general attitude about the outward form and appearance of their bodies, as measured by the Body attitude scale" (Drake, Verhutst, Fawcett and Barger, 1988).
- *Social support*: A characteristics of the social elements that buffers the effect of stress on the health of the individual as measured by the Social Support Questionnaire (Northeuse, 1998).

The terms "theory," "theoretical framework," "conceptual scheme," "conceptual model," and "model" are sometimes used synonymously in the research literature. We have been careful in the preceding discussion to restrict our terminology to theory and theoretical framework and to use these terms to refer to a well-formulated deductive system of abstract formal statements. Distinguish of theories from conceptual frameworks and models as follows:

Conceptual Frameworks or Schemes (we will use the two terms interchangeably) represent a less formal and less well-developed mechanism for organising phenomena than theories. As the name implies, conceptual frameworks deal with abstractions (concepts) that are assembled by virtue of their relevance to a common theme. Both conceptual schemes and theories use concepts as building blocks. What is absent from conceptual schemes is the deductive system of propositions that assert relationships among the concepts.

Most of the conceptual work that has been done in connection with nursing practice is more correctly designated as conceptual frameworks or schemes than as theories. This label in no way diminishes the importance and vale of these endeavours. Indeed many existing conceptual frameworks will undoubtedly serve as the preliminary steps in the construction of more formal theories. In the meantime, conceptual frameworks can serve to guide research that will further support theory development. Conceptual frameworks, like theories can serve as a springboard for the generation of hypotheses to be tested. This chapter describes a few of the major conceptual frameworks in nursing and illustrates how they have been used in nursing research.

Models, like conceptual frameworks, are constructed representations of some aspect of our environment; they use abstractions (concepts) as the building blocks. However, models attempt to represent reality with a minimal use of words. Language is, and probably always will be, a problem of scientists. A word or phrase that designates a concept can convey different meanings to different people. A visual or symbolic representation of a theory or conceptual framework often helps express abstract ideas in a more readily understandable or precise form than the original conceptualisation.

Schematic models are quite common and undoubtedly are familiar to all readers. A schematic model or diagram represents the phenomenon of interest figuratively. Concepts and the linkages between them are represented diagrammatically through the use of boxes, arrows, or other symbols. An example of a schematic model is presented in (Fig. 1.1). This model is described by its designer as "a human interaction diagram showing nurse and client interactions" (King, 1981, p. 145).

Schematic models of this type can be quite useful in the research process in clarifying concepts and their associations, in enabling researchers to place a specific problem into an appropriate context, and in revealing areas of inquiry.

In summary, it may not always prove possible to identify a formal theory that is relevant to a nursing research problem, but conceptual schemes and models of the type discussed here can also be used to clarify concepts and to provide a context for findings that might otherwise be isolated and meaningless. Conceptual schemes in nursing are very much in need of testing if theories for nursing are to be formulated.

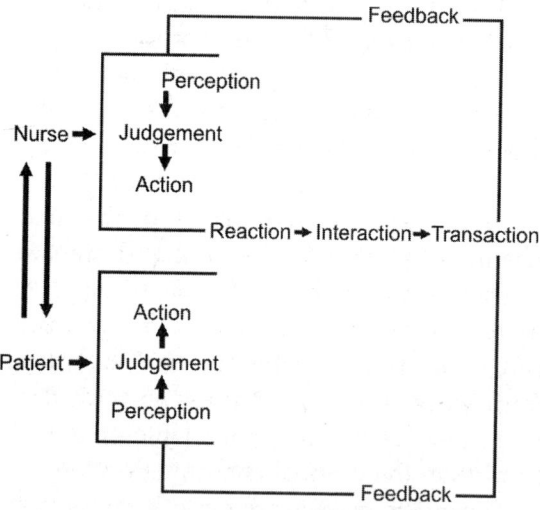

Figure 1.1: An example of schematic model

Conceptual Models in Nursing

In the past few decades, nurses have formulated a number of conceptual models of nursing and for nursing practice. These models constitute formal explanations of what the nursing discipline is according to the model developer's point of view. As Fawcett (1984) has noted, there are four central concepts of the nursing discipline; person, environment, health and nursing. However, the various models define these concepts differently, link them in diverse ways, and give different emphasis to the relationships among them. Nurse researches increasingly are turning towards these conceptual models for their inspiration and theoretical foundations in formulating research questions and hypotheses. This section briefly reviews some of the major conceptual models in nursing and gives examples of research that claimed its intellectual roots in these models.

Johnson's Behavioural Systems Model

Johnson's model focuses on a behavioural system (the patient), its subsystems, and its environment. According to this model, each individual behavioural system is a collection of seven interrelated subsystems (attachment, dependency, ingestion, elimination, sexuality, aggression, and achievement), the response patterns of which form an organized and integrated whole. Each subsystem carries out specialized tasks for the integrated system, and each is structured by four motivational elements: goal, set, choice, and action/behaviour. The model is concerned primarily with behavioural functioning that results in the equilibrium of the integrated system. In

Johnson's model, the function of nursing is to help restore the balance of each subsystem in the event of disequilibrium and to help prevent future system disturbance. Several researchers have designated Johnson's Behavioural Systems Model as their conceptual basis. For example, Derdiarian and Forsythe (1983) described the development of an instrument (the Derdiarian Behavioural System Model Instrument) to measure the perceived behavioural changes of cancer patients. Holaday (1981) focused on Johnson's concept of "behavioural set" in her study of the crying bouts of chronically-ill infants and their mothers responses.

King's Open System Model

King's conceptual model (1981) includes three types of dynamic, interacting systems; personal systems (represented by individuals); interpersonal systems (represented by such dyadic interactions such as hospitals and families). The social system provides a context in which nurses work. Within King's model, the domain of nursing includes promoting, maintaining, and restoring health. Nursing is viewed as "a process of action, reaction and interaction whereby nurse and client share information about their perceptions of the nursing situation" (King, 1981). King herself (1981) conducted a descriptive observational study of nurse-client encounters that yielded a classification of elements in nurse-client interactions. The study provided preliminary support for the proposition that goal attainment was facilitated by accurate nurse-client perceptions, satisfactory communication, and mutual goal setting.

Levine's Conservation Model

Levine's (1973) model focuses on individuals as holisting beings, and the major area of concern for nurses is maintenance of the persons wholeness. The model identifies adaptation as the process by which the integrity or wholeness of individuals is maintained. Levine's model identifies several principles of conservation the aim to facilitate patient's adaptation processes. Through these principles, the model emphasizes the nurse's responsibility to maintain the client's integrity in the threat of assault through illness or environmental influence. Newport (1984) based a study on Levine's model, she investigated two alternative methods of conserving newborn thermal energy and social integrity.

Neuman's Health Care Systems Model

Neuman's (1982) model focuses on the person as a complete system, the sub parts of which are interrelated physiological, psychological, sociocultural, and developmental factors. In this model, the person maintains balance and harmony between internal and external environments by adjusting to stress and by defending against tension-producing stimuli. Wellness is equated with equilibrium. The primary goal of nursing is to assist in the attainment and maintenance of client system stability. Nursing interventions include activities to strengthen flexible lines of defense, to strengthen resistance to stressors, and to maintain adaptation, Craddock and Stanhope (1980) applied Neuman's scheme in a study of clients' and health care provider's perceptions of stressors. Ziemer (1983) operationalized many of Neuman's concepts in a study of the effects preoperative information on the postoperative outcomes of clients who have had abdominal surgery.

Orem's Model of Self-care

Orem's (1985) model focuses on each individual's ability to perform *Self-care*, defined as "the practice of activities that individuals initiate and perform on their own behalf in maintaining life, health, and well-being." One's ability to care for oneself is referred to as *Self-care Agency*, and the ability to care for others is referred to as *Dependent-care Agency*. In Orem's model, the goal of nursing is to help people meet their own therapeutic self-care demands. Orem identified three types of nursing systems: (i) wholly compensatory, wherein the nurse compensates for the patient's total inability to perform self-care activities; (ii) partially compensatory wherein the nurse compensates for the patient's partial inability to perform these activities; and (iii) supporting-educative, wherein the nurse assists the patient in making decisions and acquiring skills and knowledge. Orem's Self-care Model has generated considerable interest among nurse researchers. For example, Chang and Colleagues (1984) examined components of nurse practitioner care in the context of Orem's model to determine what aspects of the care contributed most to the elderly patient's intentions to adhere to the care plan. Moore (1987) explored alternative strategies for promoting autonomy and self-care agency in fifth-grade students. Dodd (1984) studied the self-care behaviours of cancer patients in chemotherapy.

Roger's Model of the Unitary Person

Roger's Model (1970) focuses on the individual as a unified whole in constant interaction with the environment. The unitary person is viewed as an energy field that is more than, as well as different from the sum of the biological, social and psychological parts. In Roger's model, nursing is concerned with the unitary person as a synergistic phenomenon. Nursing science is devoted to the study of the nature and direction of unitary human development. Nursing practice helps individuals achieve maximum well-being within their potential. Examples of studies that have been based on Roger's model include Floyd's (1983) study of sleep-wake patterns with samples of rotating shift workers and hospitalised psychiatric patients and Fitzpatrick's (1980) study relating to patient's temporal experiences.

Roy's Adaptation Model

In Roy's Adaptation Model (1980), humans are biopsychosocial adaptive systems who cope with environmental change through the process of adaptation. Within the human system there are four subsystems: physiological needs, self-concept, role function, and interdependence. These subsystems constitute adaptive modes that provide mechanisms for coping with environmental stimuli and change. The goal of nursing according to this model, is to promote patients adaptation during health and illness. Nursing also regulates stimuli affecting adaptation. Nursing interventions generally take the form of increasing, decreasing, modifying, removing, or maintaining internal and external stimuli that affect adaptation. Norris, Campbell and Brenkert (1982) used Roy's concepts of focal, contextual, and residual stimuli in their study of the effect of nursing procedures on transcutaneous oxygen tension in premature infants. Shannahan and Cottrell (1985) invoked Roy's concept of manipulation of contextual stimuli in their assessment of the effects of delivering in a birth chair versus a traditional delivery table.

Types of Theory to be Tested

Theories may describe a particular phenomenon, explain relationships between or among phenomena, or predict how one phenomenon affects another. Different types of theories are tested by different approaches. For example, *descriptive theories* "describe or classify specific dimensions or characteristics of individuals, groups, situations, or events by summarizing the commonalities found in discrete observations" (Fawcett, 1989). To test descriptive theories, researchers conduct descriptive research studies. Hutchison and Bahr (1991) used a grounded theory approach to describe the types and meanings of caring behaviours in elderly nursing home residents. They observed residents and interviewed them to understand their views of caring. The commonalities that the investigators found led them to develop models of the types of cawing behaviours and their meaning as expressed by the residents.

Explanatory theories are those are that "specify relations among the dimensions or characteristics of individuals, groups, situations or events" (Fawcett, 1989), and are tested by using correlational research. Grey *et al*, (1991) conducted a correlational study to determine the influence of age, coping behaviour, and self-care on social, psychological, and physiological adaptation in adolescents and preadolescents with diabetes. Through their review of literature, they found that several factors influence adaptation to chronic illness during adolescence; however, the relative impact of these factors had not been determined.

Nursing theory is an articulated and communicated conceptualisation of invented or discovered reality (Central Phenomena and Relationships) in or pertaining to Nursing for the purpose of describing, explaining, predicting or prescribing nursing care" (Melis, 1991).

This definition adds the importance of communicating nursing theory and the purpose of prescription of nursing care.

Complete nursing theory is one that has context, content and process. (Barnum 1994). Here,

- *Context* is the environment in which the nursing acts place.
- *Content* is the subject of the theory.
- *Process* is the method by which the nurse acts in using the theory.

The nurse acts on, with or through the content elements of the theory.

Level of Theory

The level of the theory refers to the scope or range of phenomena to which the theory applies. The levels of abstraction of the concepts in the theory is closely tied to its scope.

Theory may be characteristic on micro, macro, molecular, midrange, molar, atomistic, and holistic (Chinn & Kramer 1991).

Micro, molecular and atomistic suggest relatively narrow range phenomenon where on macro, holistic and molar implies that theory covers a broader scope. *Graded theory* is the term used to mean that covers broad areas of concern within discipline. *Meta theory* is the term used to label theory about the theoretical process and theory development.

According to Dickoff, James and Wedenbach (1968) theory develops on four levels.

Level 1: Factor-isolating is descriptive in nature. It involves naming or classifying facts or events.

Level 2: Factor-relating, require correlating or associating factors in such a way that they meaningfully depict a larger situation.

Level 3: Situation-relating, explains and predicts how situations are related.

Level 4: Situation-producing requires sufficient knowledge about how and why situations are related, so that when the theory issued as a guide valued situations can be produced.

Among these levels level 4 is most powerful because it controls or does more than describe, explain or predict.

Categories of Theories

1. Needs/Problem -oriented : Nightingale, Abdellah, Henderson, Orem, Hull, Watson.
2. Interaction- oriented : Peplau, Orlando, Weidenback, King Patterson, Erickson.
3. System-oriented : Johnson, Roy, Neuman, Levine, Leininger.
4. Energyfield : Rogers, Parse, Newman.

NURSING THEORY AND KNOWLEDGE

Nursing is a unique health care discipline in which a service, based on knowledge and skill, is provided to others. Nursing therefore, has two parts—a body of knowledge through Nursing Practice. The body of knowledge, called a knowledge base, provides a rationale for nursing actions.

It is the general conception of any field of enquiry that ultimately determines the kind of knowledge that field aims to develop as well as the manner in which that knowledge is to be organized, tested and applied. Such an understanding, involves critical attention to the question of what it means to know and what kinds of knowledge are held to be most value in the discipline of nursing.

Concepts of Knowing and Knowledge

The term *'Knowing'* refers to ways of perceiving and understanding the self and the world. Knowing is an ontologic, dynamic, changing process (ontology is pertaining to ways of being in the world, perspectives on the existence and experience of being).

Knowledge refers to knowing that is in a form that can be shared or communicated with others. Knowledge is an awareness or perception of reality acquired through learning or investigation. Additionally, knowledge represents what is collectively taken to be a reasonably accurate accounting of the world as it is known by the members of the discipline. Knowledge then, is a representation of knowing that is collectively judged by standards and criteria shared within the nursing community. The ways in which knowledge and knowing are developed are epistemologic concerns that reveal how we come to know and how we acquire shared knowledge in the discipline. (Epistemology – pertaining to the 'stem' or basis of knowledge: perspectives on how knowing becomes knowledge and/or how knowledge is created.

Thus, knowing is the individual human processes of perceiving and understanding self and the world in ways that can be brought to some level of conscious awareness. Not all that is comprehended in the process of knowing can be shared or communicated, and expressed in words or in actions become knowledge of discipline.

Knowledge, is the awareness or perception of reality acquired through insight, learning or investigation expressed in a form that can be shared. Knowledge is a reasonably accurate accounting of the world as known and shared by members of a discipline. It is a representation of knowing that is collectively judged by shared standards and criteria.

As nurses practice, they know more than they can communicate symbolically or justify as knowledge. Much of what is known is expressed through actions, movements, and/ or sounds. These are the everyday actions or non-discursive expressions of knowing that always reflect the whole of knowing. Each of the patterns of knowing has nondiscursive forms of expression that give nursing its distinctive character as a healing practice and that can be recognized as arising from a particular pattern of knowing. At the time what is expressed in a nurse's action always conveys a simultaneous wholeness. Action also conveys a fuller expression of what is known than formal, discursive expression of knowledge.

It has been believed that much of what nurses know has potential to become formally expressed. Although language and other symbols will only partially reflect the whole of knowing, it is important to begin the challenge and formal expression of knowledge in order to communicate what is known within the discipline as a whole. This makes possible focus, shape, question and influence what is collectively accepted as sound, useful and valued. It is the formal expression that have potential to become the knowledge of the discipline. Sharing knowledge is important because it creates a disciplinary community, beyond the isolation of individual experience. once this happens, social purposes form, and knowledge development and shared purposes form a cyclic interrelationship that moves us toward prospective, value grounded or praxis.

Knowing and knowledge are reflections of four patterns: empirics, aesthetics, ethical and personal. Together they form an essential whole. Praxis—thoughtful reflections and action that occur in synchrony—comes from the whole of knowing and knowledge in nursing practice.

Pattern of Knowing in Nursing

Carper (1978) examined early nursing literature and named four fundamental and enduring patterns of knowing that nurses have valued and used in practice. one of the patterns is the familiar and respected patterns of empirics, the science of nursing. In addition, the identified ethics, the component of moral knowledge in nursing; aesthetics, the art of nursing; and personal knowing in nursing.

The fundamental patterns of knowing remain valuable in that they conceptualise a broad scope of knowing that accounts for a holistic practice. we retain our focus on these fundamental patterns in this text because until very recently the development of empiric knowledge has been the prevailing approach to knowledge development, and the other fundamental patterns have not been formally developed within the discipline. In part, neglect of the personal, ethical, and aesthetic patterns of knowing reflect, an overvaluing of empirics as the knowledge of the discipline. In addition methods for developing knowledge within the other patterns, particularly personal and aesthetic knowledge, are only beginning to be systematically described and developed.

In the following sections we describe each of the fundamental patterns and provide an overview of the methods we propose for developing each of the patterns.

Empirics: The Science of Nursing

Empirics is based on the assumption that what is known is accessible through the senses; seeing, touching, hearing, and so forth. Empirics can be traced to Nightingale's precepts concerning the importance of accurate observation and record keeping. The science of nursing emerged during the late 1950s. Empirics as a pattern of knowing draws on an additional idea of science in which reality is viewed as something that can be known by observation and verified by other observers.

Empiric knowing is expressed in practice through the nurse's scientific competence—embodied knowing that makes possible competent acting rounded in scientific theory. There is a cognitive component of empiric competence that involves problem-solving and logical reasoning, but much remains in the background of conscious awareness. It is also accessible to conscious reasoning when attention turns to the reasoning process itself.

Empiric knowledge is formally expressed in the form of empiric theories, statements, of fact, or descriptions of empiric events or objects. The development of empiric knowledge has traditionally been accomplished by the methods of science. Usually this has involved testing hypothesis derived from a theory that offers a tentative explanation of empiric phenomena. Although many conceptualisations of empiric knowledge in nursing are linked to this traditional view of science, ideas about what is legitimate for developing the science of nursing have broadened to include activities that are not strictly within the realm of hypothesis testing, such as phenomenologic or ethnographic descriptions or inductive means of generating theory.

Ethics: The Moral Component of Knowledge in Nursing

Ethics in nursing is focused on matters of obligation or what ought to be done. The moral component of knowing in nursing goes beyond knowledge of the norms or ethical codes of nursing, other related disciplines, and society, it involves making moment-to-moment judgements about what ought to be done, what is good and right, and what is responsible. Ethical knowing guides and directs how nurses conduct their practice, what they select as important, where loyalties are placed, and what priorities demand advocacy.

Ethical knowing also involves confronting and resolving conflicting values, norms, interests, or principles. There may be no satisfactory answer to an ethical dilemma or moral distress—only alternatives, some of which are more or less satisfactory. Ethical knowing in nursing requires both an experiential knowledge, from which ethical reasoning arises, and knowledge of the formal principles, ethical codes, and theories of the discipline and society. Like empiric knowing, ethical knowing is expressed in nursing actions —what we call moral-ethical comportment. Nursing actions based on ethical principles can be discerned and examined.

The discipline's ethical principles, codes, and theories are set forth in the philosophic ideals on which ethical decisions rest. Ethical knowledge does not describe or prescribe what a decision or action should be, rather, it provides insight about which choices are possible and why and it provides direction towards choices that are sound, good, responsible, or just.

Ethical theories are like empiric theories in that they describe some dimensions of reality and express relationships between phenomena. However, empiric theory relies on observable reality that can be confirmed by others. Ethical theory cannot be tested in this sense because the relationships of the theory rest on underlying philosophic reasoning that leads to conclusions concerning what is right, good, responsible, or just. The reasoning can include description of experience to substantiate an argument, but the conclusions are value statements that cannot be perceived or confirmed empirically.

Personal Knowing in Nursing

Personal knowing in nursing concerns the inner experience of becoming a whole, aware genuine self. Personal knowing encompasses knowing one's own self and self of others. It has been stated that "One does not know about the self, one strives simply to know the self." It is through knowing one's own self that one is able to know the other. Full awareness of the self, the moment, and the context of interaction makes possible meaningful, shared human experience. Without this component of knowledge, the idea of therapeutic use of self in nursing would not be possible.

Personal knowing is most fully communicated as an authentic, aware genuine self. What is perceived by others is the existence of a person, an embodied self. As personal knowing emerges more fully throughout life, the unique or genuine self can be more fully-expressed and becomes accessible as a means by which deliberate action and interaction take form. It is possible to describe certain things about the self in personal stories and autobiographies. These descriptions provide sources for deep reflection and a shared understanding of how personal knowledge can be developed and used in a deliberative way. Descriptions about the self are limited in what they never fully reflect personal knowing, and they are retrospective in that they can describe only the self that was. However, publicly expressed descriptions can be a tool for developing self-awareness and self-intimacy and for communicating to others valuable possibilities for developing personal knowing.

In a sense, all knowing is personal, each individual can know only through their personal senses and sensibilities. Empiric theories can be learned, but their meaning for the individual comes from personal reflection and experience with the phenomena of the theory. Aesthetic sensibilities, ethical precepts, and moral beliefs are likewise highly personal in nature. We recognise this broad meaning of personal knowing, but our focus is the aspect of personal knowing that develops into the process of knowing the self and of developing self-knowing through healing encounters with others.

Aesthetics: The Art of Nursing

Aesthetic knowing in nursing involves deep appreciation of the meaning of a situation, calling forth inner creative resources that transform experience into what is not yet real but possible. Aesthetics knowledge make it possible to move beyond the surface – beyond the limits and circumstances of a particular moment—to sense the meaning of the moment and connect with depths of human experience that are common but unique in each experience (sickness, suffering, recovery, birth, death). Aesthetic knowing in nursing is made visible through the actions, bearing, conduct attitude, narrative and interactions of the nurse in relation to others. It is also expressed in art forms such as poetry, drawing, stories, and music that reflect and communicate symbolic meanings embedded in nursing practice.

Aesthetic knowledge is what makes possible knowing what to do with and how to be in the moment instantly, without conscious deliberation. It arises from a direct perception of what is significant in the moment that is, grasping meaning in the encounter. Perception of meaning in an encounter creates artful nursing action, and the nurse's perception of meaning is reflected in the action taken. The meaning is often a shared meaning that is perceived without conscious exchange of words and may not be consciously or cognitively formed. Sometimes, meaning is brought to the situation from the nurse's own creative sensibilities, opening possibilities that would not otherwise enter into the encounter. The actions—movements and verbal expressions—of the nurse serve to transform and shape the experience into what would not otherwise exist, creating new possibilities in the encounter. The nurse's actions take on an element of artistry, creating unique meaningful deeply moving interactions with others that touch common chords of human experience. We refer to the aspect of nursing practice as the transformative art-act.

Aesthetic knowing is expressed in the moment of experience-action, in the transformative art-act. Aesthetic knowledge is formally expressed in aesthetic criticism and in works of art that symbolize experience. Aesthetic criticism is the discursive expression of aesthetic knowledge that conveys the artful aspects of the art, the technical skill required to perform the art-act, knowledge that informs the development of the art-act, the historical and cultural significance of specific aspects of nursing as an art, and the potential for the future development of the art.

Empirics

- Fundamental pattern of knowing in nursing focussed on the use of sensory experience for creation of mediated knowledge expressions, expressed as knowledge by theories and models and integrated in practice as scientific competence.
- Theory is an expression of knowledge within the empirics pattern. Creative and

rigorous structuring of ideas that project a tentative, purposeful and systematic view of phenomena.
- Models is a symbolic representative of empiric experience in words, pictorial or graphic diagram, mathematical notations or physical material (model of heart). A form of knowledge within the empirics pattern.
- Explaining—process that focuses on how concepts and variable interrelate. Interacts with the process of structuring to create empiric knowledge.
- Structuring—process that involves forming empiric concepts into formal expressions such as theories, models, or framework interact with the process of explaining to create empiric knowledge.
- Replication—process that draws on methods of science to determine the extent to which an observation remains consistent from one situation or time to another. Interacts with the process of validation to challenge and authenticate empiric knowledge.
- Validation—process that draws on methods of science to substantiate the accuracy of conceptual meaning in terms of empiric evidence. Interacts with replication to challenge and authenticate empiric knowledge.
- Scientific competence—expression of empiric knowledge and knowing in nursing practice, integrated with ethics, aesthetics and personal knowing and knowledge.

Ethics

- Fundamental pattern of knowing in nursing, focussing on matters of moral and ethical significance expressed as knowledge by principles and codes and integrated in practice as moral-ethical comportment.
- Dialogue refer to process of exchanging various points of view concerning what is right, good or responsible. Interacts with the process of justification to challenge and authenticate ethical knowledge.
- Justification is the process of developing explicit descriptions of the values of which an ethical ideal rests and the line of reasoning toward which an ethical conclusion flows. Interacts with dialogue to challenge and authenticate ethical knowledge.
- Moral-ethical component is the expression of ethical knowledge and knowing in nursing practice, integrated with personal, aesthetic, and empiric knowledge and knowing.
- Valuing is the process of examining motives, actions, outcomes and other dimensions of experience to embrace and reflect chosen values as basis for understanding moral ethical behaviour. Increases with the process of clarifying to create ethical knowledge.
- Clarifying is the process involving a deliberate focus on understanding those actions that are right and good. Interacts with the process of valuing to create ethical knowledge.
- Principles is a form of knowledge expression within the ethical pattern. They are general statements that reflect general and fundamental principles of values or truths that are followed in providing nursing care such as 'do no harm.'
- Codes are short hand expressions of prescribed professional behaviour that are

generally accepted as right and good. Codes primarily describe behaviours that represent the nursing accountability to the client as expressed in rights, duties and obligation.

Personal

- Personal pattern of knowing in nursing focussed on the inner experience of becoming a whole, aware of self. Expressed as knowledge through autobiographic stories and the genuine self and integrated in practice with other patterns as therapeutic use of self.
- Response is a process of interacting with one's own self and others to provide insight concerning the meanings conveyed in experience. Interacts with the process of reflections to challenge and authenticate personal knowledge.
- Reflection is the process that requires integrating a wide range of perceptions in order to realize what is known within the self. Interacts with the process of response to challenge and authenticate personal knowledge.
- Therapeutic use of self is the expression of personal knowledge and knowing in nursing practice, integrated with ethics, empiric and aesthetic knowledge and knowing.

Aesthetics

- Fundamental pattern of knowing in nursing related to the perception of deep meanings, calling forth inner creative resources that transform experience into what is not yet real, but possible. Expressed as knowledge through works of art and criticism and integrated in practice as transformative-art-acts.
- Appreciation is the process of focussing and reflecting on aesthetic knowledge as it is understood and valued by members of the discipline. Interacts with the process of inspiration to challenge and authenticate aesthetic knowledge.
- Inspiration is the process of responding to aesthetic knowledge to imagine new possibilities and directions. Interacts with appreciation to challenge and authenticate aesthetic knowledge.
- Envisioning is the process of imagining forms, ways of being, actions and outcomes into a possible future. Interacts with the process of rehearsing to create aesthetic knowledge.
- Rehearsing is the process of creating and recreating narrative body movements, gestures and actions in relation to an anticipated situation. Interacts with the process of envisioning to create aesthetic knowledge.

Criticism is a form of knowledge within the aesthetics pattern that is a discursive representation of meaning for expressions of aesthetic knowledge. Criticism is formed from aesthetic methods that are designed to deepen shared meanings for aesthetic knowledge (Fig. 1.2).

Above Figure 1.1 showing the practice or action expression of knowing that is associated with the pattern. The inner sphere is shown as a whole, without quadrant boundaries, representing our view that in nursing practice knowing is experienced as a whole and cannot be experienced as discrete patterns. Along the vertical axis, represented by vertical broken arrows, are the processes for developing the formal knowledge expressions. Along the horizontal axis, represented by horizontal broken arrows, are

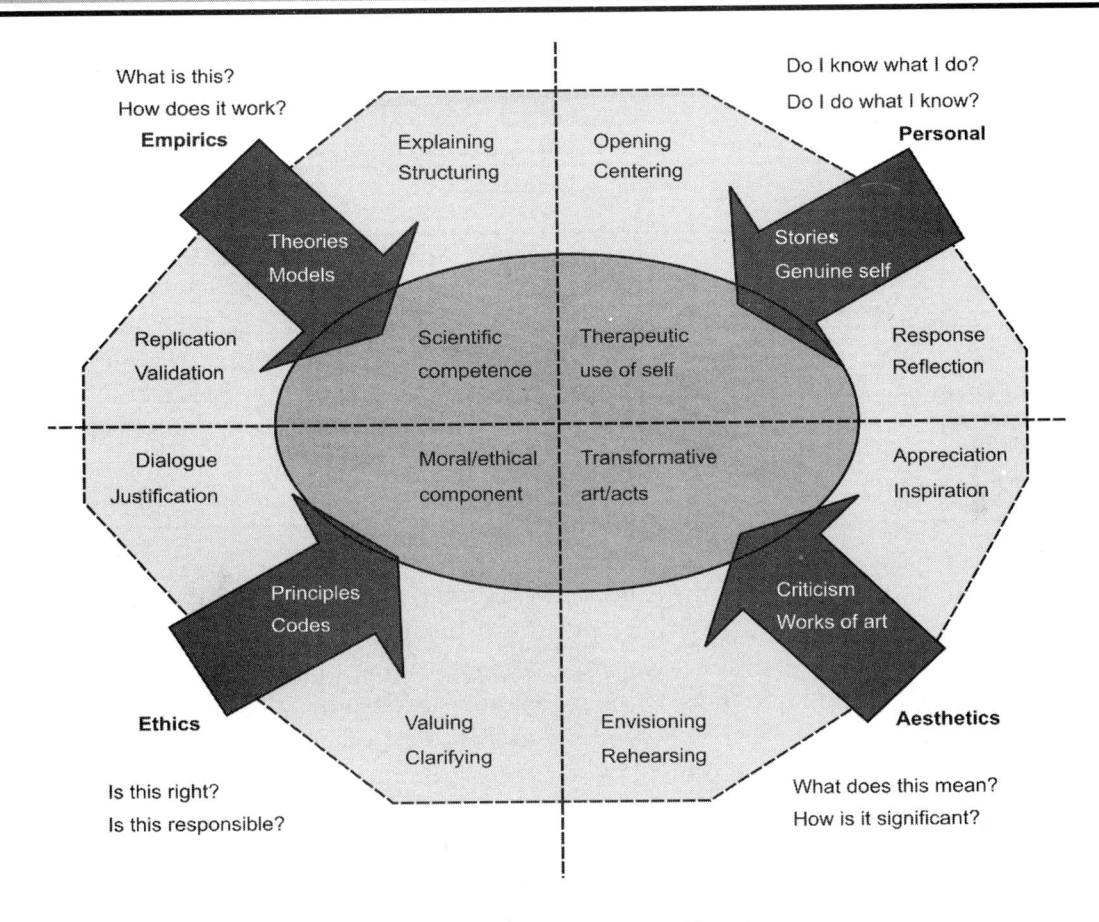

Figure 1.2: Fundamental pattern of knowing

the collective processes used within the discipline for validating or authenticating what is known.

The outer area, where the critical questions appear, and the inner sphere, showing the action expressions of knowing, represent the ontologic dimensions of knowing. The processes shown along the vertical and horizontal arrows represent the epistemologic dimensions of processes for developing and authenticating knowledge.

Another way of conceptualising these processes is shown in Table 1.1. The dimensions of the critical questions, the creative processes for developing knowledge, the formal expression of knowledge, the processes for authenticating knowledge, and the nondiscursive expressions of knowing in practice are shown for each pattern. Each of the dimensions are unique to each pattern of knowing; you cannot create empiric theory, for example, by using the creative processes of ethics, personal, or aesthetic knowing. However, in the realm of nondiscursive expression of knowing in practice, knowing is experienced as a whole, even though you can discern those aspects of practice that are possible because of each fundamental pattern of knowing.

Table 1.1: Dimensions associated with each of the fundamental patterns of knowing

Dimensions	Empirics	Ethics	Personal	Aesthetics
Critical questions	What is this? How does it work?	Is this right? Is this responsible?	Do I know what I do? Do I do what I know?	What does this mean? How is it significant?
Creative processes	Explaining, structuring	Valuing, clarifying	Opening, centering	Envisioning, rehearsing
Formal expression of knowledge	Facts, models, theories, descriptions	Principles, codes, ethical theories	Autobiographical stories, the genuine self	Aesthetic criticism, works of art
Authentication process	Replication, validation	Dialogue, justification	Response, reflection	Appreciation, inspiration
Nondiscursive expression of knowing in practice	Scientific competence	Moral-ethical component	Therapeutic use of self	Transformative art/acts

Critical questions represent the kind of understanding that emerges within the individual patterns. Empirics, the science of nursing, poses the critical questions "what is this?" and "How does it work?" Personal knowing poses the critical questions "Do I know what I do?" and "Do I do responsible?" Aesthetics the critical questions "Is this right?" and "Is this responsible?" Aesthetics poses the critical questions "what does this mean?" and "How is this significant?"

The creative inquiry processes lead toward formal expression of knowledge. Empiric knowledge development uses the reasoning processes of explaining and structuring empirical phenomena. Personal knowledge is developed by opening and centering the self. Development of ethical knowledge uses processes of clarifying and valuing issues of rights and responsibilities in practice. Aesthetic knowledge is developed by envisioning possibilities and rehearsing art-acts that can be called upon to transform experience.

From these processes, formal discursive forms of expression are created that can be presented to members of the discipline. In Figure 1.1, these are shown in the large arrows leading to the center sphere. Empiric inquiry leads to the development of theories, models, and other formal expressions, such as statements of fact and conceptual frameworks. Personal inquiry leads to the creation of autobiographic stories and the lived expression of the nurse's being in nursing care situations. This lived experience of being who we are is what we call the genuine self. Ethical inquiry leads to ethical principles and codes and to other expressions such as theories and precepts that guide ethical conduct in practice. Aesthetic inquiry leads to aesthetic criticism that reveals deep meaning embedded in nursing art-acts and works of art that symbolize nursing experience.

The formal expressions of each pattern, once they are available to the members of the discipline, make possible certain kinds of formal inquiry processes that depend on the community or on the collective efforts of several members of the discipline. These are the processes for authenticating knowledge, represented in Figure 1.1 along the horizontal axis. In the empiric pattern, statements representing empiric reality are translated into inquiry statements that can be replicated in similar but different situations, and the adequacy of the statement can be validated in these similar but different situations. Autobiographic stories and the expression of the genuine self lead to reflection and response from others in the discipline with the intent of discerning the value and adequacy of personal insights. Ethical principles and codes lead to collective dialogue and justification of the soundness of the principles in addressing nursing's ethical and moral dilemmas. Aesthetic criticism and works of art lead to formation of collective appreciation of aesthetic meanings in practice and becomes a source of inspiration for development of the art of nursing.

The innermost sphere in Figure 1.1 represents the nondiscursive forms of expression of knowing that are enacted in the practice of nursing. The nondiscursive expressions represent nursing praxis-the synchrony of thoughtful reflection and action that constitutes nursing as a human caring practice. Praxis assures, through reflections, the continual asking of critical questions associated with each fundamental pattern of knowing, as well as ongoing knowledge development.

All of these processes are interactive and nonlinear, and there is no one starting point. Nurses in practice and nurses who primarily engage in the formal inquiry processes all contribute to the activities that are involved in creating nursing knowledge. Each nurse engages in activities that make possible scientific competence, moral-ethical comportment, therapeutic use of self, and transformative art-acts.

To illustrate how these processes interact, suppose you have an empiric problem concerning what nursing approaches to relieving pain are effective in practice, and why, You might begin by planning a research program to systematically study two different approaches to pain relief. You would identify the theoretical explanations associated with each approach and plan research studies that test selected hypothetical relationships. Whereas the empiric questions are the starting point and remain the focus of your method, your approaches and methods are influenced by aesthetic meanings of experiences of relieving pain and suffering, personal meanings concerning the experience of pain, and ethical values that influence how and when pain relief is given and received.

Personal knowing is frequently the avenue through which awareness of possibilities that are not yet fully understood first emerges. For example, suppose a nurse comes to realize and appreciate the perspective of a family who is receiving care in the clinic. Something has not seemed to fit, has not felt right, and a growing appreciation of the family's perspective gradually brings a new perspective. The nurse shares her awareness with the family, and the relationship shifts to bring the family's perspective to the center. Personal knowing is the starting point to bring a situation to awareness, but as you explore your awareness, your knowledge of empiric theories also is used as a tool, within a frame of ethical and aesthetic sensibilities.

Suppose you want to address an ethical question concerning what is right. You might begin with the focused creative activities of making explicit the personal and group values (valuing) that should guide your actions, clarifying the positions you find in ethical theories and principles that inform the issue, and setting forth how the application of these principles would function with the people with whom you work. These processes would lead reasoning. When you begin to share your ideas with your colleagues, the questioning and discussion that result will bring to awareness the personal insights of others engaged in the dialogue, empiric evidence about similar situations, and the range of aesthetic meanings that are possible in this and similar situations.

Aesthetics as a starting point, like personal knowing, often begins with a nurse's own awareness, but the expression often taken an art form that shows what the nurse envisions about the situation. The art can be in the form of the nurse's action in a situation. Suppose a nurse feels a connection to a person's experience of chronic pain. In a moment of caring for the person, the nurse acts from a deeply developed knowing of the meaning of chronic pain in a way that connects with the person's own experience, bringing together empiric, personal, and ethical knowing and creating a possibility that was not previously present.

Patterns Gone Wild

When knowledge within any one pattern is not critically examined and integrated with the whole of knowing, distortion instead of understanding is produced. Failure to develop knowledge integrated within all of the patterns of knowing leads to uncritical acceptance, narrow interpretation, and partial utilization of knowledge. We call this "the patterns gone wild." When this occurs, the patterns are used in isolation from one another, and the potential for syntheses of the whole is lost.

Empirics removed from the context of the whole of knowing produces control and manipulation. Ironically, these have been explicit traditional goals of the empiric sciences. When the validity of empiric knowledge is not questioned, one danger is its potential use in contexts where it does not belong. When you recognize how all the patterns contribute to the validity of empirics, you begin to see the unquestioned goals of control and manipulation as a distortion or misuse of empiric knowledge.

Ethics removed from the context of the whole of knowing produces rigid doctrine and insensitivity to the rights of others. This happens when someone simply sets forth personal ideas concerning what is right or good and advocates a position on reasoning derived from personal perspectives. The person may present a justification for a perspective to others but not take seriously the processes of dialogue that the justification invites. In the absence of this integrating process, the person's position remains isolated, with little or no opportunity for empiric, personal, or aesthetic insights to give meaning and social relevance to the ideas.

Personal knowing removed from the context of the whole of knowing produces isolation and self-distortion. When this happens, the self remains isolated, and knowledge of self comes only from what is known internally. Self-distortions can take a wide range of forms, from aggrandizement and overestimation of self to destruction and underestimation of self.

Aesthetics removed from the context of the whole of knowing produces indulgence in self-serving expressions and lack of appreciation for the fullness of meaning in a context. Human actions emerge from and are represented by the tastes and desires of the individual alone, without taking into account the deep cultural meanings inherent in the art-act. Art-acts become self-serving, shallow, arrogant, and empty. Self-serving preferences grow out of a failure to comprehend the deeper cultural, historical, and political significance of the art-act itself. Inauthentic meanings are assigned to another's experience, or a self-serving posture is assumed with respect to another person.

To illustrate "patterns gone wild," imagine an elderly woman admitted to a nursing home. She has lived a life rich in experience and activities and loves to verbally explore her past, making sense of what it means and how it relates to her present life. Having always been physically active, she takes a nightly stroll before going to bed. In the nursing home, she climbs over the bed rails after the lights are out and, with her walker, walks the halls, unsteady but determined, smiling and peering into other rooms. Hearing other residents talking or moaning, she sometimes goes into their rooms and tells them stories or talks with them to ease their troubled nights.

Consider what you might see if any one of the patterns of knowing were isolated from the context of the whole of knowing. Empirics isolated from the other patterns of knowing might require giving a drug that would be effective in bringing sleep to the woman soon after the lights go out, thereby controlling the situation and manipulating her into compliance, regardless of any other concerns. Ethics taken alone might impose the nurse's view of what is right or good for the woman and lead to a rule that would confine the woman to her bed after the lights are out and create a rigid, rule-oriented atmosphere that is insensitive to what the woman and others see as right or good. Personal knowing in isolation would impose the nurse's perspective, with the nurse isolated in the view that the old woman is a nuisance who is interfering with the time needed to complete the charting for the night. Aesthetics alone would impose the nurse's own tastes, preferences, and meanings on the situation. The nurse might restrain the woman in her bed and use a tape recorder to play the nurse's favourite new age music without considering whether the woman can hear the music or whether she finds the music soothing or appealing.

When ethics, aesthetics, personal knowing, and empirics come together as a whole, the purposes of developing knowledge and the actions based on that knowledge become more responsible and humane and create liberating choices. A whole understanding of the woman in the nursing home would take into account the woman's own safety and the needs of other residents; her personal life history and that which gives her pleasure; the ethical dimensions of personal empowerment, moral development, and caring for others; the aesthetic meaning of her actions in the cultural context of aging; and the personal perspective of the nurses who care for her. Many choices remain open in addressing this situation, but all of these considerations together would lead to nursing approaches that would differ from any of the approaches taken from one knowing perspective alone.

Reasons for Developing Nursing's Patterns of Knowing

As is shown in Figure 1.1 and our discussion of it, the fundamental reason for developing a body of knowledge in nursing is for the purpose of creating expert nursing practice. Nursing's unique perspective and the particular contributions nurses bring to care come from the whole of knowing, a wholeness that has survived despite a cultural and contextual dominance of empiric knowing. In a sense the discipline of nursing can be viewed as the empiric pattern of knowing gone wild in that the majority of formal knowledge development efforts have focused on empiric knowledge development methods. Moreover, knowledge has been equated with empiric forms to the exclusion of any other forms of expression.

The idea that knowledge development is separate from the realities of practice can be seen as deriving from the dominance of empirics. Empiric theory is inadequate to represent the complexity of the practice world, and the methods of science traditionally have considered the uncontrolled and unpredictable contingencies in the practice realm unacceptable for the purposes of developing empiric knowledge. The practice implications of empiric theory are often not direct or immediately obvious, and empiric theory often uses a different language from that used in practice.

A shift to a balance in knowledge development to reflect each of the patterns of knowing in nursing holds potential to bring the realm of knowledge development and the realm of practice together. Methods for developing aesthetic, personal, and ethical knowing compel immersion within the realm of practice. Giving attention to these aspects of knowledge development shifts how empirics itself is viewed; empirics becomes part of a larger whole, and its value takes on different meaning other than empirics, many of the traditions and assumptions that underlie empiric methods are challenged, opening the way for creating empiric methods that better accommodate the contingencies of practice.

Formally expressed nursing knowledge provides professional and disciplinary identity, which in turn conveys to others what nursing contributes to the health care process. Professional identity that evolves from distinct disciplinary knowledge provides a basis from which nurses can create certain aspects of their practice. Nursing practice has traditionally been controlled by others, and what nurses do is often invisible. The knowledge that forms nursing practice provides a language for talking about the nature of nursing practice and for demonstrating its effectiveness. Once nursing practice is described, it is made visible. Moving to a conceptualisation of knowledge that more fully embraces the whole of practice will serve to impart value to what has been intangible. Also, when nursing's effectiveness can be shown, it can be deliberately shaped or controlled by those who practice it.

On an individual level, nursing knowledge can provide self-identity and esteem as a nurse because you will have a firmer base when your ideas are questioned. As you become familiar with the language and processes of knowledge development, you can begin to think about how assumptions, definitions, and relationships within each of the patterns of knowing can be challenged. The study and understanding of knowledge development will provide a basis on which to take risks, to act deliberately, and to improve practice.

Imagine yourself as a nurse who is using massage to ease chronic pain for a hospitalised person. A physician notices that you are using this method of care. Because this is an unfamiliar approach to the physician, she asks you about it. You explain your reasoning, which is based on nursing knowledge. You can provide research evidence of the effectiveness of massage and information about the positive results that this particular person is experiencing. You can explain the ethical dimensions of providing relief from suffering, the aesthetic components of meaning in the situation, and what you have learned about the therapeutic use of self in giving a massage. Your explanation leads to an informed discussion about various approaches to caring for people with pain and why your approach seems to be effective for this person. As other practitioners learn of your knowledge in this area, they seek your consultation in caring for people with pain. Your knowledge of empiric pain theory and what is effective in caring for people with pain, as well as your ethical, aesthetic, and personal knowledge, provides a valuable resource for developing and improving practice.

Nursing's formally expressed body of knowledge also provides the discipline with a coherence of purpose. Coherence of professional purpose is closely linked to professional identity. Coherence of purpose contributes to a collective identity when nurses agree on the general practice domain. The processes of developing nursing's body of knowledge serve as a means for resolving significant disagreements among practitioners about what is to be accomplished. Varying points of view concerning the general purpose of nursing are reflected in the following questions:

- Should nurses address prevention of illness?
- Should nurses treat human responses to illness?
- Should educational programs be structured around nursing process?
- Nursing diagnosis? Patterns of knowing? Critical thinking?
- Should nurses view health and illness as opposites?
- Can ill or diseased people also be healthy?

As nurses develop individual and collective responses to these questions, our directions for developing knowledge will be clearer, and in turn our knowledge development efforts will contribute to clarifying responses to questions such as these. Nursing knowledge facilities coherence by examining such questions as a basis for deliberate choices. When nurses examine and agree about professional purposes and develop knowledge related to those purposes, the public and other practitioners will recognize nursing's expertise in relation to that arena. The fact that nurses are responsible for certain situations will be directly and indirectly communicated to society, and professional identity and coherence of purpose will continue to evolve. By shifting to a balance in the development of all the fundamental knowledge patterns, a sense of purpose can develop that is grounded in the whole of knowing that shapes and directs nursing practice.

Chapter 2

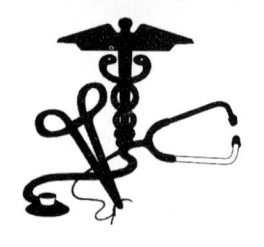

Nightingale's Environment Model

Florence Nightingale, the matriarch of modern nursing, was born May 12, 1820, while her British parents were on an extended European tour. Her parents, Edward and Frances Nightingale, named their daughter for her birthplace, Florence, Italy. The Nightingales were affluent and well-educated members of a Victorian family. So as Nightingale grew older, her father tutored her in mathematics, languages, religion, and philosophy. In her teens Nightingale was active in aristocratic society, but she felt her life should be more useful. In 1837 she confined in her diary, "God spoke to me and called me to his service."

In 1851 she went to Kaiserswerth, Germany, for her early nursing training. After leaving Kaiserswerth, she continued to examine the facilities at hospitals, reformatories, and charitable institutions. In 1853 she became Superintendent of the Hospital for Invalid Gentlewomen in London. During the Crimean War, Nightingale volunteered to go to Scutari, Turkey, where she organized a nursing department and devoted her efforts to eliminating sanitation problems in the wards. At that time, women working in hospitals were not respectable, reliable, or educated. There were no trained nurses and no British Red Cross. Consequently, Nightingale solicited and received help from the Sisters of Mercy. Conditions in the army wards were poor. In addition to their wounds, the soldiers suffered from exposure, frostbite, lice infestations, and disease. There were few chamber pots; latrines were blocked; cesspools overflowed; and the water was contaminated. Patients who could not feed themselves starved. There were no surgery tables or anaesthesia.

Nightingale's work make her popular with the men. They called her "The Lady of the Lamp," in recognition of her Turkish candle lantern, which she carried through the corridors packed with wounded soldiers. While at Scutari, Nightingale became critically ill with Crimean fever, which might have been typhus.

Nightingale returned to England following the war and established a teaching institution for nurses at St. Thomas Hospital and at King's College Hospital in London. These were established from funds received in recognition of her war service. Nightingale kept close contact with her graduates through encouraging letters. Within a few years after its foundation, the Nightingale School began receiving requests for nurses to found new schools at hospitals world-wide, and Florence Nightingale's reputation as the founder of modern nursing was assured.

During her career, Nightingale concentrated on army sanitation reform, army hospitals, and sanitation in India and among the poorer classes in England. She wrote Notes on Matters Affecting the Health, Efficiency, and Hospital Administration of the British Army (1858), Notes on Hospitals (1858), Notes on the Sanitary State of the Army in India (1871), and Life or Death in India (1874). For her efforts, Nightingale received numerous awards, including the Order of Merit from King Edward VII, Germany's Cross of Merit, and France's Secours aux Blesses Militaries.

Nightingale wrote between 15,000 and 20,000 letters to friends and distinguished acquaintances. These often displayed her beliefs, observations, and desire for change in health care. She worked into her eighties, gathering data and writing about nursing and health care. She enjoyed a robust old age before suffering a gradual loss of vision, which made reading and writing difficult. She was widely recognized for her knowledge, drive, and compassion.

Nightingale died in her sleep at the age of 90 on August 13, 1910, in London. But many of her revolutionary ideas continue to inspire contemporary nursing.

EVOLUTION OF THEORY

Many factors influenced the development of Nightingale's theory for nursing. Individual, societal, and professional values were all integral in the development of her work. She combined her individual resources with societal and professional resources to produce change.

Nightingale, who considered nursing a religious calling to be answered only by women, believed she should strive to change the things she saw as unacceptable. Chinn and Jacobs note that "When individual or professional values are in conflict with and challenge societal values, there is potential for creating change in society." Nightingale lived up to that potential. The health care system of her era used the uneducated and incompetent to care for the ill. But Nightingale transformed it into the system of professional nursing practices we value today.

Nightingale knew that contact with the professionals of her time was important. She expanded of her time was important. She expanded her philosophy of nursing through association with numerous prominent physicians and other influential members of society. The strongest influences on the development of her practice were her education, experience, and observation. She gained these through years of charitable and hospital work and military nursing. Then established the logical base for her nursing philosophy.

Florence Nightingale is viewed as founder and architect of modern nursing and also viewed as the mother of modern nursing. She synthesized informations gathered in many of her life experiences to assist her in the development of modern nursing. Many factors influenced the development of Nightingale's, theory of nursing. Individual, societal, and professional values were all integral in the development of her work. She combined her individual resources with societal and professional resources to produce change, because when individual or professional values are in conflict with and challenge societal values, there is potential for creating change in society. Nightingale lived up to that potential. The health care system her era used the uneducated and incompetent to care for the ill. Nightingale transformed it into the system of professional practice that valued at present.

Nightingale used her broad base of knowledge, her understanding of the incidence and prevalence of disease, and her acute powers of observation to develop an approach to nursing as well as to the management and construction of hospitals. Nightingale's main focus was the control of environment of individuals and families, both healthy and ill. She discussed the need for ventilation and light in sick rooms, proper disposal of sewage, and appropriate nutrition. Her work "Notes on Nursing" is a thought-provoking essay on the organization and manipulation of the environment of those persons requiring nursing care. She stated then her purpose was "everyday sanitary knowledge, or the knowledge of nursing as in other words, of how to put the constitution in show a state as thus it will have no disease, or than it can recover from disease: She viewed disease as a reparative process, a then is reflected to the policy states that "nursing is the diagnosis and treatment of human responses to actual or potential health problems. Her voluminous works provided much information on the influence of the environment in the human being and the critical nature of balance between the human and his environment.

NIGHTINGALE'S THEORY ON ENVIRONMENT

Nightingale's grand theory focussed on the environment. Environment is the surrounding matters that influence or modify a course of development, the system must interact and adjust to its environment. Environment which is capable of preventing, suppressing or contributing to disease, accidents or death, in all the external conditions and influences affecting the life and developments of all organism. Nightingale viewed the manipulations of the physical environment as a major component of nursing care. She identified ventilation and warmth, light, noise, variety, bed and bedding, cleanliness of rooms and walls, and nutrition as major areas of the environment the nurse could control. When one or more aspects of the environment are out of balance, the clients must use increased energy to canter the environmental stress. These stresses drawn the client of energy needed for healing. These aspects of the physical environment as also influenced by the social and psychological environment of the individual. In her writing, "Notes on Nursing," she discussed many aspects of environment related to nursing care which includes health of houses, ventilation and warming light, noise, variety, bed and bedding, personal cleanliness, diet, chattering of hopes and advices, and social consideration. The view on these is as follows:

Health of Houses

Nightingale discussed the importance of the health of houses as being closely related to the presence of pure air, pure water, efficient drainage, cleanliness and light. To support the hospital based nursing attending to these, she said, "badly constructed houses do for the healthy what badly constructed hospitals do for the sick. Once ensure that the air is stagnant and sickness is certain to follow." Nightingale also noted that the cleanliness outside the house effected the inside. Just as she noted that doing heaps affected the health of the houses is her time, so too can modern families are affected by toxic waste, contaminated water, and polluted air. She wanted people to use commonsense but only after these were educated to essential facts regarding health.

Ventilation and Warming

The aspect of the environment that concerned Nightingale most was providing proper ventilation for a patient. This meant the nurse was "to keep the air he breathes as pure as the external air, without chilling." She urged the caregiver to consider the source of the air in the patients room, as she believed a steady supply of fresh air was the most important principles of nursing. the air might be full of fumes from gas, mustiness, or open sewage of the source was not the freshest. Nightingale believed that the person who repeatedly breathed his or her own air would become sick or remain sick.

Nightingale was very concerned about "noxious air" or "effluvia" or four odours that came from excrement. In many public places, as well as hospitals, raw sewage could be found near patients, in ditches under or near the house, or contaminating drinking water. Her concerns about "effluvia" also included bedpans, urinals, and other utensils used to discard excrement.

Nightingale stressed the importance of room temperature. The patient should not be too warm or too cold. The temperature could be controlled by appropriate balance between burning fires and ventilation from windows. She advised nurses to constantly monitor patients body temperature by palpating the extremities to prevent the effects of vital heat loss and take measure, accordingly.

Light

Light was another element of nursing care that Nightingale believed could not be ignored. She viewed that direct sunlight was what patients wanted. Although acknowledging a lack of scientific rationale for it, she noted that light has "quite real and tangible effects upon the human body." She pointed out that people do not consider the different between light needed in a bedroom (where individual sleep at night) and light needed in a sickroom. Light, especially direct sunlight has purifying effect on the air of the room. Modern hospital may be constructed in suchaway that day light is available for patients to serve variety of purposes through properly constructed windows.

Noise

Noise was another environmental element. Nightingale believed that the nurse should manipulate. She stated that patients should never be waked intentionally or accidentally during the first part of sleep. She asserted that whispered or long conversations about patients are thoughtless and cruel. She viewed unnecessary noise, including noise from female dress, as cruel and irritating to the patient. Nurses today do not wear crinoline petticoats, but they do wear jewellery and carry keys that jingle and make other noises. Other more modern noises include the snapping of rubber gloves, the clank of stethoscope against metal bed rails, as radios and TVs. Modern health care facilities contain much equipment that issues alarms, beeps and other noises than startle or jar a patient from sleep to wakefulness. She was very critical of noises that annoyed the patient, such as a window shade blowing against the window frame. She viewed that on the nurses responsibility to assess and stop this kind of noise.

Variety

Nightingale believed that variety in the environment was a critical aspect of affecting the patients recovery. She discussed the need for changes in colour and form, including bringing the patient brightly coloured flowers or plants. She also advocated rotating 10 or 12 paintings and engravings each day, week, or month to provide variety for the patient which helps interaction between mind and body. Nightingale also advocated reading, needlework, writing, and cleaning as activities to relieve the sick of boredom. Now this is called diversion therapy.

Bed and Bedding

Nightingale viewed bedding as an important part of the environment. She stated that dirty carpets and walls containing large quantities of organic matter and provided ready source of infection, just as dirty sheets and beds did. She noted that an adult in health exhales about three pints of moisture through the lungs and skew in a 24 hours period. This organic matters enters the sheets and stays there unless the bedding is changed and aired frequently. She believed bed should be placed on the lightest part of the room and placed so that patient could se out of a window. She reminded caregiver never to lean against, sit upon, or unnecessarily shake the bed of a patient. Modern mattresses covered with plastic and other material, to remove drainage excreta and other matter. But sheets doesn't fit mattresses, leads to wrinkles may cause bedsores/pressure sores. It is important for the nurse to keep bedding clean, neat and dry and to position the patient for maximum comfort.

Personal Cleanliness

The need for cleanliness is extended to the patient, the nurse and the environment. Nightingale viewed the functions of the skin is important, believing that many diseases, "disorders" or caused breaks in the skin. She thought that was particularly true in children and that the excretions that come from the skin must be washed away. She believed that unwashed skin poisoned the patient and noted that bathing and drying the skin provided great relief to the patient, saying "just as it is necessary to renew the air round a sick person frequently, to carry off morbid effluvia from the lungs and skin, by maintaining free ventilations, so is it necessary to keep pores of the skin free from all obstructing excretions." She also believed that personal cleanliness extended to the nurse and that every nurse ought to wash her hands very frequently during the day.

Nutrition and Taking Food

Nightingale addressed the variety of food presented to the patients and discussed the importance of variety in the food presented. She found this attention provided to the patient affected how the patient ate. She noted their individual desire different foods at different times of the day and the frequent small services may be more beneficial to the patient than a large breakfast or dinner. She observed that patients may desire a different pattern of taking foods, show as eating breakfasts food at lunch and then chronically ill patient may be starved to death. Because their incapacitation can make them unable to eat food themselves. She urged that no business be done with patients while they are eating because this was distraction.

Chattering Hopes and Advices

Nightingale did not follow specially psychosocial environment as discussed to physical environment, but her writings on "chattering hopes and advices. She wrote that the chapter heading might seem "odd" but that to falsely cheer the sick by making laugh and their illness and its danger is not helpful. She considered not stressful for a patient to hear opinions after only brief observations had been made. False hope was depressing to patients, she felt, and caused them to worry and become fatigued. Nightingale encouraged the nurse to heed what is being said by visitors, believing that sick persons should hear good news that would assist them in becoming healthier.

Social Considerations

Nightingale supported the importance of looking beyond the persons to the social environments in which he or she lived. She observed that generations of families lived and died in poverty. Using her statistical data, she wrote letters and position papers and sent them to her acquaintance and the government in an effort to improve undesirable living conditions. Nightingale was a role model for political activities by nurses. She was also an excellent manager. She demonstrated management skills at Scutari and wrote about them in many of her nursing-related works. In her writing she discussed "Duty management." She believed that the nurse and hospital related to be well managed, i.e. organised, clean and with appropriate supplies show client and environment in balance and expending unnecessary energy being stressed by environment (Figs. 2.1 and 2.2).

PARADIGM OF NIGHTINGALE'S ENVIRONMENT MODEL

Paradigm is a term used to denote the prevailing network of science philosophy and theory accepted by a discipline. The term was meant to refer to what members of the community have in common.

Florence Nightingale did not discover or define the major concepts used to organize nursing theory but the analysis of her writing gives uses to identify her definitions of these concepts which include:

Nursing

Nightingale viewed medicine and surgery as remove obstructions to health to allow nature to return the person to health. What nursing has to do, **is to put the patient on the best condition for nature to act upon him.** She states the nursing "ought to signify the proper use of fresh air, light, warmth, cleanliness, quick and that proper selections paid

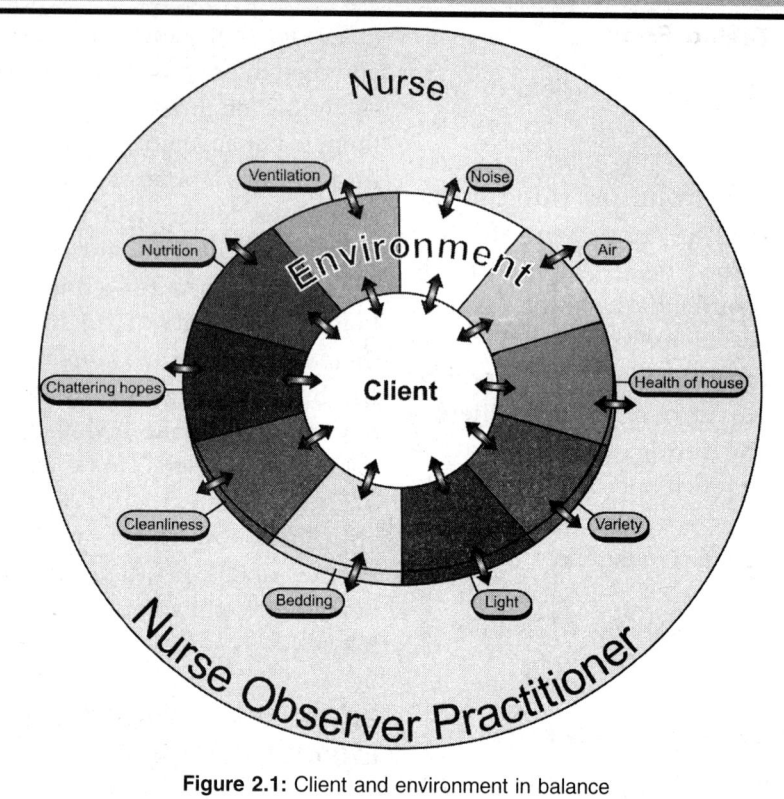

Figure 2.1: Client and environment in balance

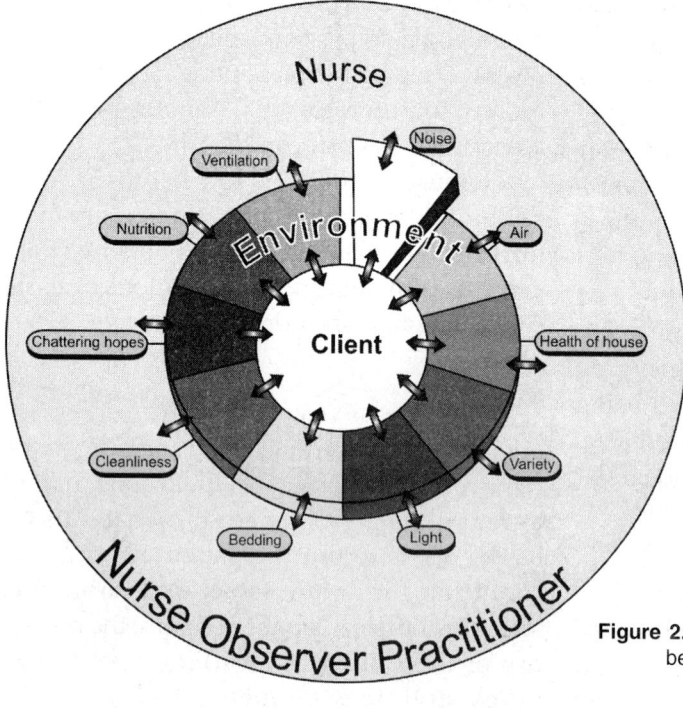

Figure 2.2: Client expending unnecessary energy by being stressed by environment (Noise)

administration of diet – all at the least expense of vital power to the patient. She reflected the art of nursing in her statement that, "the art of nursing, as now practiced, seems to be expressly constituted to unmake what God had made disease to be viz., a reparative process.

Human Being

Human being are not defined by Nightingale but they are defined on relationship to their environment and the impact of the environment upon them.

Environment

Nightingale focussed on environment then surrounding human being is considered on relation to ministrate of health, when stressed in physical environment, i.e., ventilations, warmth, noise, light and darkness. She synthesized immediate knowledge of disease with existing sanitary conditions on the environment.

Health

It is also not specifically defined. She stated "we know nothing of health, the positive of which pathology in the negative, except from observation and experience. She believed nature alone cures. Given her definition that of the art of nursing is to "unmake what God had made disease," then the goal of all nursing activities should be client health. She believed the nursing should provide care to the healthy as well as the ill and discussed health promotions as an activity in which nurses should engage.

When organizing the Nightingale environmental model, note that the client, the nurse and the major environmental concepts are in balance: that is the nurse can manipulate the environment to compensate for the clients response to it. The goal of the nurse is to assist the patient in staying balance. If the environment of an client is out of balance, the client expends unnecessary energy to adjust to unit.

NIGHTINGALE AND NURSING PROCESS

Assessment

In this stage Nightingale advocates two essential behaviours by the nurses. The **first** is to ask the client what is needed or wanted, i.e. ask many question to know the actual status of the client. Nightingale warned against asking leading questions and advocated asking precise questions with knack. The **second** area of assessment the advocates was the use of observation. She used precise observations concerning all aspects of the clients physical health and environment. First one is subjective data and second one is objective data that are used to present nursing process. An assessment guide can be structured from Nightingale environmental model.

Nursing Diagnoses

Nursing diagnoses are based on an analysis of the conclusion gained from the information to the assessment. Nightingale believed data should be used as the basis for drawing any conclusion. It is important that the diagnosis in the client response to their environment and not the environmental problem. Nursing diagnosis reflect the importance of the environment to the health and well-being of the client.

Planning

Planning includes identifying the nursing actions needed to keep clients comfortable, dry and in the best state for nature to work on. The value of informed action, based on extensive knowledge is well illustrated by Nightingale's personality. Planning focussed on modifying the environment to enhance the clients, ability to respond to the disease process.

Implementation

Implementation takes place on the environment that affects out client and involves taking action to modify that environment. All factors of the environment should be considered, including noise, air, odours, beddings, cleanliness, light—all the factors that place clients in the best positions for nature to work upon them.

Evaluation

Evaluation is based on the effects of the changes in the environment on the clients ability to regain their health at the least expense of energy. Observation is primary method of data collection based to evaluate the clients responses to the intervention.

NIGHTINGALE MODEL AND THE CHARACTERISTICS OF THEORY

1. Theories can interrelate concepts in show away as to create different way and loving at a particular phenomena.
   When nursing situations are viewed from a Nightingale perspective, using her environment model, new insights into the phenomena of interest to nursing can be identified. Examining environmental aspects, such as light, noise or warmth can provide new insights into human responses to health and illness, which means that health and illness not only influenced by the pathophysiology and also psychosocial environment.

2. *Theories must logical in nature.*
   Florence Nightingale environmental model is logical. There is nothing illogical in her discussions of the physical or psychosocial environment. She built her conclusion from observations, she made her case, drew her conclusions, and then acted. She believed that she has used logic to correct her conclusion.

3. *Theories must be relatively single yet generalizable.*
   Nightingale's writings are simple, as in the articulation of her environmental model. The beauty of her model is its generalizability, including its continued applicability to day. Her model can be applied and the most complex hospital intensive care unit, the home, a work site, or the community at large. Concepts related to air, light, noise and cleanliness can be applied across specific environment.

4. *Theories can be bases for hypothesis that can be tested or for theory to the explained.*
   Nightingale has stimulated the development of nursing science with her work. She has had a profound effect on many of the other nursing theorists. These individuals have indicated the influence of Nightingale by citing her in their work or commenting on her influence in a commemorative edition of "Notes on Nursing." The research related to the impact of the environments on client health has been influenced by Nightingale.

5. *Theories constitute to and assist in increasing the general body of knowledge within the discipline through the research implementation to validate them.*

Nightingale's theory seems to have more relevance to practitioners today than ever before. More and more data are becoming available to indicate the critical nature of the impact of the environment on the health and well-being of the individual. This information is relevant in all environment for the intensive care unit to the community.

6. *Theories can be used by practitioner to guide and improve them practice.*

Nightingale's theory has found applicability to the nurse practitioner. Reading her work raises a consciousness on the nurse about how the environment influences client outcomes. For example, controlling sound in the wards, mounting ventilation and light, put off light during nights all and all help in recovery from illness.

7. *Theories must be consistent with validated theories, laws and principles but will have open unanswered questions that need to be investigated.*

Nightingale's theory works well with ecological, systems, adaptation and interpersonal theories. Although she did not believed in germs theory, the practices she recommend did not consistent with scientific knowledge. But many of her suggestions which she based on observation of client response to their environment, have been documented on scientifically sound when tested with rigorous application of modern research methods.

"A theory in the early stage of development is characterized by discursive presentation and descriptive accounts of anecdotal report to illustrate and support its claims. The theoretical terms are usually vague and ill defined, and their meaning may be close to everyday language. A paradigm at this embryonic stage is very readable and provides a perspective rather than a set of interrelated theoretical statements. This type of formulation, the "grand theory" or "general orientation," is aimed at explaining the totality of behaviour. Grand theories tend to use vague terminology, leave the relationships between terms unclear and provide formulations that cannot be tested."

Nightingale's intention to provide a first step for the formalization and development of nursing seems to have been accomplished. Her achievements spawned the beginning of nursing as we know it today. Nightingale's theory was a lower level theory, but it sets the stage for further work in the development of nursing theories.

Evaluation of Theory

- Nightingale's theory contains three major relationships—environment to patient, nurse to environment, and nurse to patient. She viewed environment as the main factor acting on the patient to produce an illness state and regarded disease as "the reactions of kindly nature against the conditions in which we have placed ourselves." The nurse as manipulator of environment and actor on the patient is described when Nightingale said nursing "ought to signify the proper use of fresh air, light, warmth, cleanliness, quiet, and the proper selection and administration of diet–all at the least expense of vital power to the patient." Those relationships are expanded on in *Notes on Nursing*. This book is organized into chapters dealing with the components of environment, such as ventilation, warmth, light, noise, and cleanliness. Relationships between these environmental components are also described, such as when Nightingale states, "Without cleanliness, within and without your house, ventilation is comparatively useless."

- Nightingale's theory attempts to provide general guidelines for all nurses in all times. Although many of her specific directives are no longer applicable, the general concepts, such as the relationships between nurse, patient, and environment, are still pertinent. The theory is specifically directed toward the nurse, defined as a woman who at some time has charge of somebody's health, and is thus not restricted to the professional nurse. To address her audience, the proposed theory is of necessity very broad. Generality is a criterion met by Nightingale's theory.

- Concepts and relationships within Nightingale's theory are frequently stated implicitly and are presented as established truths rather than as tentative, testable statements. Little or no provision is made for empirical examination. Indeed, Nightingale suggested that the practice of nursing should be built on individual observation rather than systematic research when she advised, "Let experience, not theory, decide upon this as upon all other things."

- Nightingale's writings, to an extraordinary degree, direct the nurse to action on behalf of her patient and herself. These directives encompass the areas of practice, research, and education. Most specific are her principles attempting to shape nursing practice. She urges nurses to provide doctors with "not your opinion, however respectfully given, but your facts." She goes on to say, "If you cannot get the habit of observation one way or other, you had better give up the being a nurse, for it is not your calling, however kind and anxious you may be." Her encouragement of a measure of independence and precision previously unknown in nursing may still guide and motivate us today as nursing continues to evolve.

- Nightingale's view of humanity was consistent with her theories of nursing. She believed in creative, universal humanity with the potential and ability for growth and change. Deeply religious, she viewed nursing as a means of doing the will of her God. Perhaps it is because of this concept of nursing as a divine calling that she relegated the patient to a passive role, essentially infantile, with every want and need provided by the nurse. The excessive zeal and self-righteousness of a religious reformer might partially account for this behaviour. Although the lack of patient involvement in health seems to be a gap in Nightingale's views, it may be accounted for by the historical period in which she lived and wrote.

Basic principles of environmental manipulation and psychological care of the patient can be applied with modification in many contemporary nursing settings. Of course, many technological and societal changes have occurred since Nightingale's day, which reduce some of her fondest assertions to the ludicrous. Her unshakable disdain for the germ theory of disease and adherence to the belief that dirt and dampness are pathogenic now seems less than progressive. Likewise, her emphasis on personal observation rather than formation of a unified body of nursing knowledge has fallen into disuse.

Lack of specificity has hindered use of Nightingale's ideas for the generation of nursing research. However, her writings continue to stimulate productive thinking for the individual nurse and the nursing profession. Nightingale was brilliant and creative. She gave nursing much food for thought–food that continues to nourish us over 130 years later.

Chapter 3

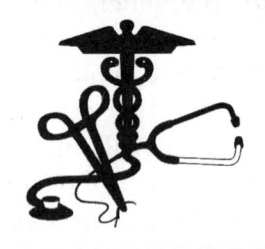

Abdellah's Typology of 21 Problems

Faye Glenn Abdellah was born in New York City. A 1942 Magna Cum Laude graduate of Fitkin Memorial Hospital School of Nursing (now Ann May School of Nursing), she received her BS, MA, and EdD from Teacher's College at Columbia University. She completed her doctoral work in 1955.

Recognized as "one of the country's leading and best known researchers in health and public policy" as well as an "international expert of health problems," Abdellah has practiced in many settings. She has been a staff nurse, a head nurse, a faculty member at Yale University and at Columbia University, a public health nurse, a researcher, and an author of more than 146 articles and books. Since 1949, Abdellah has held various positions in the U.S. Public Health Service, including nurse consultant to the states, chief of the nurse education branch, senior consultant of nursing research, principle investigator in the progressive patient care project, chief of the research grants branch, director of nursing home affairs, and director of long-term care.

Abdellah was appointed Chief Nurse Officer of the USPHS in 1970, and served in that position for 17 years. Concurrently, in 1982 she was selected as Deputy Surgeon General, the first nurse and first woman to hold the post until her retirement in 1989. In this position, she was the focal point for nursing and a chief advisor on long-term care policy within the Office of the Surgeon General. Abdellah represented the interests of health professionals in all categories in the Public Health Service. She was advisor on matters related to nursing, long-term care policy, mental retardation, the developmentally disabled, home health services, aging, hospice, and AIDS. Because her efforts were directed toward improvement of the quality of health care for all Americans, she supervised the activities in both health and nonhealth agencies. She is the recipient of over 60 academic honors and professional awards. These include selection as a Charter Fellow of the American Academy of Nursing; 10 honorary degrees, including an honorary Doctor of Laws degree from Case Western Reserve University for pioneering nursing research and being responsible for the advent of the nurse-scientist scholar; an honorary degree from the University of Bridgeport for devoting her career to advancing the quality of health care through research and being an innovative and inspirational leader for nursing professionals; the Federal Nursing Service Award for the advancement of professional nursing; and the Distinguished Service Honor Award of the US Department of Health, Education, and Welfare for exceptional leadership and professional commitment and the first presidential award of Sigma Theta Tau International. In 1989, she receive the prestigious Allied-Signal Achievement Award for research in aging, and in 1992 she received the Gustav O. Lienhard Award, given by the Institute of Medicine, NAS, in recognition of her contributions to the betterment of the health of all Americans.

In 1988 and 1989, Abdellah received the Surgeon General's Medallion, which was presented by former Surgeon General Koop in recognition of contributions as Chief Nurse Officer, US Public Health Service and for exemplary service to the Surgeon General.

Abdellah's international involvement is extensive, and includes consultation to the Portuguese government in the development of programs for the care of the elderly and disabled. While in the People's Republic of China, she studied the care of the elderly and mentally retarded. She was assigned direct responsibility for developing a resolution to organize the World Assembly on the Elderly in 1982.

Abdellah was instrumental in the implementation of exchange programmes for US/USSR and US/France US scientists and health professionals with their counterparts in the then USSR and France, as well as exchange programmes for nurses in developing countries. Her leadership assistance in Yugoslavia resulted in the enactment of a law requiring the establishment of training programs for hospital managers. Her expertise and consultation led to the establishment of nursing research programs at Tel Aviv University in Israel and the development of a pre-screening examination used for foreign nurses. She served as consultant to the Japanese Nursing Associations in setting up graduate programs in nursing education and research. Abdellah also participated in a seminar series for nursing home leaders in Australia and nursing education and research meetings in New Zealand. She was Chairperson of the task force to establish the first Federal College of Nursing, to include the Army, Navy, Air Force, and US Public Health Service.

Evolution of Theory

Abdellah realized that for nursing to gain full professional status and autonomy, a strong knowledge base was imperative. Nursing also needed to move away from the control on medicine and toward a philosophy of comprehensive patient-centered care. Abdellah and her colleagues conceptualized 21 nursing problems to teach and evaluate students. The typology of 21 nursing problems first appeared in the 1960 edition of *Patient-centered Approach to Nursing* and had a far-reaching impact on the profession and on the development of nursing theories (Fig. 3.1).

The patient or family presents with nursing problems that the nurse helps them address through her professional function. The nurse addresses 21 problem categories: (i) hygiene and physical comfort, (ii) activity and rest, (iii) safety, (iv) body mechanics, (v) oxygena-

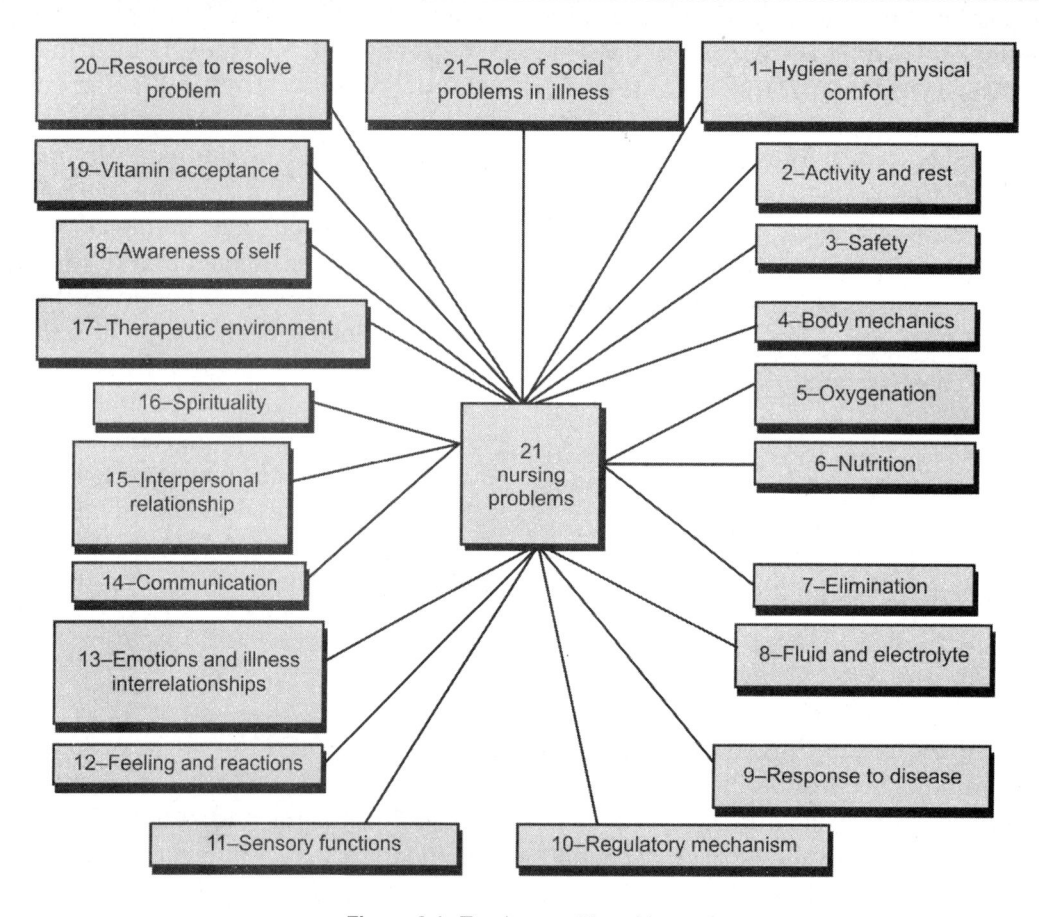

Figure 3.1: Typology or 21 problems

21 nursing problems:

1. Hygiene and physical comfort
2. Activity and rest
3. Safety
4. Body mechanics
5. Oxygenation
6. Nutrition
7. Elimination
8. Fluid and electrolyte
9. Response to disease
10. Regulatory mechanism
11. Sensory functions
12. Feeling and reactions
13. Emotions and illness interrelationships
14. Communication
15. Interpersonal relationship
16. Spirituality
17. Therapeutic environment
18. Awareness of self
19. Vitamin acceptance
20. Resource to resolve problem
21. Role of social problems in illness

tion, (vi) nutrition, (vii) elimination, (viii) fluid and electrolytes, (ix) responses to disease, (x) regulatory mechanisms, (xi) sensory function, (xii) feelings and reactions, (xiii) emotions and illness interrelationships, (xiv) communication, (xv) interpersonal relationships, (xvi) spirituality, (xvii) therapeutic environment, (xviii) awareness of self, (xix) limitation acceptance, (xx) resources to resolve problems, and (xxi) role of social problems in illness.

Nursing problems are both overt or obvious and covert. Nurses must be aware of covert problems to meet care requirements. Overt and covert problems must be identified to make a nursing diagnosis. Identification of problems precedes solution. The nursing process is the method nurses-use to establish and focus on a nursing diagnosis. The overall goal is a client's fullest possible functioning.

Individualized patient care is important for nursing. Both patients and nurses should be aware of the wholeness of clients and the need for continuity of care from before hospitalization to afterward. Individualized care will require changes in the organization and administration of nursing services and education.

Abdellah was influenced by the desire to promote client centred comprehensive nursing care and described nursing as "service to individuals and families and therefore, to Society." Nursing is based on an art and science that mould the attitudes, intellectual competencies, and technical skills of the individual nurse into the desire and ability to help people, sick or well, cope with their health needs. Nursing may be carried out under general or specific medical direction.

Abdellah's theory was derived from the following premises of comprehensive nursing care. As a comprehensive service, nursing includes the following:
- Recognizing the nursing problem of the patient (client).
- Deciding the appropriate courses of action to talk in terms of relevant nursing principles.
- Providing continuous care to relieve pain and discomfort a}nd provide immediate security for the in difficult.
- Adjusting the total nursing care plan to meet the patients (clients) individual needs.
- Helping the individual to become more-self-directing in attaining or maintaining a healthy state of mind and body.
- Instructing nursing personnel and family to help the individual do for himself that which he can within his limitations.
- Helping the individual to his limitations and emotional problems.
- Working with allied health professional in planning for optimum health on local, state, national and international level.
- Carrying out continuous evaluation and research to improve nursing techniques and to develop new techniques to meet the health needs of people.

These original premises have undergone an evolutionary process. For example, "providing continuous cares of the individual's total needs, was eliminated without any reason, but may be than it is impossible to provide continuous and total care.

CONCEPTS USED BY ABDELLAH

Nursing

Abdellah defined nursing as "Service to individuals. It is based upon an art and science which mould the attitudes, intellectual competences, and technical skills of the individual nurse into the desire and ability to help people sick or well cope with their health needs and may be carried out under general or specific medical direction.

Abdellah was clearly promoting the image of the nurse who was not only kind and caring, but also intelligent, competent and technically well prepared to provide service to the patient.

Health

Abdellah never defined health *per se*, her concept of health may be defined as the dynamic pattern of functioning, whereby there is a continued interaction with internal and external forcer, that result in the optimal use of necessary resources that serve to minimize vulnerabilities. Emphasis should be placed upon prevention and rehabilitation with wellness as a lifetime goal. By performing nursing services through a holistic approach to the client, the nurse helps the client achieve a state of health. However, effectively performs these service the nurse must accurately identify the lacks or deficits are the client's health needs.

Nursing Problem

The client's health needs can be viewed as problems. The nursing problem presented by the patients is condition faced by the patient or family which the nurse can assist him or them to meet through the performance of her professional functions. The problem can be either an **overt** or **covert** nursing problem. An **overt** nursing problem is an apparent conditions faced by the patient or family which the nurse can assist him or them to meet through the performance of her professional functions. The **covert** nursing problem is a concealed or hidden condition faced by the patient or family which the nurse can assist him or them to meet through the performance of her professional functions. Covert problems can be emotional, sociological and interpersonal in nature. They are often missed or perceived incorrectly. Yet many instances solving covert problems may solve the overt problem as well. Use of the term 'nursing problem' is more consistent with "nursing functions" or "nursing goals" than with client-control problems. Although Abdellah spoke of the patient-centred approaches she wrote nurses identifying and solving specific problems. This identification and classification of problems was called the "typology of 21 nursing problems as listed below:

1. To maintain good hygiene and physical comfort.
2. To promote optimal activity, exercise, rest, sleep.
3. To promote safety through prevention of accident, injury or other trauma and through the prevention of the spread of infection.
4. To maintain good body mechanics and prevent and correct deformities.
5. To facilitate the maintenance of a supply of oxygen to all body cells.
6. To facilitate the maintenance of nutrition to all body cells.
7. To facilitate the maintenance of elimination.
8. To facilitate the maintenance of fluid and electrolytes balance.
9. To recognize the physiological responses of the body to disease conditions—pathological, physiological and compensatory.
10. To facilitate the maintenance of regulatory mechanisms and functions.
11. To facilitate the maintenance of sensory function.
12. To identify and accept positive and negative expressions, feelings and sanctions.
13. To identify and accept interrelatedness of emotions and organic illness.
14. To facilitate the maintenance of effective verbal and non-verbal communication.
15. To promote the development of productive interpersonal relationship.
16. To facilitate progress towards achievement of personal spiritual goals.
17. To create and/or maintain a therapeutic environment.
18. To facilitate awareness of self as an individual with varying physical, emotional and developmental needs.
19. To accept the optimum possible goals in the light of limitations, physical, emotional.
20. To use community resources as an aid in resolving problems arising from illness.
21. To understand the role of social problems as influencing factors in the cause of illness.

Abdellah, typology was divided into three areas:
1. The physical, sociological and emotional needs of the patients (clients).
2. The types of interpersonal relationships between of the nurse and the patients (clients).
3. The common elements of patient (client) care.

In the process of identifying overt and covert nursing problems and interpreting, analyzing and selecting appropriate course of action to solve these problems. "Quality professional nursing care requires that nurses be able to identify and solve overt and covert nursing problems. These requirements can be met by the problem-solving pertinent data, formulating hypotheses, testing hypotheses, through the collections of data, and revising hypothesis when necessary on the basis of conclusion obtained from the data.

Many of these steps parallel to the steps of the nursing process. The problem-solving approach was selected because of the assumption that the correct identification of nursing problems influences the nurse's judgment in selecting the next steps in solving the client's nursing problems. The problem-solving approaches is also consistent with such basic elements of nursing practice espoused by Abdellah as observing, reporting and interpreting the signs and symptoms that comprise the deviations from health and constitute nursing problems and with analyzing the nursing problems and selecting the necessary course of action.

An examination of the 21 problems yields similarity to other viz., Virginia Henderson (1991), Abraham Marsow theory of hierarchy of needs (1954).

PARADIGM OF ABDELLAH'S TYPOLOGY

Abdellah does not clearly specify each of the four major concepts: human being, health, environment/society and nursing.

Human Being

She does describe the recipient of nursing as individuals (and families) although she does not delineate her beliefs or assumption about the nature of human beings. She describes people as having physical, emotional and sociological needs. These needs may be overt, consisting largely physical needs, or covert, such as emotional and social needs. The typology and nursing problem is said to evolve from the recognition of a need for patient-centred approach to nursing. The patient is described as the only justification for the existence of nursing. People are helped by the identification and alleviation of problems they are experiencing.

Health

As Abdellah discusses in "patient-centred" approaches to nursing in a state mutually exclusive of illness. Health is defined implicitly as a state when the individual has no unmet needs and no anticipated or actual impairments. Achieving of health is the purpose of Nursing Services. Although Abdellah does not give a definition of health, she speaks of 'total health needs" and 'a healthy state of mind and body' in her description of nursing as a comprehensive nursing service.

Environment

The environment is the least-discussed concept in her model. Nursing problem number 17 from the typology is "to create and/or maintain a therapeutic environment and she also states that if the nurses reaction to the patient is hostile or negative, the atmosphere in the room may be hostile, or negative. This suggests that patient interest and respond to their environment. Society is included in the premises of comprehensive nursing care, i.e. planning for optimum health on local, state, national and international.

Nursing

Nursing is a helping profession. Nursing care is doing something to or for the person or providing information to the person with goal meeting needs, increasing or restoring self-help-ability, or alleviating an impairment.

Nursing is broadly grouped into the 21 problems areas to guide care and promote the use of nursing judgment. Abdellah considers nursing to be a comprehensive service that is based on an art and science and aims to help people sick or well, cope with these health needs.

NURSING PROCESS AND ABDELLAH

Abdellah's typology of 21 nursing problems helps nurses practice in an organized systematic way. The use of this scientific base enables the nurse to understand the reason for her actions. Their use in the nursing process is primarily to direct the nurse indirectly to the client's benefits.

In **assessment phase**, each of the identified 21 nursing problems relevant data are collected. The overt or covert nature of the problems necessitates a direct or indirect approach, respectively For Example the overt problem of nutritional status can be assessed by direct measures of weight, food intake and body size, whereas the covert problem of maintaining a therapeutic environment requires more indirect approach to data collected. The nursing problems can be divided into those that are basic to all clients and those that reflect sustainable, remedial or restorative care needs.

Nursing diagnosis: is the result of data collection would determine the client's specific overt and/or covert problems. These specific problems would be grouped under one or more of the broader nursing problems.

In *planning phase* of nursing process, her statements of nursing problems most closely resemble goal statements. Therefore, once the problem has been diagnosed, the goals have been established. Many of the nursing problems statements can be considered goals for either the nurse or the client.

In implementation, nurse using the goals as the framework, a plan is developed and appropriate nursing intervention are determined. Again holism tends to be negated in implementation because of the isolated particular nature of the nursing problems.

Evaluation: The plan is evaluated in terms of client's progress or lack of progress toward the achievement of the goals.

Abdellah's Work and Characteristics of Theory

Theories can interrelate concepts in such a way as to create a different way of looking at a particular phenomena.
1. Abdellah, theory has interrelated concepts of health, nursing problems and problem solving as she attempts to create a different way of viewing nursing phenomena. The results the statement that nursing is the

use of the problem-solving approach with key nursing problems related to the health needs of the people.
2. Theoretical statement places heavy emphasis on problem-solving an activity that is inherently logical in nature.
3. Theory is appearing to be limited to use which seems to focus quite heavily on nursing practice with individuals. Theory does not provide the framework on human and society in general. This somewhat limits the ability to generalize, although the problem solving approach readily generalizable to clients with specific health needs and specific nursing problem.
4. One of the most important questions that arises when considering her work is the role of the client within the framework, a question that could generate hypotheses for testing. The results of testing such hypothesis would contribute to the general body of nursing knowledge.
5. Abdella's problem-solving approach can easily be used by practitioners to guide various activities within their nursing practice. This is especially true when considering nursing practice that deals with clients who have specific needs and specific problem.
6. Abdellah theory consistent with other validated theories, such as those of Maslows and Henderson. Although the consistency exists, many questions remain unanswered.

Evaluation of Theory

- The typology is very simple and is descriptive of nursing problems thought to be common among patients. The concepts of nursing, nursing problems, and the problem-solving process, which are central to this work, are defined explicitly. The concepts of person, health, and environment, which are associated with the nursing paradigm today, are implied. There are no stated relationships between Abdellah's major concepts or those of the nursing paradigm in her writing. This model has a limited number of concepts, and its only structure is a list. A somewhat mixed approach to concept definition is present in this work. Nursing and nursing problems are connotatively defined, while the problem-solving process is defined denotatively. These approaches to definitions do not seem to detract from the clarity of definitions. The typology does not yet constitute a theory because it lacks sufficient relationship statements.
- The 21 nursing problems are general and linked to neither time nor environment. "She acknowledges that her list is neither exhaustive nor listed according to priorities." Assuming that persons experience similar needs, the nursing goals stated in the list of 21 problems could be used by nurses in any time frame to meet patients' needs. However, according to this model, some persons do not need nursing.

Other service professions could use the typology of 21 nursing problems to focus on the psychosocial and emotional needs presented by patients. The goals of this model vary in generality. The broadest goal is to positively affect nursing education, while subgoals are to provide a scientific basis on which to practice and to provide a method of qualitative evaluation of educational experiences for students. The goals are appropriate for nursing.

- The concepts are very specific with empirical references that are easily identifiable. The concepts are within the domain of nursing. Ready linkage of the concepts and the typology to reality is secondary to an inductive approach to theory development. Validation of the typology was done by the faculty of 40 collegiate schools of nursing.
- The typology provided a general framework in which to act, but continued neither specific nursing actions nor patient-centered outcomes, despite the title of the book. However, two subsequent publications did address outcome measures (effect variables) and suggested models for organizing curricula to emphasize patient-centered outcomes. Except for stating the importance of nursing the whole patient, today's idea of holism is not apparent in this work. The skills list includes skills thought necessary for nurses to meet patients' needs but is not prescriptive. Abdellah suggests nursing research as a method for validating treatments toward resolution of patients' needs.

The emphasis on problem-solving is not limited by time or space and therefore provides a means for continued growth and change in the provision of nursing care. The problem-solving process and the typology of 21 nursing problems can be respectively considered precursors of the nursing care process and classification of nursing diagnoses in evidence today.

In *Patient-centrered Approaches to Nursing Care*, Abdellah addressed nursing education problems linked to the use of the medical model. Her typology provided a new way to qualitatively evaluate experiences and emphasized a practice based on sound rationales rather than note.

"She proposes that nurses could take a leadership role in making the public aware that quality nursing health care is available. Quality is defined as the care that the patient needs. Need is determined by a classification system that identifies the medical treatment and nursing care essential for that individual."

Abdellah has made significant contributions to patient care, education, and research in nursing and health care in this country and throughout the world.

Chapter 4

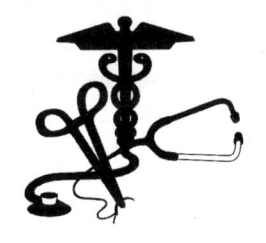

Henderson's Unique Function of Nurses

Virginia Henderson was born in 1897, the fifth of eight children in her family. A native of Kansas City, Missouri, Henderson spent her developmental years in Virginia because her father practiced law in Washington, D.C.

During World War I Henderson developed an interest in nursing. So in 1918 she entered the Army School of Nursing in Washington, D.C. Henderson graduated in 1921 and accepted a position as a staff nurse with the Henry Street Visiting Nurse Service in New York. In 1922 Henderson began teaching nursing in Norfolk Protestant Hospital in Virginia. Five years later she entered Teacher's College at Columbia University, where she subsequently earned her BS and MA degrees in nursing education. In 1929 Henderson served as a teaching supervisor in the clinics of Strong Memorial Hospital in Rochester, New York, She returned to Teacher's college in 1930 as a faculty member, teaching courses in the nursing analytical process and clinical practice until 1948.

Henderson has enjoyed a long career as an author and researcher. While on the Teacher's college faculty she rewrote the fourth edition of Bertha Harmer's *Textbook of the Principles and Practice of Nursing,* followed by the author's death. This edition was published in 1939. The fifth edition of the textbook was published in 1955 and contained Henderson's own definition of nursing. Henderson has been associated with Yale University since the early 1950s, and has done much to further nursing research through this association. From 1959 to 1971 Henderson directed the Nursing Studies Index Project sponsored by Yale. The Nursing Studies Index was developed into a four volume annotated index to nursing's biographical, analytical, and historical literature from 1900 to 1959. Concurrently, Henderson authored or coauthored several other important works. Her pamphlet, Basic *Principles of Nursing Care,* was published for the International Council of Nurses in 1960 and translated into more than 20 languages. Henderson's 5-year collaboration with Leo Simmons produced a national survey of nursing research that was published in 1964. Her book, The *Nature of Nursing,* of Nursing, was published in 1966 and described her concept of nursing's primary, unique function. It was reprinted by the National League of Nursing in 1991. The sixth edition of *The Principles and Practice of Nursing*, published in 1978, was coauthored by Henderson. This textbook has been widely used in the curricula of various nursing schools. Her classic textbooks have been translated into more than 25 languages. Through the 1980s. Henderson remained active as a Research Associate Emeritus at Yale. Henderson's achievements and influence in the nursing profession have brought her more than nine honorary doctoral degrees and the first Christiane Reimann Award. Henderson has been given the Mary Adelaide Nutting Award from the U.S. National League for Nursing, honorary Fellowship in the American Academy of Nursing, honorary membership in the Association of Integrated and Degree Courses in Nursing, London, and an honorary Fellowship in the Royal College of Nursing in England. In 1983, she received Sigma Theta Tau International's Mary Tolle Wright Founders Award for Leadership, one of the honour society's highest honours. At the 1988 American Nurses Association Convention, she received a special citation of honour for her lifelong contributions to nursing research, education, and professionalism. Sigma Theta Tau International named its international electronic computer nursing library in her honour.

EVOLUTION OF THEORY

Henderson first published her definition of nursing in the 1955 revision of Harmer and Henderson's, *The Principles and Practice of Nursing*. There were three major influences on Henderson's decision to synthesize her own definition of nursing. First, she revised *Textbook of Principles and Practice of Nursing* in 1939. Henderson identifies her work for this text as the source that made her realize "the necessity of being clear about the function of nurses. A second source was her involvement as a committee member in a regional conference of the National Nursing Council in 1946. Her committee work was incorporated into Esther Lucile Brown's 1948 report, Nursing for the Future. Henderson says this report represented" my point of view modified by the thinking of others in the group." Finally, the American Nurses Association's 5-year investigation of the function of the nurse interested Henderson, who was not fully satisfied with the definition adopted by the ANA in 1955.

Henderson labels her work a definition rather than a theory because theory was not in vogue at that time. She describes her interpretation as the "synthesis of many influences, some positive and some negative. In the Nature of Nursing she identifies the following sources of influence during her early years of nursing.

The patient is an individual who requires help toward independence. The nurse assists the individual, whether ill or not, to perform activities that will contribute to health, recovery, or peaceful death- activities that the individual who had necessary strength, will, or knowledge would perform unaided. The process of nursing strives to do this as rapidly as possible, and the goal is independence. The nurse manages this process independently of physicians. Help toward indecent dance is given autonomously by the nurse in relation to (i) breathing, (ii) eating and drinking, (iii) elimination, (iv) movement and posture, (v) sleep and rest, (vi) clothing, (vii) maintenance of body temperature, (viii) cleaning and grooming of the body and integument protection, (ix) avoidance of environmental dangers and injury of other, (x) communication, (xi) worship, (xii) work, (xiii) play and participation in recreation, and (xiv) learning and discovery. Nursing can be evaluated as a profession on the basis of the extent to which it enables the individual to achieve each of these functions autonomously.

The role and functions of professional nursing vary with the situation, If the total health care team comprises a pie graph in health care situation, in some situations no role exists for certain health care workers. Although there is always a role for family and patients, the pie wedges for team members vary in size according to (i) the problem of the patient, (ii) the patient's self-help ability, and (iii) the help resources. Central to nursing that seeks to help patients toward independence is empathetic understanding and unlimited knowledge. Empathetic understand what a patient needs. The ultimate goal for the nurse is to practice autonomously in helping patients who lack knowledge, physical strength, or strength of will in growth toward independence. Because of this function, nurses seek and promote research, education, and work settings that facilitate this goal.

EVOLUTION OF DEFINITION OF NURSING

Virginia Henderson was the nurse-theorist who devoted her career to defining nursing practice. She believed that an occupation that affects human life must outline its function, particularly if it is to be regarded as professions. Her ideas about the definition of Nursing were influenced by her nursing education and practice by her students and colleagues at Columbia University School of Nursing, and by distinguished nursing leaders of her time. Two events are the basis for her development of definition of nursing. First, she participated in the revision of a nursing textbook. Second, she was concerned that many states had no provision for nursing licensure to ensure safe and competent care for the consumer.

In the revision of the **'Textbooks of the Principles and Practice of Nursing**, written with Bertha Harmer (1922) Henderson recognized the need to be clear about the functions of the nurse. She believed a textbook that serves, as main learning source for nursing practice should present a sound and definitive description of nursing. Furthermore, the principles and practice of nursing must be built upon and derived from the definition of the profession.

Henderson was committed to the process of regulating nursing practice through licensure by each state. She believed that to accomplish this, nursing must be explicitly defined in Nurse Practice Act that would provide the legal parameters for the nurses' functions in caring for consumers and safeguard the public from unprepared and incompetent practitioner.

She examined the earlier statements of the nursing functions by American Nurses Association (1932, 1937) and viewed these statements as non-specific and unsatisfactory definition of nursing practice.

In 1955, Henderson's first definition of nursing was published in Bertha Harmer's revised Nursing Text work. It reads as:

"Nursing is primarily assisting the individual (sick or well) in the performance of those activities contributing to health or its recovery (or peaceful death) that he would perform unaided if he had the necessary strength, will, or knowledge. It is likewise the unique contribution of nursing to help the individual to be independent of such assistance as soon as possible."

In this, some similarities are found with the earlier definition of nursing by Bertha Harmer. It reads as follows:

"Nursing is rooted in the needs of humanity and is found on the ideal of service. Its object is not only to cure the sick and heal the wounded but to bring health and ease, rest and comfort to mind and body to shelter, nourish and protect and to minister to all those who are helpless or handicapped, young, aged, or immature. Its object is to prevent disease and to preserve health. Nursing is, therefore, linked with every other social, which strives for the prevention of disease and the preservation of health. The nurse finds herself not only concerned with the care of the individual but with the health of a people."

Henderson definition abbreviated and consolidated portions of Harmer's belief about nursing. Harmer's definition highlighted disease prevention, health preservation and the need for linkages with other social agencies to strive for preventive care and stressed that nursing role in society was oriented toward the community and wellness. Henderson placed more emphasis on the care of the sick and well individuals and did not mention nursing concern for the health and welfare of the aggregate.

CONCEPTS USED BY HENDERSON

Henderson viewed human being, health, environment and Nursing as follows:

- *Human being*: The patient as an individual who requires assistance to achieve health and independence or peaceful death. The mind and body are inseparable. The patient and his family are viewed as a unit.
- *Health*: She views health in terms of the patient's ability to perform unaided the 14 components of nursing care. She says it is "the quality of health rather than life itself, that margin of mental physical vigor that allows a person to work most effectively and to reach his highest potential of satisfaction in life. She does not state her own definition of health.
- *Environment*: She used Webster Dictionary, which defines environment as "the aggregate of all the external conditions and influences affecting the life and development of an organism.
- *Nursing*: In 1966, Henderson's ultimate statements in the definition of nursing were published of her ideas. It reads as follows:

"The unique function of the nurse is to assist the individual, sick or well, in the performance of those activities contributing to health or its recovery (or to peaceful death) that he would perform unaided if he had the necessary strength, will or knowledge. And to do this, in such a way as to help him gain independence as rapidly as possible."

Needs (Fig. 4.1)

Henderson does not give any definition of need. Her focus on individual care is evident in that she stressed assisting individuals with essential activities to maintain health, to recover, or to achieve peaceful death. She proposed 14 basic needs of patient. For basic Nursing care to augment her definitions, which comprise the components of nursing care, Theses include the need to:

1. Breathe normally.

2. Eat and drink adequately
3. Eliminate body wastes.
4. Move and maintain desirable position.
5. Sleep and rest.
6. Select suitable clothes—dress and undress.
7. Maintain body temperature within normal range by adjusting clothing and modifying the environment.
8. Keep the body clean and well groomed and protect integument.
9. Avoid dangers in environment and avoid injuring others.
10. Communicate with others in expressing emotions, needs, and fears of opinions.
11. Worship according to one's faith.
12. Work in such a way that there is a sense of accomplishments.
13. Play or participate in various forms of recreations.
14. Learn, discover, or satisfy the curiosity that leads to normal development and health and use the available health facilities

These needs were considered on basic principles of nursing care.

Henderson does not directly cite what she feels, Her underlying assumption includes, but following assumptions have been adapted from her publication which include assumption of Nursing, person, health and environment.

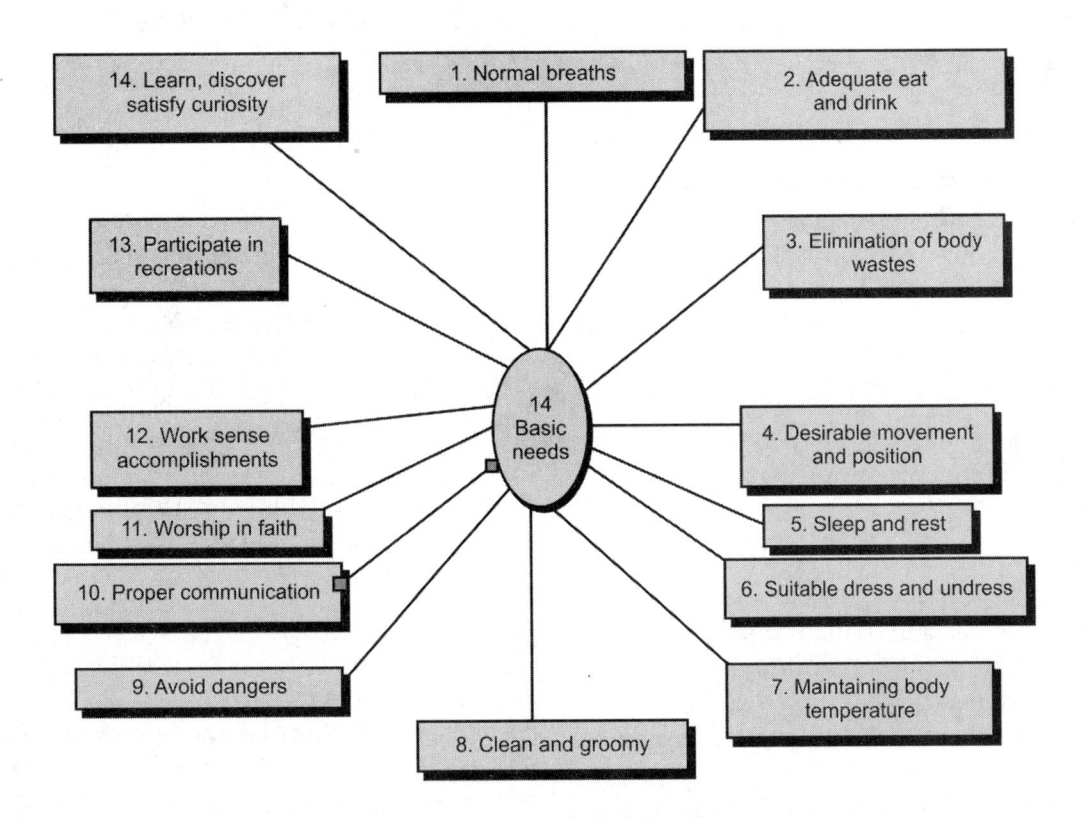

Figure 4.1: Henderson's 14 basic needs

Nursing

- The nurse has a unique function to help well or sick individual.
- The nurse functions as a member of a medical team.
- The nurse functions independently of the physician, but promotes his or her plan, if there is physician in attendance.
- The nurse can and functions independently and must if he or she is the best-prepared health worker in the situation.
- The nurse can and must diagnose and treat if the situation demands it.
- The nurse is knowledgeable in both biologic al and social sciences.
- The nurse can assess basic human needs.
- The 14 components of nursing care encompass all possible functions of Nursing.

Person

- The person must maintain physiological and emotional balance.
- The mind and body of the person are inseparable.
- The patient requires help toward independence.
- The patient and his family are a unit.
- The patient needs are encompassed by the 14 components of nursing.

Health

- Health is a quality of life.
- Health basic to human functioning.
- Health requires independence and interdependence.
- Promotion of health is more important than care of the sick.
- Individual will achieve or maintain health if they have the necessary strength, will or knowledge.

Environment

- Healthy individuals may be able to control their environments, but illness may interfere with that ability.
- Nurses should have safety education.
- Nurses should protect patients from mechanical injury.
- Nurses should minimize the chances of injury through recommendation regarding construction of building, purchase of equipment and maintenance.
- Doctors like nurses observations and judgments upon which to base prescriptions for protective devices.
- Nurses must know about social customs and religious practices to assess dangers.

METAPARADIGM OF HENDERSON THEORY

In viewing the concept of human or individual she considers the biological, psychological, and sociological and spiritual components. Her 14 (Fourteen) components of nursing functions can be categorized in the following manner.

- First nine components are physiological.
- The tenth and fourteenth are psychological aspects of communicating and learning.
- The eleventh component is spiritual and moral, and
- The twelfth and thirteenth components are sociologically oriented to occupation and recreation.

Human

Henderson refers to *humans* as having basic needs that are included in the 14 components. She goes on to state, "It is equally important to realize, that these needs are satisfied by infinitely varied patterns of living no two of which are alike." She also believes that mind and body are inseparable. It is implied that the mind and body are interrelated.

Environment

Henderson views of *environment* are that she sees individuals in relation to their families but minimally discusses the impact of the community on the individual and family. She supported the tasks of the private and public agencies in keeping people healthy. She believes that society wants and expects the nurse's service of acting for individuals who are unable to function independently. In turn, she expects society to contribute to nursing education for preparation of good nurses to society.

Health

Henderson beliefs about *Health* are related to human functioning independently goal for the individuals; she argues that it is difficult for the nurse to help the person reach it. She also refers to nurses stressing promotion of health and prevention and cure of disease and explains how the factors of age, cultural background, physical and intellectual capacities and emotional balance affect one's health. These conditions are always present and affect basic needs.

Nursing

She believes that nurses should be in the forefront of those who work for social justice, for healthful environment, for access to adequate food, shelter, and clothing and universal opportunities for education and employment, realizing that all of these as well as preventive and creative health care are essential to the well-being of citizens (Henderson 1989). By working on various social issues, nurses can have an impact on people's health.

Henderson believes that the function the nurse performs is primarily and independent one that of acting for the patient when he lacks knowledge, physical strength, or the will to act for himself as he would ordinarily act in healthy, or in carrying out prescribed therapy. This function is seen as complex and creative, as offering unlimited opportunity for the application of the physical, biological and social sciences, and the development of skills on them. For Henderson the nurse must be knowledgeable. Has some base, for practicing individualized and human care, and be a scientific problem solver. It is important that nursing care be improved by implementing valid ideation and improvement of nursing practice.

Virginia Henderson's definition is of the 'unique function' of the nurse, which she deliberately calls not a definition, but a 'personal' that this is not all there is, to nursing and this statement was never intended to define the entire discipline. This statement is about the unique function of the nursing... the aspect of her work. She initiates and counties; of this she is master. For Henderson, this unique function is the core of nursing from which all other things spring and which must be protected. "No one should make such heavy demands on another member (of the Medical Team) that any of them is unable to perform his or her unique function." In a passage so lovely that it is almost poetry Henderson translates this unique function.

"(The nurse) is temporarily the conscious of the unconscious, the love of life for the suicidal, the leg of the amputee, the eyes of the newly blind, a mean of locomotion for the infant, knowledge and confidence of the young mother, the voice for those too weak or with drawn to speak." This indicates nurse-patient relationship, and role of nurse as substitute for helper to and partner of patient.

In these activities the nurse is independent practitioner, and able to make independent treatment for disease or making the prognosis, for these is physician functions. But today the roles of the nurses as givers of "Primary health care" as those who diagnose and treat when a doctor is unavailable, even as the midwife functions in the absence of an obstetrician. Nurse may be general (Medical) practitioners of tomorrow.

HENDERSON ON NURSING PROCESS

Henderson (1980) views the nursing process as "really the application of the logical approach to the solution of a problem. The steps are those of the scientific method." Even though Henderson's definition and explanation of nursing process, a relationship between the two can be demonstrated. Although she does not refer directly to assessment, to but imply it in her description of the 14 components of basic nursing care. The nurse uses the 14 components to *assess* the individual needs. Following the analysis of the data collected, the nurse then determines the *nursing diagnosis*. Ones the nursing diagnosis is made, the nurse proceeds to the *planning* phases of the nursing process, ass stated by Henderson that " all effective nursing is planned some extent A written plan forces those who make it to give some thought and the individual needs-unless simply fit the person's regimen into the institution's routine.

For Henderson, nursing *implementation* is based on helping the patient meet the 14 components. One primary function of the practicing nurse, of course, must be performed in such a way, that it promotes the physician's therapeutic plan." So the nurse needs to carry out the physician's levels of functioning need to be observed and recorded. A comparison of data provides evaluation of nursing care provided.

Evaluation of each person according to the speed with which, he performs independently the activity that makes for him, a normal day for evaluation purpose, and changes in person's levels of functioning need to be observed and recorded. A comparison of data provides evaluation of nursing care provided.

The stages of the nursing process as applied to Henderson's definition of nursing and to the 14 components of basic nursing care are as follows.

Nursing Assessment

- Assess needs of human being based in the 14 components of basic nursing care.
  - Breathe normally
  - Eat and drink adequately
  - Eliminate body wastes.
  - Move and maintain posture.
  - Sleep and rest.
  - Suitable clothing, dress or uniform.
  - Maintain body temperature.
  - Keep body clear and well groomed.
  - Avoid dangers in environment.
  - Communicate.
  - Worship according to one's faith.
  - Recreation.
  - Learn, discover of satisfy curiosity.
- Analysis: compare data to knowledge base of health and disease.

Nursing Diagnosis

- Identify individuals ability to meet own needs with or without assistance, taking into consideration strength will or knowledge.

Nursing Plan

- Document how the nurse can assist the individual stick or well.

Nursing Implementation

- Assist the sick or well individual in the performance of activities in meeting human needs to maintain health, recover from illness or to aid in peaceful death. Implementation based on principles age, cultural background, emotional balance and physical and intellectual capacities carry out treatment prescribed by the Doctor.

Nursing Evaluation

- Use the acceptable definitions of nursing and appropriate laws related to the practice of nursing. The quality of care distinctly affected by the preparation and native ability of the nursing personnel rather than the amount of hours of care. Successful outcomes of Nursing care is based on the speed with then which the patient performs independently ADL.

Henderson's Work and Characteristics of Theory

Prior to development of concepts and theories of nursing, Henderson formulated the definition of nursing. Her intent was to identify the specific functions the nurse performs, rather than to describe the theoretical basis for nursing practice. But, her work can be applied to nurse and characteristics of theory as given below.

1. *Theories can interrelate concepts in such a way as to create a difference.* Henderson uses the concepts of fundamental human needs, biopsychology, and culture, and interaction, communication. Their concept being borrowed from other disciplines rather than being unique to nursing. Maslow (1970) hierarchy of human need fits well with the 14 basic components. The first nine components are physiological and safety needs. The remaining five components deal with love and belonging, social esteem and self-acknowledgment needs. She uses the biophysical concepts in making decisions about nursing care i.e., physiology and its balances. The concept of culture on it affects human needs learned from the family and other social groups. She believes in sensitivity to non-verbal communication is essential to encourage the expression of feelings. Furthermore, a prerequisite to validate patient needs is a constructive nurse-patient relationship.

2. *Theories must be logical in nature.* Henderson's definition and components are logical. The nurse assists the individual to perform those activities contributing to health or its recovery or peaceful death and encourages independences as quickly as possible. The fourteen components are a guide for the individual and nurse in reaching the chosen goals. The components start with physiological functioning and moves to the psychosocial aspects, which conveys the idea that bodily, operation is a priority to emotional and or cognitive status.

3. *Theories should be relatively simply yet generalize.* Henderson's work is relatively simple yet generalizable with some limitations. Her work can be applied to health of the individuals of all ages. A nurse functioning at various levels and in diverse cultures has used her definition.

But it is lacking in empirical testing to generalizability of the definition and 14 components.

4. *Theories can be the bases for the hypothesis that can be tested or for theory to be explained.* It is impossible to generate hypothesis from the Henderson definition of nursing. Although she is an advocate of conducting research, in nursing, favours studies directed to improving nursing practice rather than those conducted as an academic or theoretical endeavour. She believes that research is not a substitute for instinctive and intuitive reactions to situations but that these reactions are influenced by the nurse's knowledge of science that guides human behaviour in the society of which nursing is an integral part.

5. *Theories contribute to and assist in increasing body of knowledge within discipline through research.* To validate in Henderson's ideas of nursing practice are well accepted throughout the world as a basis of nursing care. However, impact of the definition and components has not been established through research. Well designed empirical\studies are needed to determine Henderson's contribution to worldwide knowledge about nursing practice and patient out comes. This would help validate her beliefs about the unique functions of Nursing.

6. *Theories can be used by practitioner to guide and improve their practice.* Ideally, the nurse would improve nursing practice by using the definition and 14 components of nursing given by Henderson to improve the health of the individuals and thus reduce illness. The final desirable outcome would be measure of recovery rate, health promotion and eminence or a peaceful death.

7. *Theories must be consistent with other validated theses, laws, principles, but leave open unanswered questions that need to be investigating.*

There is a potential for comparison of Henderson's definition and components with validated theories, laws and principles. The concepts of fundamental human needs, culture, Independence and interaction-communication are widely investigated by nurse-researchers as well as those in the social and psychological disciplines.

EVALUATION OF THEORY

Before one attempts to evaluate Virginia Henderson's theory of nursing with respect to the generally accepted criteria of simplicity, generality, empirical precision, and derivable consequences, one must understand that she did not intend to develop a definitive nursing theory. Instead, she developed a personal concept or definition in an attempt to clarify what she considers to be the unique function of nursing. She states, "My interpretation of the nurse's function is the synthesis of many influences, some positive and some negative. I should first make clear that I do not expect everyone to agree with me. Rather, I would urge every nurse to develop her own concept."

Henderson's definition can be considered a grand theory or philosophy within the preparadigm stage of theory development in nursing. Her concept is descriptive and easy to read. It is defined in common language terms. Her definitions of nursing and enumeration of the 14 basic nursing functions presents a perspective aimed at explaining a totality of nursing behaviour. Because she had no intention of developing a theory, Henderson does not develop the interrelated theoretical statements or operational definitions necessary to provide the theory testability. However, that can be done.

- Henderson's concept of nursing is complex rather than simplistic. It contains many variables and several different descriptive and explanatory relationships. It is not associated with structural organizations within a framework or model from to enhance simplicity, although some work has been done in this area. Diagrams of Henderson's and Orem's concepts of nursing from the Nursing Developmental Conference Groups's book, *Concepts Formation* in Nursing, have been reproduced in Henderson and Nite's book. In addition, the 14 basic needs appear simple as stated, but they become complex when an alteration of a need occurs and all the parameters relating to that need are considered. The sixth edition of Principles and Practices of Nursing is extremely comprehensive and well illustrated to add clarity.
- Generality is present in Henderson's definition since it is broad in scope. It attempts to include the function of all nurses and all patients in their various interrelationships and interdependencies.
- Henderson's perspective has been useful in promoting new ideas and in furthering conceptual development of emerging theorists. In her many published works she has discussed the importance of nursing's independence from, and interdependence with, other branches of the health care field. She has also influenced curriculum development and made a great contribution in promoting the importance of research in the clinical practice of nursing. She has made extensive use of other theorists' research in her own work. Evans states that *Principles and Practice of Nursing* has made "a revolutionary change in one's thinking about nursing research." He states that the revolutionary thesis of the book is:

"The habits of minds which inform the everyday tasks of a nurse are exactly the same as those which undergird the very finest published research; in this way, every nurse ought not just to do simple research tasks as part of her work, but she ought also always to be a researcher, whether or not she writes or speaks a word in print or public."

Since Henderson's definition of the unique function of nursing has been widely read, it has functioned as a major stepping-stone in the emergence of nursing as a professional scientific discipline.

She continues to be cited in current nursing literature and publications in all areas of nursing practice from holistic nursing to the nursing process.

Chapter 5

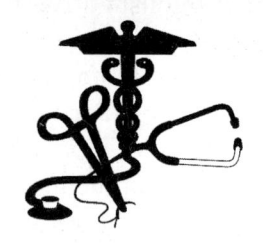

Orem's Self-care Theory

Dorothea Elizabeth Orem, one of America's foremost nursing theorists, was born in Baltimore, Maryland. Her father was a construction worker who liked fishing, and her mother was a homemaker who liked reading. The younger of two daughters, she began her nursing career at Providence Hospital School of Nursing in Washington, DC, where she received her diploma certificate of nursing in the early 1930s. Orem continued her education and received a BSN from Catholic University of America in 1939 and an MS in nursing education in 1945 from the same university.

Her nursing experience included private duty nursing, hospital staff nursing, and teaching. Orem held directorship of both the nursing school and the department of nursing at Providence Hospital, Detroit, from 1940 to 1949. After leaving Detroit, Orem spent seven years (1949-1957) in Indiana working in the Division of Hospital and Institutional Services of the Indiana State Board of Health. While there her goal was to upgrade the quality of nursing in general hospitals throughout the state. During this time, Orem developed her definition of nursing practice.

In 1957 Orem moved to Washington, DC, where she was employed by the Office of Education, US Department of Health, Education, and Welfare, as a curriculum consultant from 1958 to 1960. During this time she began to see deficits in the training of practical nurses. While at HEW she worked on a project to up grade practical nursing training that stimulated a need to address the question, what is the subject matter of nursing? As a result, she published *Guidelines for Developing Curricula for the Education of Practical Nurses.*

In 1959, Orem became an assistant professor of Nursing Education at Catholic University of America. She subsequently served as acting dean of the School of Nursing and as associate professor of Nursing Education. She continued to develop her concept of nursing and self-care while at Catholic University. While there, she wrote "The Hope of Nursing" (1962), which was published in the *Journal of Nursing Education.* In 1970 Orem left Catholic University and began her own consulting firm of Orem and Shields, Inc., of Chevy Chase, Maryland. Orem's first book, published in 1971, was

Nursing: Concepts of practice. Georgetown University conferred Orem with the honorary degree of Doctor of Science in 1976. "Levels of Nursing Education and Practice" was published in the alumnae magazine of Johns Hopkins School of Nursing in 1979. She received the Catholic University of America Alumni Association Award for Nursing Theory in 1980. The second edition of Nursing: *Concepts of Practice* was published in 1980, and the third edition followed in 1985. Orem retired in 1984 and resides in Savannah, Georgia, where she enjoys reading, travelling, consulting, and attending nursing conferences to discuss her theory. Work on her fourth edition of Nursing: *Concepts of Practice* was completed in 1991. Orem has been working alone and with colleagues on the continued conceptual development of Self-care Deficit Nursing Theory (SCDNT). She participates in conferences and prepares papers about various conceptual elements of the theory. She continues to contribute to the work of her colleagues through discussions about the structure of the theory and its use in nursing.

EVOLUTION OF THEORY

Although Orem cites Eugenia K. Spaulding as a great friend and teacher, she indicates that no particular nursing leader was a direct influence on her work. She believes association with many nurses over the years provided many learning experiences, and she views her work with graduate students and collaborative works with colleagues as valuable endeavours. While crediting no one as a major influence, she does cite many other nurses works in terms of their contributions to nursing including, but not limited to, Abdellah, Henderson, Johnson, King, Levine, Nightingale, Orlando, Peplau, Riehl, Rogers, Roy, Travelbee, and Wiedenbach. She also cites numerous authors in other disciplines including, but not limited to, Gordon Allport, Chester Barnard, Rene Dubos, Erich Fromm, Gartly Jaco, Robert Katz, Kurt Lewin, Ernest Nagel, Talcott, Parsons, Hans Selye, and Ludwig von Bertalanffy.

In 1958, Orem experienced a spontaneous insight about why individuals required and could be helped through nursing. This knowledge enabled her to formulate and express her concept of nursing. Her knowledge of the features of nursing practice situations was acquired over many years.

Orem's self-care deficit theory of nursing includes theories of (i) self-care deficit, (ii) self-care, and (iii) nursing system. Self-care deficit theory postulates that people benefit from nursing in that they have health-related limitations in providing self-care. Self-care theory postulates that self-care and care of dependents are learned behaviours that purposely regulate human structural integrity, functioning, and development. Nursing systems theory postulates that nursing systems form when nurses prescribe, design, and provide nursing that regulates the individual's self-care capabilities and meets therapeutic self-care requirements.

Assumptions basic to the general theory are as follows:
1. Humans require deliberate input to self and environment to be alive and to function.
2. The power to act deliberately is exercised in caring for self and others.
3. Mature humans sometimes experience limitations in their ability to care for self and others.
4. Humans discover, develop, and transmit ways to care for self and others.
5. Humans structure relationships and tasks to provide self-care.

Human need continuous self-care maintenance and regulation and provide this by caring for self, which enables purposeful action. Self-care activities maintain life, health, and well-being. Health refers to the state of a person, which is characterized by soundness or wholeness of developed human structures and bodily and mental functioning. Well-being refers to a person's perceived condition of existence, which is characterized by experiences of contentment, pleasure, happiness, movement toward self-ideals, and continuing personalization.

Three kinds of self-care requisites are universal, development, and health deviation. Universal requirements relate to meeting common human needs. Developmental self-care requisites relate to conditions that promote developmental processes throughout the life cycle. Health deviation self-care requisites relate to self-care that prevents defects and deviations from normal structure and integrity and those that control the extension and effects of such defects.

Adults care for themselves, whereas infants, the aged, the ill, and the disabled require assistance with self-care activities. When self-care action is limited because of the health state or needs of the care recipient, nursing responds and provides a legitimate service. Thus patients are people with health-related self-care deficits. Two variables affect these deficits: self-care agency (ability) and self-care demands.

Self-care agency is a learned ability and is deliberate action. Given their focus on care of patients with health-related limitations in self-care abilities, nurses must accurately diagnose self-care agency. Thus they must have information about deficits and their reasons for existing. Such information is basic to selecting helping methods.

Nursing agency regulates or develops patient's self-care agency and ability to meet therapeutic self-care demand. Nursing is a helping service that involves acting or doing for another, guiding and supporting another, providing a developmental environment, and teaching another. Nursing agency varies with educational preparation, orientation to practice situations, mastery of technologies of practice, and ability to accept, work with, and care for others.

Nursing systems may be wholly compensatory, partially compensatory, or supportive-educative. Wholly compensatory systems are required for patients unable to monitor their environment and process information. Such patients are unable to control their movement and position and are unresponsive to stimuli. Partially compensatory systems are designed for patients with limitations in movement as a result of pathology or injury or who are under medical orders to restrict their movements. Supportive-educative systems are designed for patients who need to learn to perform self-care measures and need assistance to do so. Nursing systems are formed to regulate self-care capabilities and meet therapeutic self-care requirements.

Dorothea E. Orem participated in a project to improve practical or vocational Nurse theory, as a consultant to the office of Education at the US Department, Health, Education and Welfare. This work stimulated to consider the question: What condition exists in a person when that person or other, determine that person should be under Nursing Care? Her answer encompassed the idea that a nurse is "another self." The idea evolved into her nursing concept of "self-care." That is, when they are able: individuals care for themselves. When the person is unable to provide self-care, for the nurse provides the assistance needed. For children, nursing care is needed when the parents or guardians are unable to provide the amount and quality of care needed.

In 1958, Orem experienced a spontaneous insight about why individuals required and could be helped through nursing. This knowledge enabled her to formulate and express her concept of nursing. In 1959, Orem's concept of nursing on the provision of self-care was first published. She further developed her nursing concepts of self-care and in 1971 published "Nursing: Concepts of Practice." The 2nd, 3rd, 4th editions of the work were published in 1980, 1985 and 1991. The first edition focused on the individual, the second edition was expanded to include multi person units (families, group and communities). The third edition presented Orem's **General Theory** of Nursing as it is constituted from three related theoretical constructs; Self-care, deficit, and nursing systems. In the 4th edition, her writing incorporates a greater emphasis on the child, groups and society; Her knowledge of the features of nursing practice situations was acquired over many years.

GENERAL THEORY OF NURSING

Orem labels her self-care deficit theory of nursing as general theory and states that:

"The condition that validates the existence of a requirement for nursing in an adult is the absence of the ability to maintain continuously that amount and quality of self-care which is therapeutic in sustaining life and health in recovering from disease or injury or in coping with their efforts. With children, the condition is the inability of the parent (or guardian) to maintain earnestly for the child the amount and quality of care that is therapeutic.

Orem's general theory composed of three interrelated theories which includes:
1. The theory of self-care (describes and explains self-care).
2. The theory of self-care deficit (describes and explains why people can be helped through nursing); and
3. The theory of nursing systems (describes and explains relationships that must be brought about and maintained for nursing to be produced).

Concepts Used by Orem

The major concepts used by Orem are:

Theory of Self-care

Self-care is learned, goal oriented activity of individual.

Self-care Requisition

This is an additional concept incorporated within the theory of self-care. Self-care requisites are "expressions of purposes to be attained results desired from deliberate engagement in self-care. These are the reasons for doing actions that constitute self-care. Self-care requisites can be defined as actions directed toward the provisions of self-care.

Orem (1991) presents three categories of self-care requisites or requires any universal, developmental and health deviation.

Universal Self-care Requisites

These are common to all human beings and include the maintenance of air, water, food, eliminations, activity and rest, and solitude and social interaction, prevention of hazards and promotion of human functioning. They are associated with life processes and the maintenance of the integrities of human structures and functioning. Since they are common to all human beings during all stages of the life cycle and should be viewed as interrelated factors, each affecting the others. There are activities of daily living (ADL).

Orem identifies these self-care requisites as follows:

- The maintenance of sufficient intake of air.
- The maintenance of sufficient intake of water.
- The maintenance of sufficient intake of food.
- The provision of care associated with elimination process and excrements.
- The maintenance of balance between activity and rest.
- The maintenance of a balance between solitude and social interactions.
- The prevention of hazards to human life, human functioning and human well being.
- The promotion of human functioning and development within social groups and accord with human potential, known human limitations and human desire to be normal.

Developmental Self-care Requisites

These were separate from universal self-care requisites, which promote processes for life and maturation and prevent conditions deleterious to maturation or mitigate those effects. Developmental self-care requisites are "either specialized expression of universal self-care requisites, that have been particularized for developmental process or they are new requisites derived from a condition or associated with an event. For example, adjusting to new job or adjusting to body changes such as facial lines or hair loss.

Health Deviation Self-care Requisites

Health deviation self-care requisites is required in condition of illness, injury, or disease or may result from medical measures required to diagnose and correct the condition (For example: light upper quadrant abdominal pain when food with a high fat content are eaten, or, learning to walk using crutches following casting of a fractured leg). According to Orem, health deviation self-care requisites are as follows:

- Seeking and securing appropriate medical assistance.
- Being aware of and attending to the effects and results of pathologic conditions and states.
- Effectively carrying out medically prescribed diagnosis, therapeutic and rehabilitative measures.
- Being aware of attending to or regulating the discomforting or deleterious effects of prescribed medical care measures.
- Modifying the self-concept and self-image in accepting oneself as being in a particular state of health and in need of specific forms of health care.
- Learning to live with the effects of pathologic conditions and states and the effects of medical diagnostic and treatment measures in a life style that promotes continued personal development.

THEORY OF SELF-CARE DEFICIT

Self-care deficit is a relation between the human properties of therapeutic self-care demand and self-care agency in which constituents developed self-care capabilities within the self-care agency are not operable or not adequate for knowing and meeting some or all components of the existent or projected therapeutic self-care demand (Fig. 5.1).

- The theory of self-care deficit is the core of general theory of nursing because it delineates when nursing is needed. Nursing is required when an adult (or in the case of a dependent, the parent or guardian) is incapable of or limited in the provision of continuous effective self-care. Nursing may be provided if the 'care abilities are less than those required for meeting a known self-care demand or self-care or dependent-self-care abilities exceed or are equal to those required for meeting the current self-care demand, but a future deficit relationship can be foreseen because of predictable decreases in care abilities, qualitative or quantitative increase in the care demand or both; when individual need "to incorporate newly prescribed, complex, self-care measures in to that self-care systems, the performance of which required specialized knowledge and skills to be acquired through training and experience or the individual needs help in recovering from disease or injury, or in coping with their effects.' Here first category includes universal development and health-deviation self-care.

Orem (1991) identifies the following five methods of helping.
- Acting for or doing for another.
- Guiding and directing.
- Providing physical or psychological support.
- Providing and maintaining an environment that supports personal development.
- Teaching.

The nurse may help the individual by using any or all of these methods to provide assistance with self-care.

Orem presents a model to show the relationship between her concepts. From this model, it can be seen that any given time, an individual has specific self-care abilities as well as therapeutic self-care demands. If there are more demands than abilities, nursing is needed. The activities in which nurses engage when they provide nursing care can be used to describe the domain nursing.

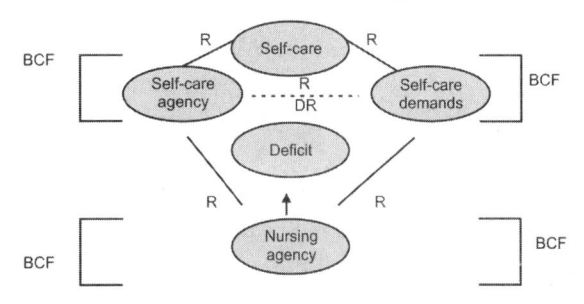

Figure 5.1: Conceptual framework of nursing (R = Relationship, DR = Deficit relationship, BCF = Basic conditioning factor)

Orem (1991) has identified five areas of activity for nursing practices as given below:
- Entering into and maintaining nurse-patient relationship with individuals, families or groups until patients can legitimately be discharged from nursing.
- Determining if and how patients can be helped through nursing.
- Responding to patients' requests, desires, and needs for nurse contacts and assistance.
- Prescribing, providing and regulating direct help to patients (and their significant others) in the form of nursing.
- Coordinating and integrating nursing with the patients daily living, other health care needed or being received, and social and educational services needed or being received.

THEORY OF NURSING SYSTEM

Nursing system is a "continuing series of actions produced when nurses link one way or a number of ways of helping to their own actions or the actions of persons under care that are directed to meet these persons' therapeutic self-care demands or to regulate their self-care agency."

The nursing system, designed by the nurse is based on the self-care needs and abilities of the patient to perform self-care activities. If there is self-care deficit, that is, if there is deficit between what the optimum functioning (self-care demand) then nursing is required.

Nursing Agency is the complex property or attribute of persons educated and trained as nurses that is enabling when exercised for knowing and helping others meet or in meeting their therapeutic self-care demands, and helping others regulate the exercise or development of their self-care agency - or their dependent care agency. In short, the nursing care agency, the property of nurses that enables them to act, to know, then to act and help others meet their therapeutic self-care demands by exercising and developing their own self-care agency. Nursing agency is analogous to self-care agency in that both symbolize characteristics and abilities for specific types of deliberate action. They differ in their Nursing agency is exercised for the benefit and well-being of others, and self-care agency is developed and exercised for the benefit of oneself.

Orem (1991) has identified three classifications of nursing system to meet self-care requisites of the patient (Fig. 5.2). These systems are:
- The wholly compensatory system.
- The partial compensatory system.
- The supportive educative system.
  This design and elements of nursing systems define
- The scope of the nursing responsibility in health care situations;
- The general and specific roles of nurses, patients and others.
- The reasons for nurses relationship with patients; and
- The kind of action to be performed and the performance patterns and nurses and actions in regulating patients' self-care agency and in meeting their therapeutic self-care demand.

The three types of nursing system identified as shown in Figure 5.2. Whether the nursing system wholly compensatory. partly compensatory or supportive educative, depends on who can or should perform those self-care actions.

Wholly Compensatory Nursing System

Wholly compensatory nursing system is needed when the "nurse should be compensating for a patient's total inability for (or prescriptions against) engaging in self-care activities that require ambulation and manipulation movements."

This system is represented by a situation in which the individual is unable to engage in those self-care actions requiring self-directed and controlled ambulation and manipulative movement or the medical prescription to refrain from such activity. Persons with these limitations are socially dependent on others for their continued existence and well-being.

Subtypes of the wholly compensatory are nursing systems for people who are:
- Unable to engage in any form of deliberate action. Example: person in coma.
- Aware and who may be able to make observations, judgments and decisions about self-care and other matters but cannot or should not perform actions requiring ambulation and manipulative

Wholly Compensatory System

```
Nurse action → Accomplishes patient's therapeutic self-care.
Nurse action → Compensates for patients inability to engage in self-care
Nurse action → Support and protects patients
                                                    ← Patient action limited
```

Partly Compensatory System

```
Nurse action → Performs some self-care limitations of patients
Nurse action → Compensates for self-care limitations of patients.
Nurse action → Assist patients as required
Nurse action → Performs some self-care measures.
Nurse action → Regulates self-care agency         ← Patient action
              Accepts care and assistance from nurse.
```

Supportive-educative System

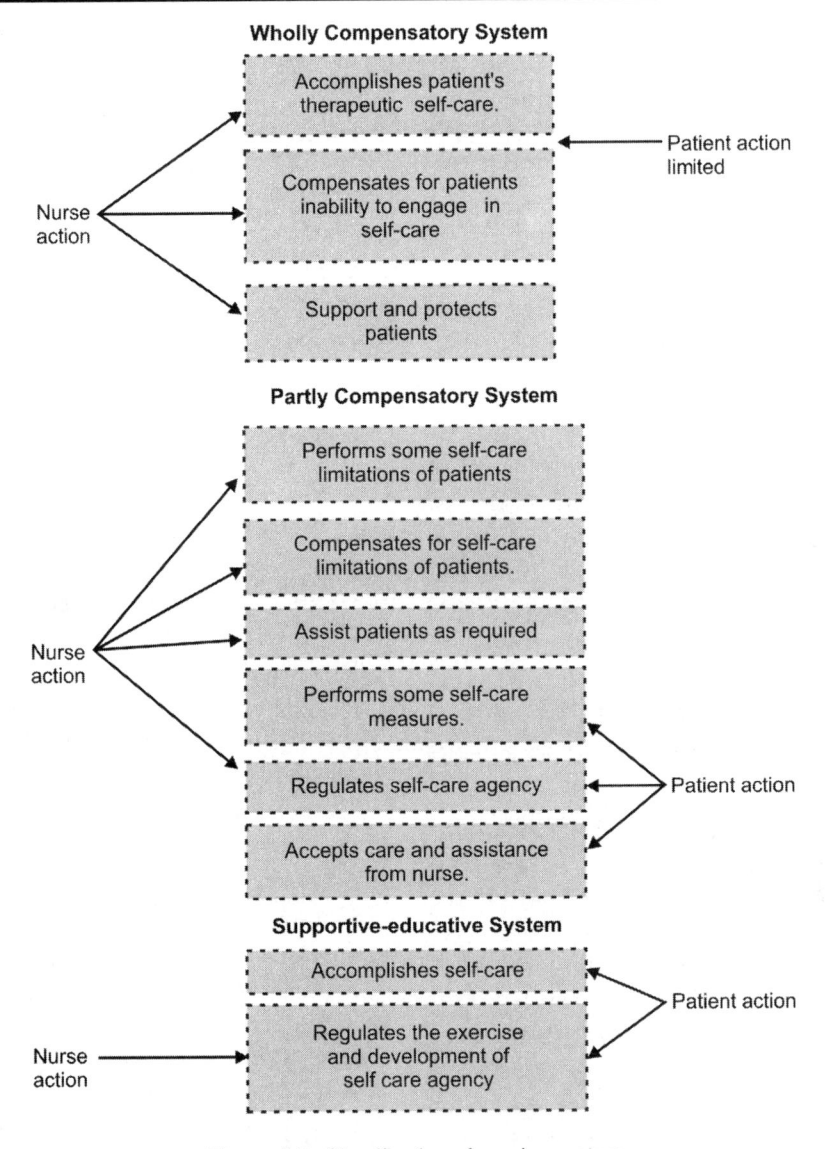

```
                Accomplishes self-care            ← Patient action
Nurse action → Regulates the exercise and development of self care agency
```

Figure 5.2: Classification of nursing system

movements. For example, persons with C3-C4 vertebral fractures.

- Unable to attend to themselves and make reasoned judgments and decisions about self-care and other matters but who can be ambulatory and may be able to perform some measures of self-care with continuous guidance and supervision, e.g. persons who are severely mentally retarded.

Partly Compensatory Nursing System

This system exists when both nurse and perform care measures or other actions involving manipulative tasks or ambulation. It is represented by a situation in which the patient or the nurse may have the major role in the performance of care measures. For example, patients who have undergone abdominal surgery might be able to wash his or her face and brush his or her teeth but needs the nurse for help in ambulating and in changing the surgical dressing.

Supportive-educative Nursing System

Supportive-educative systems are "for situations where the patient is able to perform or can and should learn to perform required measures of externally or internally oriented therapeutic self-care, but cannot do so without assistance." This is also known as supportive-developmental system. Here, the patient is doing all the self-care. The patient's requirements for help are confined to decision making, behaviour control, and acquiring, knowledge and skills. The nurses' role, then is to promote the patient as self-care agent, the nurse's role in this system is primarily that for reaches or consultant.

The above three systems may be utilized for one patient For example woman in labour—when required a cesarean delivery, her care might-require wholly compensatory, if normal delivery is required, partly compensatory care, and or after canal delivery progress to partly compensatory when she recovers from anesthesia. And later she should require supportive-educative, when she prepares to go home.

In the theory of self-care, Orem explains **what** is meant by self-care and lists the various factors that affect its provision. In the self-care deficit, theory, she specifies **when** nursing is needed to assist the individual in the provision of self-care and in third theory of nursing systems, she outlines how the patients self-care needs will be met by the nurse, the patient or both.

PARADIGM OF OREM'S THEORY

Orem discusses each of the four major concepts of human beings, health, society/environment in her work.

Human being: She identifies the five assumptions underlying the theory of nursing.
- Human beings require continuous deliberate inputs to themselves and their environments to remain alive and function in accord with natural human endowments.
- Human agency, the power to act deliberately is exercised in the form of care of self and others in identifying needs for and in making needed inputs.
- Mature human beings experience privations in the form of limitation for actions in care of self and others involving the making of life sustaining and function regulating inputs.
- Human agency is exercised in discovering, developing and transmitting to other ways and means to identify needs for and make inputs to self and others.
- Groups of human beings with structured relationships cluster tasks and allocate responsibilities for providing care to group members who experience privations for making deliberate input to self and others.
- Human beings are distinguished from other living things by that capacity to:
  – Reflect upon themselves and their environment.
  – Symbolize what they experience, and
  – Use symbolic creations (ideas, worth) in thinking, communicating and in guiding efforts to do and to make things that are beneficial for themselves or others.

Integrated human functioning includes physical, psychological, interpersonal and social aspects. Orem believed that individuals have the potential for learning and developing. The way an individual meet self-care needs is not instinctual but is a learned behaviour. That affects learning include age, mental capacity, culture, society and the emotional state of the individual. If the individual cannot learn self-care, measures, others must learn and the care and provide to perform.

Health

Orem (1991) supports the definition of health as the state of physical, mental and social well being and not merely the absence of disease or infirmity (WHO). She states that the physical, psychological, interpersonal and social aspects of health are inseparable in the individual. She also presents health based on the concept of preventive health care which includes promotion and maintenance of health (Primary prevention.

Nursing

Orem speaks to several factors related to the concept of nursing. These are the art and prudence of nursing, nursing as a service, role theory related to nursing and the technologies in nursing.

The **art of nursing** is the quality of individual nurses that allows them to make creative investigations and analyzing and synthesizes of the variables and conditioning factors within nursing situations in order to work toward the goal of the production of effective systems of nursing assistance for individual or multi person units. These decisions require a theoretical base in the discipline of nursing and in the Sciences, arts and humanities. This base directs decision when designing nursing systems within the nursing process.

Nursing prudence: It is the quality of nurses that enables them:
- to seek and take counsel on new or difficult nursing situations.
- to make correct judgments.
- to decide to act in a particular way and
- to take action.

The development of the individual nurse's art and prudence is affected by unique life and nursing experiences.

Further, Orem defines nursing as a human service, Nursing is distinguished from other human services by its focus on persons with inabilities to maintain the continuous provisions of health care.

Environment

The nurse and patient's roles define the expected behaviours for each in the specific nursing situation. Various factors that influence the expected role behaviours are culture, environment, age, sex, the health setting and finance. The roles of nurses and patients are complementary to each other, both work together to accomplish goals of self-care. For example, in nurse patient relationship, may experience role conflict, to solve them both should play differently in their environment.

Nursing Technologies

Orem recognizes that specialized technologies are usually developed by the members of the health professions. She emphasizes the need for social and interpersonal technologies with regulatory technologies promotes quality professional nursing.

Treatment or regulatory operations are practical activities through which what is prescribed is executed and through which the diagnosed conditions or problem is treated in order to remove it, to control it, or to keep it within boundaries compatible with human life, health and well-being.

OREM'S ON NURSING PROCESS

Nursing process is a term used by nurses to refer to the professional-technologic operations of nursing practice and to associated planning and evaluative operations; (Orem 1991). Process is a continuous and regular action or succession of actions taking place or carried out in a definite manner. She discusses a three-step nursing process which she labels the technologic process operation of nursing practice.

Step 1: Nursing diagnosis and prescription—that is determining why nursing is needed, analysis and interpretation—making judgment regarding care, also labeled case management operations. This step can be comparable to present nursing process steps, i.e. assessment and nursing diagnosis.

Step 2: Designing the nursing system and planning for delivery of care. This can be comparable to planning step of present nursing process.

Step 3: The production and management of nursing system also labeled planning and controlled. This can be compared to implementation of evaluation phases of present nursing process.

The little details of these steps are as follows:

Nursing Diagnosis and Prescription

The nursing diagnosis necessitates investigation and accumulation of facts about patients self-care agency and their therapeutic self-care demand and existent or projected relationships between them. The goal defines the direction and nature of the actions. Prescriptive operations specify the means (course of actions, care measures) to be used to meet particular self-care requisites or to meet all components of the therapeutic self-care demand. Orem emphasizes that in nursing diagnostic and prescriptive operations and in the regulatory or treatment operations, patients and families' abilities and interests in collaboration affect what nurses can do.

Designing for Regulatory Operation

Designing is an effective and efficient system of nursing involves selecting valid ways of assisting the patient. This design includes nurse and patient roles in relation to which self-care tasks will be performed when adjusting the therapeutic self-care demands, regulating the exercise of self-care agency, protecting the already developed powers of self-care agency and assisting with new developments in self-care agency.

Planning is the movement from the design of nursing system to ways and means of their production. A plan set forth the organization of essential tasks to be performed in accordance with role responsibilities. The planning for implementation of the design and related procurement activities determine when nurses should be with patients and when essential materials and equipments will be available and ready for use to perform the tasks.

Production and Managing Nursing System

Regulatory nursing systems are produced when nurses interact with patients and take consistent action to meet their prescribed therapeutic self-care demands and regulate the exercise or development of their capabilities for self-care. In this third step of the technologic nursing process, nurses act or produce and manage nursing systems. During the interactions of nurses and patients, nurse acts as follows:

1. Perform and regulate the self-care tasks for patients or assist patients with their performance of self-care tasks.
2. Co-ordinate self-care tasks performance so that a unified system of care is produced and coordinated with other components of health care.
3. Help patients, that families and others bring about systems of daily living for patients that supports the accomplishment of self-care, and are at the same time, satisfying in relation to patient's interest, talents and goals.
4. Guide, direct and support patients in their exercise of or in withholding the exercise of their self-care agency.
5. Stimulate patients interest in self-care by raising questions and promoting discussions of care problems and issues when condition permits.
6. Support and guide patients in learning activities and provide cues for learning as well as instructional sessions.
7. Support and guide patients as they experience illness or disability and the effects of medical care measures and as they experience the need to engage in new measures of self-care or change their ways of meeting on going self-care requisites.
8. Monitor patients and assist patient to monitor themselves to determine if self-care measures were performed and to determine the effects of self-care, the results of efforts to regulate the exercise or development of self-care agency, and the sufficiency and efficiency of nursing action direction to these ends.
9. Make characterizing judgments about the sufficiency and efficiency of self-care, the regulation of the exercise or development of self-care agency, and nursing assistance.
10. Make judgments about the meaning of the results derived from nurses performance of the preceding two operations for the well-being of the patient and make or recommend adjustments in the nursing care systems through changes in nurse and patient roles.

In the above actions, first seven operations constitute direct nursing care. The last three are for the purpose of deciding if the care rises the evaluation component of the nursing process.

OREM'S WORK AND CHARACTERISTICS OF THEORY

1. Orem's theoretical constructs of self-care, self-care deficits and nursing systems are interrelated in her general comprehensive theory of nursing. This interrelationships provide a view of the practice of nursing (a particular phenomenon) that is unique.
2. Orem's theory follows a logical thought process. She states her general theory, that presents the central idea of each of the three interrelated theories. In her discussion of each interrelated theories she presents presuppositions or statements that describe a concept or explain and predict relationship between two concepts.

3. Orem's theory has been used in both nursing education and practice. The theory is used by several school and colleges of nursing as a theoretical foundation for students' basic preparation for practice. Her concepts of self-care with its prepositions of universal self-care needs is easily understood by beginning and advanced nursing practitioners, as the activities of daily living. The theories of self-care deficit and nursing systems can be comprehended and applied to all individual patients and, with further adaptation, to multiperson units.
4. Orem's theory of self-care has been used to generate testable hypothesis in a variety of settings. Several researchers tested Orem's theory in the area of self-care agency including studies focused on the development of tools to measures aspects of self-care.
5. Orem's focusses yon nursing a helping art that assists an individual to meet self-care needs and that is the foundation for nursing practice. Research on self-care needs and the assistance to meet them adds to nursing's body of knowledge. Orem's theory is being tested by many researchers.
6. Orem's theory is used by nurses in varieties of settings. These settings include that of an independent practitioner of nursing, rehabilitation, haemodialysis, bone marrow transplant, psychiatric care, and public and community health. Others have documented self-care in relation to children in pain and with leukaemia. Women with gestational diabetes, persons receiving enterstomal therapy, adult diabetes, the elderly and the terminally ill.
7. Orem's theory is consistent with role theory, need theory, field theory and health promotional concepts. For example, she discusses the important of an understudy of the roles of nurse and patient which determining the patient's need for nursing care.

Orem's work has been used most often with ill adults. However, Orem defined dependent care agent as the provider of infant or child care and identified early on developmental as one of the three types of self-care requisites. She added a section on "age-specific factors in nursing children" in the 1980 edition of her book Nursing: *Concepts of Practice* and a section on multiperson units in the 1985 edition. She has addressed the multiperson unit in a table in the 1980 edition. Orem discussed her conceptual model and community health nursing at the eighth annual community health nursing at the eighth annual community health nursing conference at the University of North Carolina at Chapel Hill and has addressed the relationship of her model to rehabilitation in Cincinnati. The fourth edition of Nursing: Concepts of practice expanded on the self-care agency concept and the factors influencing development of the individual's ability for self-care.

EVALUATION OF THEORY

- Orem identified six major concepts in the self-care deficit theory of nursing: self-care, therapeutic self-care demand, self-care agency, self-care deficit, nursing agency, and nursing system. She uses these six concepts to express the three constituent theories of the general theory of nursing. The conceptual framework

appears simple. Subconcepts are identified to express the substantive structure of the six broad conceptual elements of the theory.
- The self-care deficit theory of nursing as expressed is universal. It is a theory of nursing as nursing regardless of time or place. Its use as a guide to practice was initially and at present most commonly applied in the care of ill adults. From the beginning, it has been applied in the care of both well and sick children. The universality of the theory should be differentiated from its application in terms of time, place, and individuals.
- This theory identifies concepts, provides definitions, describes relationships, and states assumptions. It can be, and has been, used for research.
- Orem's self-care deficit theory of nursing provides a general framework to direct nursing action. Orem views nursing within the framework of the theory as related to patients' therapeutic self-care demands, their self-care agency, and the relationships between them. She sees three types of nursing systems: doing self-care for the individual (wholly compensatory), assisting the individual (wholly compensatory), assisting the individual with self-care (partially compensatory), and educating and supporting the individual to help him or her better perform self-care.
- Orem believes her self-care theory applies to other groups in addition to nurses.

The self-care theory component of the general theory of nursing is common to the health professions and to all members of social groups. Physicians as well as paramedical groups help people with aspects of self-care and with development of capabilities to engage in self-care. Persons helped may or may not be in need of nursing or may or may not be under nursing care.

The assumptions used in this theory are logically sound and accepted by the nursing community. The concepts are relevant for nursing. The relationships explained and implied are useful in explaining patiency and the nurse-patient relationship.

Orem's theory directs nursing practice, the stated goal. Her nursing systems provide a framework for nursing practice, based on the amount and kind of nursing agency needed. In her books, Orem also addresses educational needs for nurses to be able to practice as well as the use of various levels of nursing practice.

Chapter 6

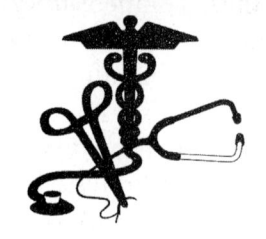

Hall's Core, Care and Cure Models

Lydia Hall began her prestigious career in nursing as a graduate of the York Hospital School of Nursing in York, Pennsylvania. She then earned her B.S. and M.A. degrees from Teacher's College, Columbia University in New York, like many other contemporary nursing theorists.

Hall had faculty positions at the York Hospital School of Nursing and the Fordham Hospital School of Nursing and was a consultant in Nursing Education to the nursing faculty at State University of New York, Upstate Medical Center. She also was an instructor of Nursing Education at Teacher's College.

Hall's career interests revolved around public health nursing, cardiovascular nursing, pediatric cardiology, and nursing of long-term illnesses. She authored 21 publications, with the bulk of articles and addresses regarding her nursing theories published in the early to middle 1960s. In 1967 she received the Award for Distinguished Achievement in Nursing Practice from Columbia University.

Perhaps Hall's greatest achievement in nursing was her design and development of the Loeb Center for Nursing at Montefiore Hospital in New York. Established to apply her theory to nursing practice, the center opened in January 1963. It demonstrated extreme success and provided empirical evidence to support the major concepts in Hall's theory. Hall served as Administrative Director of the Loeb Center for Nursing from its opening until her death in February 1969.

EVOLUTION OF THEORY

Hall drew extensively from the schools of psychiatry and psychology in theorizing about the nurse-patient relationship. She was a proponent of Carl Rogers' philosophy of "client-centered therapy." This method of therapy entails establishing a relationship of warmth and safety, conveying a sensitive empathy with the client's feelings and communications as expressed. A major premise Hall borrowed from Rogers is that patients achieve their maximal potential through a learning process. Rogers states that psychotherapy facilitates significant learning by (i) pointing out and labelling unsatisfying behaviours, (ii) exploring objectively with the client the reasons for the behaviours, and (iii) establishing through reeducation more effective problem-solving habits. In client-centered therapy, changes occur when:

1. The person accepts himself and his feelings more fully.
2. He becomes more self-confident and self-directing.
3. He changes maladaptive behaviours, even chronic ones.
4. He becomes more open to evidence of what is going on both inside and outside of himself.

Extensive documentation indicates the result of this treatment is that physiological and psychological tensions are reduced and that the change lasts.

The major therapeutic approach advocated by Hall is also Rogerian. This approach is the use of reflection, a nondirective method of helping the patient clarify, explore, and validate what he says. Rogers states, "The therapist procedure what (clients) had found most helpful was that the therapist clarified and openly stated feelings which the client had been approaching hazily and hesitantly."

Hall derived her postulates regarding the nature of feeling-based behaviour from Rogers, who repeatedly speaks to the interaction of known feelings and feelings out-of-awareness. Rogers hypothesizes that in a client-centered relationship the patient: Will re-organize himself at both the conscious and deeper levels of his personality in such a manner as to cope with life more constructively. He shows more of the characteristics of the healthy, well-functioning person. He is less frustrated by stress, and recovers from stress more quickly.

Hall also adopted Rogers' theory on motivation for change. In this theory Rogers asserts that although the therapist does not motivate the client, neither is the motivation supplied by the client. Alternatively, motivation for change "springs from the self-actualizing tendency of life itself." In the proper psychological climate, this tendency is released.

In addition to utilizing Rogers' theories, Hall also integrated educational and interpersonal theories into her theory. Hall developed her ideas regarding interpersonal behaviour from Harry Stack Sullivan and also utilized teaching and learning ideas integrated from John Dewey. Hall did not utilize ideas of the contemporary nursing theorists. The influence of Dewey can be seen in Hall's emphasis on the teaching-learning process with the nurse's primary responsibility as one of teacher. Sullivan's influence was evidenced in the role of the nurse as nurturer for the patient within the "Core" circle.

The patient is a unity composed of three overlapping parts: a person (the core aspect), a pathology and treatment (the cure aspect), and a body (the care aspect). The nurse is a bodily caregiver. Provision of bodily care allows the nurse to comfort and learn the patient's pathology, treatment aspect, and person. Understanding, resulting from the integration of all three areas, allows the nurse to be an effective teacher and nurturer. The patient learns and is nurtured in the person (that is, in the core aspect). Nurturance leads to effective rehabilitation, greater levels of self-actualization, and self-love.

Nursing occurs during one of two phases of medical care. Phase 1 medical care is the diagnostic and treatment phase; phase 2 is the evaluative, follow-up phase. The professional nurse's role is in phase 2, and professional nursing practice requires a setting in which patients are free to learn. In phase 2 the nurse's goal is to help the patient learn. Motivation to learn is assured by advocating the patient's learning goals and not the doctor's curative goals. Once patient learning goals are codetermined with the nurse and motivation therefore assured, the patient will learn, and nurturance, rehabilitation, and self-love follow. The overall goal for the client is rehabilitation, which inspires a greater measure of self-actualization and self-love.

As a nurse theorist, Lydia Hall is unique in that, her beliefs about nursing were demonstrated in practice with relatively little documentation in the literature. Hall's greatest achievement in Nursing was her design and development of the Lobe Center for Nursing at Montefiore Hospital, Brona, New York. Established to apply the theory of nursing practice, the center opened in January 1963. The purpose of establishment of this center was to provide professional nursing care to persons past the acute stage of illness. The center, functioning concepts was that the need for professional nursing care increases as the need for medical cure decreases. It demonstrated extreme success and provided empirical evidence to support the major concepts in Halls Theory.

Hall drew extensively from the schools of Psychiatry and Psychology in theorizing about the nurse-patient relationship. She was a proponent of Carl Roger's philosophy of "Client-centred therapy. In addition, to utilizing Roger's theories, Hall also integrated educational and interpersonal theories into her theory. She developed her ideas regarding interpersonal behaviour from Harry Stack Sullivan and also utilized teaching and learning ideas integrated form John Dewey. Dewy's influence was evidenced in the role of the nurse as teacher and Sullivan influence was evidenced in the role of the nurse as "nurture" for the patient within the 'core circle'.

Concepts Used by Hall

- *Behaviour:* refers to everything that is said or done. Behaviour is dictated by feelings, both conscious and unconscious.
- *Reflection:* refers to a method of communication in which selected verbalizations for the patient are repeated back to him using different phraseology, to invite him to explore his feelings further.
- *Self-awareness:* refers to the state of being that nurses endeavor to help their patient's achieve. The more self-awareness a person has of his feelings, the more control he has over his behaviour.
- *Phases of medical care:* Hall divides medical care into two phases; biologically critical and evaluative follow-up. During first phase, the patient receives intensive medical care and multiple diagnostic. The second phase starts when doctors begin giving only follow-up care. Hall defines second stage of illness as the non-acute recovery phase of illness. This stage is conducive to learning and rehabilitation. The need for medical care is minimal although the need for nurturing and learning is great. Therefore, this is the ideal time for wholly professional nursing care.
- *Wholly professional nursing:* It implies nursing care given exclusively by RNS educated in the behavioural sciences who take the responsibility and opportunity to co-ordinate and deliver the roles of nurturing, teaching and advocacy in the fostering of healing.

- *Care, Core and Cure:* Nursing circles of care, core and cure are the central concepts of Hall's theory. Care alludes to the 'hands on' intimate bodily care of the patient implies a comforting, nurturing relationship. Core involves the therapeutic use of self in communicating with the patient. The nurse reflects questions appropriately and helps the patient clarify motives and goals facilitating the process of increasing the patient's self-awareness. Cure is the aspect of nursing involved with administration of medications and treatments. The nurse functions in this role as an investigator and potential 'painer'. The diagrammatic representation of these concepts shown.

Presentation of Theory

Lydia Hall presented her theory of nursing visually by drawing three interlocking circles, each circle presenting a particular aspect of nursing. The circles represents care, core and cure (Fig. 6.1).

Care

The Body Natural and Biological Sciences Intimate bodily care aspects of nursing 'The Care'. The care circle represents the nurturing components of nursing and exclusive to nursing. Nurturing involves using the factors that make up the concept of mothering (Care and comfort of the person may provide for teaching-learning activities. The professional nurse provides bodily care for the patient and helps the patient to complete such basic daily biological functions as eating, bathing, elimination, and dressing. When providing this care, the nurse's goal is to comfort of the patient, while providing care, the nurse gets an opportunity for closeness. This closeness gives an opportunity to explore feelings,

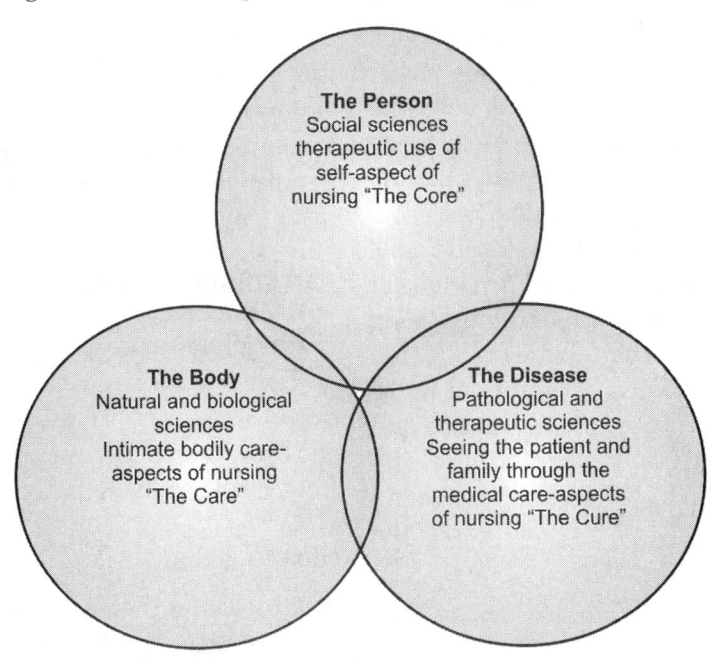

Figure 6.1: Core, Care, and Cure Models

represents the teaching-learning aspect of nurturing. When functioning the care circle, the nurse applies knowledge of the natural and biological sciences to provide a strong theoretical base for nursing implementation. In this, patient views the nurse as a potential comforter.

Core

The person social security therapeutic use and self-aspect of nursing. The core circle of patient care is based in the social sciences involves the therapeutic use of self and is shared with other members of the health team. The professional nurse, by developing an interpersonal relationship with the patient, is able to help the patient verbally express feelings regarding the disease process and its effect. Through such expression the patient is able to gain self-identity and further develop maturity. The professional nurse by use of the reflective technique (acting as a mirror for the patient) helps the patient look at and explore feelings regarding his or her current health status and related potential changes in life-style. The nurses use a freely offered closeness to help the patient bring into awareness the verbal and non-verbal messages, being sent to others. Motivations are discovered through the process of bringing into awareness of the feelings being experienced with the awareness. This awareness the patient is now able to make conscious decisions based on understood and accepted feelings and motivations. The motivations and energy necessary for healing exist within the patient, rather than in the health care team.

Cure

The 'cure' circle of patient care is based on pathological and therapeutic sciences and is shared with other members of the health team. The professional nurse helps the patient and family through the medical, surgical, and rehabilitative prescriptions made by the physician. During this aspect of nursing care, the nurse is an active advocate of the patient. The nurse's role during the cure aspect is different from the care circle because many of the nurses action take on a negative quality of avoidance of pain rather than a positive quality of comforting. For example, giving injection, preparing and performing diagnosing procedure on patients. Pathological and Therapeutic Sciences Seeing the patient and family through the Medical Care aspects of nursing 'The Cure.'

Hall emphasizes the importance of a total person approach, it is important that the three aspects of nursing not viewed as functioning independently but as interrelated. Here, the professional nurse functions most therapeutically when patients have entered the second stage of their hospital stay (i.e. they are recuperating and are past the acute stage of illness. During this recuperation stage, the care and core aspects are the most prominent and the core aspect is less prominent.

PARADIGM OF HALL

Although the concept of nursing is identified by Hall, she does not speak directly to other three concepts of human health and environment. However, inferences made from her work is noted below:

Human Being

Hall viewed a patient in composed of three aspects, body, pathology and person. She emphasizes the importance of the individual as unique, capable of growth and learning, and requiring total person approach. Patients achieve their maximal potential through learning process, therefore, the chief therapy they need is teaching.

Health

Hall viewed becoming ill is behaviour. Illness is directed by one's feelings-out-of-awareness, which are the roots adjustment difficulties. Heal can be inferred to be a state of self-awareness with conscious selection of behaviours that are optimal for that individual. She stresses the need to help the person explore the meaning of his or her behaviour to identify and overcome problems through developing self-identify and maturity.

Environment

Hall said 'any career that is defined around work that has to be done and how it is divided to get it done is a trade.' She vehemently opposed the ideas of any one other than educated, professional nurses taking direct care of patients and decried the fact that nursing has trained non-professionals to function as practical nurses, so that professional nurses can function as practical doctors.

The concept of environment is dealt with in relation to the individual. Hall is credited with developing the concept of **Loeb Center** because she assumed that the hospital environment during the treatment of acute illness creates a difficult psychological experience for the ill individual. Loeb Center focuses on providing an environment, i.e. conducive to self development; in which any action of the nurses is for assisting the individual in attaining a personal goal.

Nursing

Nursing is identified as consisting of participation in the **care, core** and **cure** aspects of patient care. Care is the sole function of nurse, whereas core and cure are shared with other members of the Health Care Team. However, the major purpose of care is to achieve an interpersonal relationship with the individual that will facilitate the development of core, i.e. the development of self-identity and self-direction by the patient.

Nursing Process and Hall

According to Hall, the motivation and energy needed for healing within the patient.' This aspect of her theory influences the five phases of nursing process as follows:

- *Assessment:* involves data collection about health status of the person. Hall viewed the process of data collection is directed for the benefit of the patient rather than benefit the nurse. It should be directed towards increasing the patient self-awareness. Through the use of observation and reflection, the nurse is able to assist the patient in becoming aware of both verbal and non-verbal behaviours. In the individual, increased awareness of feelings and needs in relation to health status increases the ability of self-healing. This phase helps guiding patients through the cure aspects of nursing.
- *Nursing diagnoses:* is the statement of the patient needs or problems. Analysis and interpretations of data collects help identify nursing diagnoses, viewing the patient as the power of self-healing directs conclusions differently than if the healing power rests in the doctor or nurse. The patient is the one in control than one who identifies the need.

- *Planning:* involves setting priorities and mutually establishing patient centered goals. The patient decides what is of highest priority and what goals are desirable. The core is involved in planning. The role of the Nurse is to use reflection to help the patient become aware of and understand needs, feelings and motivations. Once motivation are clarified, the patient is the best person to set goals and arrange priorities. The nurse seeks to increase patient awareness and to support decision making based on the patient's new level of awareness. The nurse works with patient to help keep the goals consistent with the medical prescriptions.
- *Implementation:* involves actual institution of the plan of care. This phase is the actual giving of nursing care. In this care and core circles, the Nurse works with the patient, helping with bathing, dressing, eating and other care of comfort needs. The professional nurses use a permissible non-directive teaching-learning approach to implement nursing care, then helping the patients reach the established goals. This includes 'helping the patient with his feelings, providing requested information and supporting patient-made decision. The nurse also helps the patient and family through the cure aspects of nursing. Working with patient and family to help them understand and implement the medical plan.
- *Evaluation:* is the process of assessing the patient's progress toward the health goals. This phase is directed toward the health goals. This phase is directed towards deciding whether or not the patient is successful in reaching the established goals, and according to Hall, whether or not a person is growing in self-awareness regarding his or her feelings and motivations can be recognized through changes in his or her outward behaviour.

Hall's Work and Characteristics of Theory

Hall's work may be considered a theory, because it meets each of the characteristics of theories.

1. The use of the terms: care, core cure is unique to Hall. She interrelated these concepts.
2. Hall's theory is formulated using inductive logic moves from specific observations to a generalized concept. For example,
   - Nursing care shortens patient recovery time.
   - Nursing care facilitates patient recovery.
   - Professional nursing improves patient's care.
   - Therefore, wholly professional nursing will hasten recovery.

   Her work appears to be completely and singly logical. She indicates that care, the bodily laying on of hands, is the only aspect that is solely nursing—implying that it is the major focus for nursing—her major emphasis on core. The care aspects is a means for achieving core rather than end in itself.
3. Hall's works is simple in its presentation. However, the openness and flexibility required for its application may not be simple. For nurses whose personality, educational preparation and experience have not prepared them to function with minimal structure.
4. Hall's work has been demonstrated in the research conducted to evaluate the

effectiveness of Loeb Center. This evidenced that hypothesis can be developed and tested and also shown evidence of an increase in the general look and knowledge.
5. Hall's work was designed for practice and has been implemented successfully Loeb center and their centers.
6. Hall recognized the importance of knowledge of validation theories, laws and principles. She indicated the theoretical basis for each aspect of nursing care. The care aspect based in the natural and biological sciences, the core in the social sciences and cure in the pathological and therapeutic sciences.

Hall's theory delineates definite ideas regarding nursing care being provided for by a professional nursing staff. The acceptance of this philosophy can be seen in the current shift toward professional staffing in many health care facilities, and in the growing trend toward the BSN as the minimum entry level requirement for professional practice. Hall also emphasized the concept of nurses practicing nursing while completing their educational programmes, instead of practicing as practical doctors. Today's issues of narrowing the divide between nursing education and service, and of using nursing diagnoses as a guide for patient care instead of medical diagnoses support Hall's concepts from her theory.

Until the late 1980s, research testing Hall's theory had been done only at Loeb Center. Now two different facilities in Europe are utilizing the ideas of Hall to develop nursing care units. Pearson, Durand, and Punton (1988) compared patients in an acute care hospital with patients receiving care at a nursing unit. All patients were over 65 and had suffered femur neck fractures. The researchers compared length of acute stay, quality of nursing care, and life satisfaction 6 months after discharge. Those patients who received care on the nursing unit spent less time in acute care, received more consistent quality of nursing care, and reported improvements in level of life satisfaction after 6 months.

Pearson, Durant, and Punton again conducted a larger scale study similar to the 1988 study. They found the same results of increased satisfaction for patients who received care on a nursing unit. Hall's theory is also being implemented in Oxford, England. No specific research studies were done, but McMahon (1989) wrote two articles detailing the use and success of the Oxford Nursing Development Unit. Implementation of Hall's theory in nursing units within the United States was not found outside of the Loeb Center.

Much research and testing of Hall's theory is needed before it can be applicable and useful to areas of nursing other than long-term illnesses and rehabilitative nursing. In particular, the theory needs to be adapted to health care facilities that differ from the Loeb Center for Nursing before its true impact and contribution to nursing can be judged. This step would require flexibility and change in several of Hall's main concepts and relationships, particularly those relating to the age and illness orientation of the client. It would be interesting to further develop in a variety of settings the concept of increased nursing care as a means to hasten patient recovery. This tenet has been highly successful at the Loeb Center in reducing both patient days and health care costs.

Home health care is one domain of nursing in which testing could be done to see if utilizing Hall's ideas could decrease readmissions to the hospital. With the instillation of diagnostic related groups, patients leave the hospital as soon as the acute phase of illness is resolved. Home health nurses could utilize Hall's ideas of teaching-learning by using reflection to increase self-awareness. Since the patient was ill while hospitalised, the patient would not have learned all needed information for proper care at home. Home health nurses can intervene to assure the patient learns all needed information for proper care.

EVALUATION OF THEORY

- Hall's theory is simple and easily understood. The major concepts and relationships are limited and clear. The three aspects of professional nursing are identified both individually and as they relate to each other in the total process of patient care. Hall designed basic models to represent the major concepts and relationships of her theory, using individual and interlocking circles to define the three aspects of the patient and their relationships to the three aspects of nursing. The language used to define and describe the theory is easily understood and is indigenous to nursing.
- Perhaps the most serious flaw in Hall's theory of nursing is its limited generality. Hall's primary target in nursing theory is the adult patient who has passed the acute phase of his or her illness and has a relatively good chance at rehabilitation. This concept severely limits application of the theory to a small population of patients of specific age and stage of illness. Although the ideas of core, care and cure can possibly be applied to patients in the acute phase of their illness, the theory would be most difficult to apply to infants, small children, and comatose patients. In addition, Hall devotes her theory to adult individuals who are ill. The function of the nurse in preventive health care and health maintenance is not addressed, nor is the nurse's role in community health, even though the model could be adapted. Hall viewed the role of the nurse as heavily involved in the care and core aspects of patient care. Unfortunately, this concept provides for little interaction between the nurse and the family, because her theory delineates the family aspect of patient care only in the cure circle.

The use of therapeutic communication to help the patient look at and explore his feelings regarding his illness and the potential changes the illness might cause is discussed in the core aspect of nursing care. Therapeutic communication is also thought to motivate the patient by making him aware of his true feelings. However, the only communication technique Hall described in her theory as a means to assist the patient toward self-awareness was reflection. This is very limited approach to therapeutic communication because not all nurses can effectively use the technique of reflection, and it is not always the most effective and successful communication tool in dealing with patients.

- Hall's concept of professional nursing hastening patient recovery with increased care as the patient improves has been subjected to a great amount of testing at the Loeb Center for Nursing. The fact that the theory is identified with empirical reality cannot be disputed. Evidence obtained through research at the Loeb Center demonstrates that Hall's theory does in fact obtain its goal of shortening patient recovery time through concentrated, professional nursing efforts. Currently, the available literature supports the results obtained at the Loeb Center in testing the theory. Although research support has been demonstrated by the success of the Center, a wider range of testing in various settings is necessary to allow for increased empirical precision of the theory.

Hall's theory has been tested at two other facilities and has been found to be successful. These two facilities still only care for adults, mainly those over 65 years of age. Therefore empirical precision of Hall's theory continues to be limited and further testing in facilities not caring for adults will still be needed.

- The theory provides a general framework for nursing, and the concepts are within the domain of nursing, although the aspects of cure and core are shared with other health professionals and family members. Although the theory does not provide for the resolution of specific issues and problems, it does address itself to the pertinent and contemporary issues of accountability, responsibility, and professionalism. Application of the theory in practice has produced valued outcomes in all three areas. In addition, the theory demonstrates a great impact on the educational preparation of nursing students. Hall stated, "With early field experience in a center where nursing rather than medicine is emphasized, the student may emerge a nurse first." Hall believed that in nursing centers the student would benefit from experiencing nursing as it is taught to them in the classroom.

Despite the shortcomings of Hall's theory of nursing, her contribution to nursing practice is tremendous. Her insight into the problems of nursing in the 1960s has provided a base for professional practice in the multidimensional modern domain of nursing in the 1990s.

Chapter 7

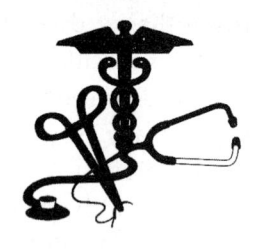

Watson's Philosophy and Science on Caring

(Margaret) Jean Harman Watson was born in southern West Virginia and grew up during the 1940s and 1950s in the small town of Welch, West Virginia, in the Appalachian Mountains. As the youngest of eight children, she was surrounded by an extended family-community environment.

After graduating from high school in West Virginia, she attended the Lewis-Gale School of Nursing in Roanoke, Virginia, graduating in 1961. After graduation she married her husband, Douglas, and moved west to his native state of Colorado. They have two grown daughters, Jennifer (1963) and Julie (1967). Watson and her husband have continued to live in Boulder, Colorado, since 1962.

After moving to Colorado, Watson continued her nursing education and graduate studies at the University of Colorado. She earned a B.S. in Psychiatric-Mental Health Nursing in 1966 at the Health Sciences campus; and a Ph.D. in Educational Psychology and Counselling in 1973 at the Graduate School, Boulder campus.

After Watson completed her Ph D degree, she joined the School of Nursing faculty of the University of Colorado Health Sciences Center in Denver, where she has served in both faculty and administrative positions. She has been chair and Assistant Dean of the undergraduate program and she was involved in early planning and implementation of the Nursing Ph D program in Colorado, which was initiated in 1978. She was Coordinator and Director of the Ph D programme between 1978 and 1981. In 1981 and 82 she pursued sabbatical studies and upon her return was Dean of the University of Colorado School of Nursing and Associate Director, Nursing Practice, University Hospital from 1983 to 1990. Currently she is professor of Nursing and Director of the Center for Human Caring at the University of Colorado Health Sciences Center in Denver.

During her deanship she was instrumental in the development of a post-baccalaureate nursing curriculum in human caring, health, and healing, which leads to a career professional clinical doctoral degree (ND). This pilot ND programme has been selected and funded as a national demonstration programme by the Helene Fuld Health Trust in New York and Colorado clinical agencies. The program was implemented in 1990 as a partnership between nursing education and practice, whereby clinical and academic agencies in Colorado work jointly to simultaneously restructure nursing education and nursing practice for the future.

Dr. Watson has also helped to establish the Center for Human Caring at the University of Colorado, which is the nation's first interdisciplinary center with an overall commitment to develop and use knowledge of human caring and healing as the moral and scientific basis of clinical practice and nursing scholarship, and as the foundation for efforts to transform the current health care system. The center develops and sponsors numerous clinical, educational, and community scholarship activities and projects in human caring, including national and international scholars in residence.

During her career, Watson has been active in community programmes, having served as one of the early founders, clinical consultants, and members of the Board of Boulder County Hospice. The recipient of several research and advanced education federal grants and awards, Watson also has received numerous University and private grants and extramural funding for her faculty and administrative projects and scholarships in human caring. Other honors include two honorary doctorate degrees from Assumption College, Worcester, Massachusetts (1985), and from the University of Akron (1987).

Dr. Watson's national and international work includes distinguished lectureships throughout the United States and in other countries, including Boston College, Catholic University, Adelphi University, Columbia University-Teacher's College, State University of New York, and the University of Montreal in Canada.

Her international activities include an International Kellogg Fellowship in Australia (1982) and a Fulbright Research and Lecture Award to Sweden, and other parts of Scandinavia (1991) and a lecture tour in the United Kingdom. She has also been involved in international projects and invitations in New Zealand, India, Thailand, Taiwan, Israel, and Japan.

Watson is also featured in several national videos on nursing theory. These include "Circles of Knowledge" and "Conversations on Caring with Jean Watson and Janet Quinn" from the National League for Nursing (NLN), "Portraits of Excellence-Nursing Theorists and their Work" form the Helene Fuld Health Trust, "Theory in Practice," from the NLN, which features the Denver Nursing Project in Human Caring, a nurse-directed Caring Center for persons with AIDS. The Denver Nursing Project in Human Caring is a clinical (caring theory based) demonstration project of the University of Colorado Center for Human Caring/School of Nursing.

Dr. Watson's publications reflect the evolution of her theory of caring. Her writings have been geared toward educating nursing students and providing them the ontological and epistemological basis for their praxis and research directions. Much of her current work began with the 1979 publication, *Nursing; The philosophy and Science of Caring*, which she says began as class notes for a course she was developing. Although Watson refers to this book as a treatise on nursing, the nursing community considers this book a theory for nursing.

Her second major work, *Nursing: Human Science and Human Care, A Theory of Nursing* was published in 1985 (re-released in 1988). The purpose of this book was to address some of the conceptual and philosophical problems that still existed in nursing. She hoped that others would join her as she seeks to "elucidate the human care process in nursing, preserve the concept of the person in our science, and better our contribution to society."

EVOLUTION OF THEORY

The discrepancy in nursing between theory and practice is well known. To reduce this dichotomy, Watson proposes a philosophy and science of caring. She refers to caring as the essence of nursing practice. It is a moral ideal rather than a task-oriented behaviour and includes such elusive aspects of the actual caring occasion and the transpersonal caring relationship between the nurse and the client. The goal is the preservation of human dignity and humanity in the health care system. Watson believes professional nursing care is developed through a combined study of the sciences and the humanities and culminates in a human care process between nurse and client that transcends time and space and has spiritual dimensions.

According to Watson, the goal of nursing is to facilitate individuals gaining "a higher degree of harmony within the mind, body, and soul which generates self-knowledge, self-reverence, self-healing, and self-care processes while allowing increasing diversity." She states that the goal is attained through the human-to-human caring process and caring transactions.

One way Watson has attempted to bridge the gap between theory and practice is through the development of the Center for Human Caring and the ND program at the University of Colorado Health Science Center. Both the center and the ND programme provide opportunities to "integrate the arts, humanities, and social and behavioural sciences into human care and the healing process."

In addition to traditional nursing knowledge and the works of Nightingale, Henderson, Krueter, and Hall, Watson acknowledges the work of Leininger and Gadow as background for her work. In her more recent work, Watson refers to the works of others such as Maslow, Heidegger, Erikson, Seyle, and Lazarus. In developing her Framework, Watson drew heavily on the sciences and the humanities, thereby providing a more phenomenological, existential, and spiritual orientation.

Watson attributes her emphasis on the interpersonal and transpersonal qualities of congruence, empathy, and warmth to the views of Carl Rogers and recent transpersonal psychology writers. Rogers describes several incidents leading to the formulation of his thoughts on human behaviour. One such episode involves his learning "that it is the client who knows what hurts and that the facilitator should allow the direction of the therapeutic process to come from the client." Rogers believed that through understanding the client would come to accept himself, an initial step toward a positive outcome. The therapist helps by clarifying and stating feelings about which the client has been unclear. To accomplish this goal, the therapist must be able to understand the meaning, feeling, and attitudes of the client. A warm interest facilitates understanding.

Assumptions underlying human care values in nursing are (i) care and love comprise the primal and universal psychic energy and (ii) care and love are requisite for survival and the nourishment of humanity. Caring for and loving self is requisite to caring for others. Curing is not the end to be sought but is a means to care. Nursing's ability to sustain its caring ideology and translate it into practice will determine its contribution to society. Nursing has traditionally held a caring stance in relation to patients with health and illness concerns, and caring is the unifying focus for practice in nursing caring has received little emphasis in the health care system, and the caring values of nursing are critical to sustaining care ideals in practice. Practiced only interpersonally and nursing's social, moral, and scientific contributions lie in its commitment to human care ideals. The foregoing assumptions provide a rationale for developing nursing as a human science.

Human are capable of transcending time and space, and each possesses a spirit, oil, or essence that enables self-awareness, higher degrees of consciousness, and a power to transcend the usual self. Human life is a continuous (with time and space) being in the world. Caring, an intersubjective human process is the moral ideal of nursing. Human care processes have an energy field and involve engagement of mind-body-soul with another in a lived moment. Illness, not necessarily decrease, is a state of subjective turmoil in which self as "I" is separated from self as "me". Conversely, health is a harmony within mind-body-soul in which the "I" and "me" are aligned. A healthy person is open to increased diversity. The goal of nursing is to help people increase harmony within mind-body-soul, which leads to self-knowledge, self-reverence, self-healing and self-care.

Theoretic premises identified include the following. At nursing's highest level, the nurse makes contact with the person's emotional and subjective world as the route to inner self; mind and soul are not confined in time and space and to the physical universe; a nurse can access inner self through the mind-body-soul, provided the physical body is not perceived separate from the higher sense of self. The gist (Spirit or inner self) exists in and for it and relates to the human ability to be free; love and caring are universal givens; illness may be hidden from the "eyes" and requires finding meaning in inner experience. Finally the totality of experiences at the moment constitutes a phenomenal field or the individual's frame of reference.

Human strive to satisfy needs experienced in the perceived phenomenal field, including being cared for, loved, and valued and experiencing positive regard, acceptance, and understanding. People also strive to achieve union, transcend individual life, and find harmony with life. All needs are subservient to a basic striving toward actualizing spiritual self and establishing harmony within mind-body-soul. Harmony is consistent with a sense of congruence between "I" and "me" between self as perceived and self as experienced, and between subjective reality (Phenomenal field) and external reality (world as is).

Caring occasions involve action and choice by nurse and individual. If the caring occasion is transpersonal, the limits of openness and human capacities are expanded. Transpersonal caring relationships depend on (i) moral commitments to enhance human dignity to allow people to determine their own meaning, (ii) the nurse's affirmation of the subjective significance of the person, (iii) the nurse's ability to detect feelings of another's inner condition and feel a union with another, and (iv) the nurse's history of living and experiencing feelings and human conditions and imagining others feelings (that is personal growth, maturation, and development of the nurse's self).

Nursing interventions related to human care are referred to as curative factors and include nurturing, forming, cultivating, and using (i) a humanistic-altruistic system of values;(ii) faith-hope, (iii) sensitivity to self and others; (iv) helping-trusting human care relationship; (v) expressed positive and negative feelings;(vi) a creative problem-solving caring processes; (vii) transpersonal teaching-learning;(viii) supportive, protective, and or corrective mental, physical, societal, and spiritual environment; (ix) human needs assistance; and (x) existential-phenomenological spiritual forces. Captive factors are actualized in the human care process.

Dr. Watson's publication reflects the evolution of her theory of caring most of her current work began with the 1979 publications Nursing: The philosophy and science of caring, laid the foundation of her theory. She believes that main focus in nursing is on creative focus in nursing is on creative factors that are derived from a humanistic perspective combined with scientific knowledge base. For nurses to develop humanistic philosophies and value systems, a strong liberal arts background is necessary. This philosophy and value system, in turn provides a solid foundation for the science of caring. A liberal arts base can assist nurses to expand their vision and views of the world and to develop critical thinking skills. An expanded world view and critical thinking skills are needed in the science of caring. Which focusses on health promotion rather than on cure of disease? According to Watson, curing disease is the domain of medicine. She asserts that caring stance that nursing always held in being threatened by the tasks and technology demands of the curative factors. In her works, one finds the reference to existential humanists such as Erickson, Maslow and Roger, sleeve, Lazarus, Lining and Henderson.

THEORY OF CARING

Jean Watson stated the following assumptions of the science of caring in Nursing and primary curative factors. The basic assumptions are as given below:
1. Caring can only be effectively demonstrated and practiced interpersonally.
2. Caring consist of curative factors that result in the satisfaction of certain human needs.
3. Effective caring promotes health and individual or family growth.
4. Caring responses accept a person not only as he or she is now but on what he or she may become.
5. A caring environment is one that offers the development of potential while allowing the person to choose the best action for himself or herself at given point of time.
6. Caring is more 'healthogenic' than is curing. The practice of caring integrates biophysical knowledge with knowledge of human behaviour to generate or promote health and to provide ministrations to those who are well. A

science of caring therefore is complementary to the science of curing.

7. The practice of caring is central to nursing.

In 1981, she views caring as the most valuable attributes nursing has to offer to humanity, yet caring has over time, received less emphasis than other aspects of the practice of nursing. At present, nursing seems to be responding to the various demands of the machinery witless consideration of the needs of the person attached to the machine. She also viewed-thus, disease might be cured, but illness would remain because without caring, health is not attained. Caring is the essence of nursing and connotes responsiveness between the nurse and the person; the nurse co-participates with the person. She contends that caring can assist the person to gain control, become knowledgeable, and promote health changes. In her humanistic value system there is high regard for autonomy and freedom of choice, which leads to an emphasis on client self-knowledge and self-control and client as the person in charge.

Watson says that nursing education and the health care delivery system must be based on human values and concern for the welfare of others. To further define the social ethical responsibilities, and to explicate the human care concepts, she proposes the following 11 assumptions related to human care value (1985).

1. Care and love comprise the primal and universal psychic energy.
2. Care and love, often overlooked, are the cornerstones of our humanness; nourishment of these needs fulfill our humanity.
3. The ability to sustain the caring ideal and ideology in practice will affect the development of civilization and determine nursing's contribution to society.
4. Caring for ourselves is perquisite caring for others.
5. Historically nursing has held a human care and caring stance in regard to people with health-illness concerns.
6. Caring is the central unifying focuses of nursing practice the essence of nursing.
7. Caring at the human level has been increasingly deemphasized in the health car delivery system.
8. Nursling's caring foundation has been sublimated by technological advancement, and institutional constraints.
9. A significant issue for nursing today and in the future is the preservation and advancement of human care.
10. Only through interpersonal relationships can human care be effectively demonstrated and practiced.
11. Nursing social, moral and scientific contributions to human kind and society lie in its commitments to human care ideals in theory practice and research.

Watson bases her theory nursing practice or the structure for the science of caring is built upon the following **Ten Curative Factors**. Each has a dynamic phenomenological component that is relative to the individuals involved in the relationship as encompassed by nursing:

1. The formation of humanistic altruistic system of values.
2. The instillation of faith-hope.
3. The cultivation of sensitivity to one's self and to others.
4. The development of helping-trust relationships.
5. The promotion and acceptance of the expression of positive and negative feelings.

Nursing Theories

6. The systematic use of the scientific problem solving method for decision-making.
7. The promotion of interpersonal teaching learning.
8. The provision for supportive, protective and or corrective mental, physical, sociocultural and spiritual environment.
9. Assistance with the gratification of human need.
10. The allowance for existential phenomenological forces.

Of these ten curative factors, the first three form the "philosophical foundation for the science of Nursing. The details of the above curative factors are as follows:

1. Humanistic-altruistic System of Values (Maturity)

Humanistic-altruistic system of values are learned early in life but can be greatly influenced by the nurse educators. This factor can be defined as satisfaction through giving and extension of the sense of self. Formation of this value system begins developmentally at an early age with values shared with parents. This is mediated through one's own life experiences, the learning one again, and exposure to the humanities. Watson suggests that caring that is based on humanistic values and altruistic behaviour can b e developed through examination of ones own views, beliefs, interactions with various cultures, and personal growth experiences. These are all perceived as necessary to the nurses' own maturation, which then promote altruistic behaviour towards others.

2. Instillation of Faith-hope

This factor incorporating humanistic and altruistic values facilitated the promotion of holistic nursing care and positive health with the client population. It also does cribs nurses role in developing effective nurse-patient interrelationships and in promoting wellness by helping to client adopt health-seeking behaviour. It is essential to both the curative and curative processes. Nurses need to transcend the push towards acceptance of only medicine and assist the person to understanding of alternatives, such as meditations or the healing power of belief in self or in the spiritual. When modern science has nothing to offer the person, the nurse can continue to use faith-hope to provide a sense of well being through those beliefs that are meaningful to the Individual.

3. Cultivation of Sensitivity to Self and Others

The recognitions of feelings lead to self-actualization and thorough self-acceptance for both the nurse and the client. As nurses acknowledge their sensitivity and feelings, they become more genuine, authentic, and sensitive to others. This factor explores the need of nurse to begin to feel an emotion as it presents itself. It is only through developments of one's own feelings that can genuinely and sensitively interact with others. As nurses strive to increase their own sensitivity they become more authentic. Becoming authentic encourages self-growth and self-actualization in both the nurse and those with whom the nurse interacts. The nurse promote health and as opposed to manipulative relationship.

4. Helping-trust Relationships

The development of helping-trust relationship between the nurse and the client is crucial for transpersonal caring. A trusting relationship promotes and accepts the expression of both a positive and negative feelings. The characteristics needed in the trusting relationship are congruence, empathy, warmth and effective communication. **Congruence** involves being real, honest, genuine, and authentic. **Empathy** is the ability to experience and there by understand others persons perceptions and feelings and to communicate those understandings. Non-possessive **warmth** is demonstrated by a moderate speaking volume, a relaxed, open, positive and facial expressions that are congruent with others communication. **Effective communication** has cognitive, affective and behaviour response components.

Congruence implies that nurses are genuine in their interactions and do not put up facades; the nurses act in an open and honest manner. Empathy refers to the attempt that nurses make a tune into the feeling of their clients. Warmth refers to the positive acceptance of another. It is expressed often by open body language, touch and tone of voice. It is through the intense focus on communication (verbal or nonverbal) that the nurse can center on clues and themes that can lead to an even greater depth of awareness for the person.

5. Promotion and Acceptance of the Expression of Positive and Negative Feelings

The expression of feelings both positive and negative ought to be facilitated because such expression improves one's level of awareness. The sharing of feelings is a risk-taking experience for both nurse and client. The nurse must be prepared for either positive or negative feelings. The nurse must recognize that intellectual and emotional understandings of a situation differ. Feelings alter troughs and behaviour and they need to be considered and they need to be considered and allowed for in a caring relationship. Indeed, if one can become aware of the feelings, one can often understand the behaviour it engenders.

6. Use of Scientific Problem-solving for Decision-making

Systematic use of the scientific problem-solving method for decision making of the nursing process brings a scientific problem solving approach to nursing care, dispelling, the traditional image of nurses as the "doctor's hand maiden." The nursing process is similar to the research process in that it is systematic and organized. The issue of research and systematic problem solving presented, because nurse are occupied with the tasks of nursing (i.e., treatment, procedures, charting) they often fail to address the larger issues of conducting research, defining the discipline, or developing a scientific base for nursing. The body of knowledge serves us. Foundation for practice: requires theories and scientific method.

7. Promotion of Interpersonal Teaching Learning

This factor is an important concept for nursing in that it separates caring from curing. It allows the client should be informed and thus shift the responsibility for one's wellness and health to the client. The nurse facilitates the process with teaching-leaning techniques that are designed to enable the client to provide self-care, determine personal needs and provide opportunities for their personal growth.

This is the factor which affords people the most control over their one health because it provides them men with information and alternatives the caring nurse focuses on the learning process as much as the teaching process, for learning offers the best way to individualize the information to be disseminated. Understanding the person's perceptions of the situation assists the nurse to prepare cognitive plan that works within the person's framework and alleviate the suffering.

8. Provision of Suitable Conducive Environment

This factor deals with the daily routine function that the nurse uses to promote health, restore to health or prevent illness. This factor includes the provisions of supportive, protective and or corrective, mental, physical, sociocultural and spiritual environment. Nurses must recognize the influence of internal and external environments both on the health and illness of the individual. Concepts relevant to the internal environment include the mental and spiritual well-being. And sociocultural beliefs of an individual. In addition to epidemiological variable other external variable includes comfort, privacy, safety, and clean aesthetic surrounding. Nurses manipulate both internal and external environment in order to provide support and protection for the person's psychological and physical well-being.

9. Assistance with the Gratification of Human Needs

These needs are similar to that of Maslows (1954). Watson created a hierarchy that she considered to be the science of caring in nursing.

Watson (1979) ordering of needs is as follows:

i. Lower order needs (Biophysical needs) — Survival needs
   - The need for food and fluid.
   - The need for elimination
   - The need ventilation.

ii. Lower order needs (psychophysical needs) — Functional needs
   - The need for activity and inactivity.
   - The need for sexuality.

iii. Higher order needs (psycho-social needs) — Integrative needs
   - The need for achievement.
   - The need for affiliation.

iv. Higher order needs (inter and inter-personal needs) — Growth seeking needs
   - The need for self-actualization.

The nurse recognizes the biophysical, psycho physical, psychosocial and intrapersonal need of self and client. Client must satisfy lower order needs before attempting to attainment of higher order one's as stated above.

10. Allowance for Existential-phenomenological Factors

Phenomenology is way of understanding people from the way things appear to then, from their frame of reference. Phenomenology describes data of the immediate situation that help people understand the phenomena in question. Existential psychology is a science of human existence that uses phenomenological analysis. For the Nurse this factor helps to reconcile and mediate the incongruity of viewing the person holistically while at the same time attending to a hierarchical ordering of needs. By using this factor nurse may assist the person to find the strength and of courage to confront life or death.

Paradigm of Watson Theory

Human Being

By using nursing's heritage, Watson adopts a view of the human being as "a valued person in and of him or herself to be cared for, respected, nurtured, understood and assisted; in general philosophical view of a person as a fully functional integrated self. She believes that humans are best viewed in developmental conflicts of individuals and their family is necessary for health care". The nurse must understand human being when they are sick, well or under stress.

Health

Watson acknowledges the WHO definition of Health and believes that others factors needed to be included in health which includes the adding of following three elements.
  i. A high level of over all-physical, mental and social functioning.
  ii. The General adapting maintenance level of daily functioning.
  iii. The absence of illness (or the presence of efforts that lead to its absence).

She states that what has traditionally been called health care is a myth. That which has been called health care, the diagnosing the disease, treatment of illness and prescription of drugs in medical care. The health care focuses on lifestyle, social conditions and environment. For which she adds that "Health refers to unity and harmony within the mind, body and soul. Health is also associated with the degree of congruence between the self as perceived and self as expressed.

Environment

Watson (1979) states, "Caring (and nursing) has existed in every society. Every society has had some people who cared for others a caring attitude is not transmitted by the culture of the profession as a unique way of coping with its environment." In this way, she viewed environment and which helps the person to meeting their need accordingly.

Nursing

Nursing is concerned with promoting health, preventing illness caring for the sick, and restoring health." Nursing focus on health promotion as well as treatment of disease. She sees nursing as having to move educationally in the two areas of stress and developmental conflict to provide holistic health care, which she believes central to the practice of caring in nursing. One of the assumptions of hers is "nursing's social, moral, and scientific contribution to humankind and society life in its commitment to human care ideals in theory, practice and search.

Watson defines nursing as "a human science of persons and human health-illness experiences that are mediated by professional, personal, scientific, aesthetic and ethical, human care transaction." In this context nursing is rooted in the humanities as well as natural sciences and its goal through the caring process, is to help people gain a higher of harmony within the self in order to promote self-knowledge and self healing, or to gain insight into the meaning of happenings in life.

Nursing Process and Watson

Broad approach to nursing in their searches out connections rather than separation between the parts that make up the whole of the person. To accomplish this, nurses employ scientific problem-solving method by which they can draw from a database and basic nursing principles to make nursing judgment and decision. Watson points out that the nursing process contains the same steps as the scientific research process. Both the process is identical and try to solve a problem or answer, or to discover the best solution. Watson (1979) elaborates the nursing process and research process as follows.

Table 7.1: Nursing process and research processes (Watson, 1979)

Nursing process	Scientific research process
Assessment	• Assessment involves observation, identification and review of problems, use of the applicable
	• Knowledge in literature.
	• It includes conceptual knowledge for the formulation and conceptualization of a framework in which to view and assess the problem.
	• It also includes the formulation of hypothesis about relationships and factors that influence problem.
	• Assessment also includes defining variable that will be examined in solving-problem.
Plan	• The plan helps to determine how variables will be examined or measured.
	• It includes a conceptual approach or design for solving problems that is referred to as the nursing care plan.
	• It also includes determining what data will be collected and on what person and how data will be collected.
Intervention	• Interventions direct action and implementation of the plan.
	• It includes the collection of data.
Evaluation	• Evaluation is the method of and the process of analyzing data as well as the examination of the effects of intervention based on the date.
	• It includes interpretation of the results, the degree to which a positive outcome occurred and whether the results can be generalized beyond that situation.
	• In addition-evaluation also generates additional hypothesis or possibly even lead to the generation of horsing theory based on the problem studied by solution.

Characteristic of Theory and Watson's Work

A theory is an imaginative grouping of knowledge ideas and experience that are represented symbolically and seek to illuminate given phenomenon. Although Watson rejects traditional, quantifiable methodology, when such methodology scarifies the pursuit of new knowledge of human behaviour, her work has been developed within the traditional contact and can be compared to the characteristics of theory:

1. The use of the term 'caring' is not unique in Watson what is unique in her basic assumptions for the structure for this concept. She describes caring in both philosophical and scientific terms. Caring is placed in hierarchical context, meeting lower order biophysical needs first, and moving towards higher order psycho-social and intrapersonal needs. She also said that needs are interrelated.

2. Watson work is logical in that curative factors are based on the board assumption that provides a supportive framework. She uses these curative factors to help delineate nursing from medicine. The curative facts are logically derived from the assumptions and related to the hierarchy needs.
3. Watson theory is relatively simple, because it does use theories from others disciplines that are familiar to nurses. It is simple because the fact that it de-emphasizes the pathophyological for the psychosocial diminishes it, ability to be generalizable.
4. Her work is based upon phenomenological studies that generally ask questions rather than state hypothesis. Its purpose is to describe the phenomena, to analyze and to gain an understanding.
5. Watson suggested that the best method of testing her theory is through field study. For example, her work in area of loss and caring that place in Western Australia and involved tribe of aborigines after analysis. She found that loss creates a disharmony in three spheres: mind, body, and spirit. The nurse can other into the process of transpersonal caring by comforting. Listening and allowing for norms of the person. Because the curative factors expand on theories learned from other disciplines and mould them into uniquely nursing knowledge, continued research that involves the curative factors should increase the body of knowledge in nursing.
6. Watson's work can be used to guide and improve practice. It can provide the nurse with the most satisfying aspects of practice and can provide the client with holistic cure so necessary for human growth and development.
7. Watson work supported by the theoretical work of numerous humanists, philosophers, develops mentalists and psychologists. She clearly designates the theories of stress, development, communication, teaching learning, humanistic psychology and existential phenomenology that provide the foundations for the science of caring. She presents these in a way into provide a uniquely nursing view that leads to further questions to be studied.

EVALUATION OF THEORY

- Watson's theory is easily read and uses nontechnical language that provides clarity. In *Nursing; Human Science and Human Care*, Watson expands the philosophical nature of her theory. The reader's comprehension of her theory is enhanced by an understanding of philosophy.
- Watson draws on a number of disciplines to formulate her theory. The reader must have an understanding of a variety of subject matters to understand the theory as it is presented. It is seen as complex when considering the existential-phenomenological nature of her work, due in part to the limited liberal arts background of many nurses and the limited integration of liberal arts in baccalaureate nursing curricula.
- The theory seeks to provide a moral and philosophical basis for nursing. The scope of the framework encompasses all aspects of the health-illness continuum. In addition, the theory addresses aspects of preventing illness and experiencing a peaceful death, thereby in creasing its

generality. The carative factors, described by Watson, have provided important guidelines for nurse-client interactions; however, some critics have stated that the generality is limited due to the emphasis placed on the psychosocial aspects rather than on the physiological aspects of caring.

- Although the framework is difficult to study empirically, Watson draws heavily on widely accepted work from other disciplines. This solid foundation strengthens her views. Watson describes her theory as descriptive. She acknowledges the newness of the theory. She welcomes input by others as she continues to develop her theory.

- The theory does not lend itself to research conducted using traditional scientific methodologies. In her second book, Watson addresses the issue of methodology. The methodologies relevant to studying transpersonal caring and developing nursing as a human science and art can be classified as qualitative, naturalistic, or phenomenological. Watson does acknowledge that a combination of qualitative quantitative inquiry may also be useful.

- Although further testing is necessary, Watson's theory continues to provide a useful and important metaphysical orientation for the delivery of nursing care. Watson's theoretical concepts, such as use of self, client-identified needs, the caring process, and the spiritual sense of being human, may help nurses and their clients find meaning and harmony in a period of increasing complexity.

Chapter 8

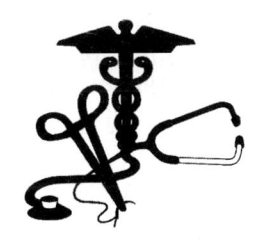

Peplau's Interpersonal Relations Theory

Hildegard E. Peplau was born September 1, 1909, in Reading, Pennsylvania. She graduated from Pottstown, Pennsylvania, Hospital School of Nursing in 1931. She received a B.A. in interpersonal psychology from Bennington College, Vermonr, in 1943, an M.A. in psychiatric nursing from Teachers College, Columbia, New York, in 1947, and an Ed.D. in curriculum development from Columbia in 1953.

Peplau's professional and teaching experiences have been broad and varied. She was operating room supervisor at Pottstown Hospital and later headed the staff of the Bennington infirmary while pursuing her undergraduate degree. She did clinical work at Bellevue and Chestnut Lodge psychiatric facilities and was in contact with renowned psychiatrists Freida Fromm-Riechman and Harry Stack Sullivan. A member of the Army Nurse Corps during World War II, she worked in a neuropsychiatric hospital in England.

After obtaining her master's degree at Columbia, she was invited to develop and teach in the graduate program in psychiatric nursing. She remained on the faculty 5 years. In 1954 Peplau went to Rutgers, where she developed and chaired the graduate psychiatric nursing programme until her retirement in 1974.

Peplau's contribution to nursing and the speciality of psychiatric nursing has been enormous, beginning in 1952 with her book *Interpersonal Relations in Nursing*. Throughout the 1950s and 1960s she conducted workshops, "abundantly sharing her knowledge and clinical skills and encouraging nurses to use their competence in a continuous, experiential and educative process." She analysed verbatim notes of sessions with medical and psychiatric patients to develop numerous lectures, articles, and workshops. She has maintained a part-time private practice since 1960 and has given many lectures throughout the United States, Canada, Africa, and South America. During the 1970s William E. Field, Jr., took copious notes on the numerous lectures Peplau delivered to psychiatric nurses. He published them for his mentor in "The Psychotherapy of Hildegard E. Peplau." Peplau's theory and method was presented as investigative psychotherapy as it developed from 1948 to 1974.

In 1969 Peplau became executive director of the American Nurses' Association. She served as president of the ANA from 1970 to 1972, and as second vice-president from 1972 to 1974. She has also served as director of the New Jersey State Nurses' Association; a member of the Expert Advisory Council of WHO; the National Nurse Consultant to the Surgeon General of the Air Force; and a nursing consultant to the United States Public Health Services, the National Institute of Mental Health, and various foreign countries. She chaired the editorial board of *Perspectives in Psychiatric Care* when the journal was founded and served as chief advisor of *Nursing 74*. She is on the editorial board of the Journal of *Psychosocial Nursing*.

Peplau's archives are deposited in the Arthur and Elizabeth Schlesinger Library on the History of Women in America, Radcliffe College, Cambridge, Massachusetts.

The patient is an individual with a felt need, and nursing is a process that is both interpersonal and therapeutic. Nursing is the simultaneous application of art and science. The overall goal or purpose of nursing is to educate and be a maturing force so that personality development (a new view of self) occurs. This purpose is achieved when the nurse, as a medium for change, enters into a personal relationship with an individual, the patient, when a felt need presents itself. The personal relationship in nursing provides for meeting the individual patient's needs and assists the two persons (nurse and patient) with different goals to develop or assume congruent goals. The nurse-patient relationship occurs in phases, during which the nurse functions as a resource person, a counselor, and a surrogate. There are four phases: orientation, identification, exploitation, and resolution. When a person with a need seeks help, the nurse assists in orientation to the problem. During phase 1 the illness event is integrated. The person learns the facets of the difficulty and the extent of need for help. Orientating to use of services, productively exploiting anxiety and tension, and learning the limits of necessary space and freedom also occur. This helps to ensure that the illness event is not repressed. When orientation is completed to a given degree, the phase of identification begins. In phase 2 the patient assumes a posture of interdependence, dependence, or independence in relation to the nurse. The nurse assists the patient during this phase by taking into consideration the services needed and the patient's history. Identification helps assure the patient that the nurse can understand the interpersonal meaning of the patient's situation. When identification is accomplished, phase 3, exploitation, begins. In this phase, the patient derives full value from the relationship by using the services available on the basis of self-interest and needs. Resolution; the final phase, occurs as old needs are met. With resolution of older needs, newer and more mature needs emerge. When needs are resolved, the person is freed from dependence on others. The maturing force of nursing is realized as the personality develops through the educational, therapeutic, and interpersonal process of nursing. The phases of the relationship are serial, and the patient assumes an active role.

During the dyadic nurse-patient relationship and the more extensive nursing relationships with communities, nurses assume many roles, including stranger, teacher, resource person, surrogate, leader, and counselor. Multiple roles occur as a result of multiple client problems and needs in individual interpersonal relationships, team functions, and varying social and professional expectations. The overall goal for professional nursing is the same as for the nurse-patient dyads: to implement a process that facilitates personality development by helping people use forces and experiences to ensure maximum productivity.

EVOLUTION OF THEORY

A Hildegard Peplau has been a pioneer in nursing throughout her career. Her contribution to nursing and the specialty of psychiatric nursing has been enormous, beginning in 1952 with her book *Interpersonal Relations in Nursing*. It is quite remarkable that she referred to her book as a *Partial Theory for the Practice of Nursing*. In this book, she discussed the phases of interpersonal process, roles of nursing and methods for studying nursing as an interpersonal process.

The nature of science in nursing refers to the 'body of verified knowledge found within the discipline of nursing, that is mainly knowledge from the biological and behavioural science. The synthesis, reorganization or extension of concepts drawn from the basic and applied science, which in their reformations and tend to become new concepts. Thus the evolution of Peplau's theory of interpersonal relations resulted. Theories available when she developed her theory described behaviour within the prospectives of psychoanalytical theory, the principles of social learning, the concept of human motivation and the concept of personality development.

Peplau used knowledge borrowed from behaviour sciences and what can be termed the "Psychological mold." This enabled the nurse to begin to move away from a disease orientation to one whereby the psychologic meaning of events, feelings, and behaviours could be explored and incorporated into nursing interventions. It gave nurses and opportunity to teach patients how to experience their feelings while developing conceptual frame work of 'interpersonal relations. She used the theory of Harry Stack Sullivan, Percival Symonds, Abraham Maslow, Bela Mittleman, and Neal Elgar Miller. Some of these theorists therapeutic concepts devised, arose directly from the works.

Concepts Used by Peplau's

Peplau's model evolves through the "Psychodynamics of Nursing." She defines "Psychodynamic nursing is being able to understand one's own behaviour to help others identify felt difficulties and to apply principles of human relations to the problems that arise at all levels of experiences." She develops the model by describing the structural concepts of the interpersonal process, which are the phases of nurse-patient relationship. This is to be the basic to psychodynamic nursing.

Peplau identifies Four sequential steps in interpersonal relationship–orientation, identification, exploitation and resolution. Each of these phases overlaps, interrelates and varies in duration as the process evolves toward a solution (Fig. 8.1).

Peplau's model evolves through the "Psychodynamics of Nursing. The different roles are assumed during the various phases

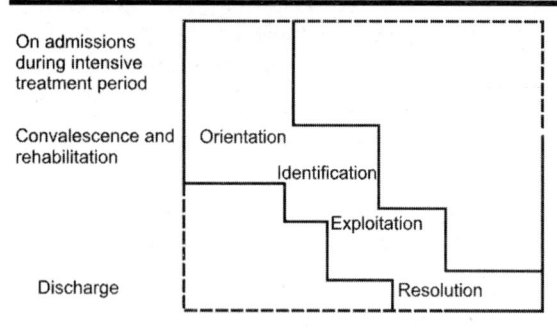

Figure 8.1: Overlapping phases in nurse-patient relationship

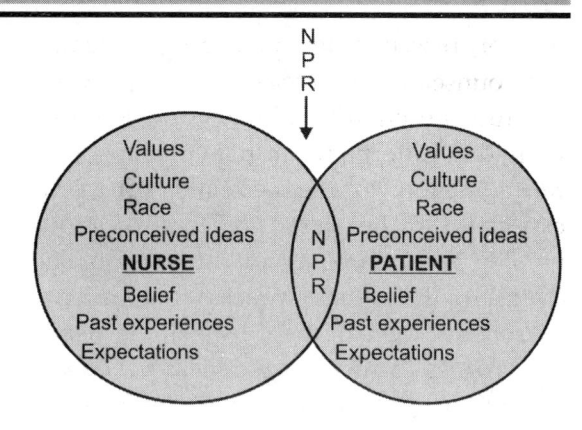

Figure 8.2: Factors influencing NPR

which includes Teacher, Resource, Counselor, Leader, Technical experts and Surrogate

Phases of Interpersonal Relationship

As stated earlier (Fig. 8.1) although the four phases separate, they overlap and occur over the time of the relationship. The factors influencing the blending Nurse-Patient-Relatioships (NPR) shown in Figure 8.2.

Orientation

During the orientation phases, the individual has a 'felt need' and seeks professional assistance. The nurse helps the patient recognize and understand his problem and determine his need for help. In this initial phases of orientation the nurse and patient and/or family has a felt need; therefore professional assistance is sought. It is the phase that the nurse needs to assist the patient and family to realize what is happening to the patient. It is of the utmost importance that the nurse works collectively with the patient and family in analyzing the situation, so that they together can recognize clarifies and defines the existing problem. Mutually clarifying and defining the problems in orientation phase, the patient can direct the accumulated energy from anxiety above unmet needs and begin working with the presenting problem. Nurse-patient rapport is established and continues to be strengthened while concerns are being identified. And mutual decisions need to be made regarding what type of professional assistance the patient and family need.

Orientation phase is directly affected by the patients and nurse's attitude about giving or receiving aid from a reciprocal person. In this initial stage, the nurse needs to be aware of her or his personal reaction to the patient. The nurses as well as the patient's, culture, religion, race, educational background, experiences and preconceived, ideas and expectations all influence the nurse's reaction to the patient. In addition, the same factors influence the patient reactions to the nurse.

Nursing is an interpersonal process, and both the patient and nurse have an equally important part in the therapeutic interactions. The nurse, the patient and the family work together to recognize, clarify, and define the existing problem. This in turn decreases the tension and anxiety associated with the felt need and the fear of unknown. Decreasing tension and anxiety prevents future problems that might arise as a result of repressing or not-resolving significant events. Stress full situations are identified through therapeutic interaction. It is imperative that the patient recognizes and begin to work through feelings connected with events before an illness.

To sum up, in this initial phase, the nurse and the patient meet as strangers, but at the end they are concurrently striving to identify the problem and are becoming more comfortable with one another. Patient becomes more comfortable in the helping environment. The nurse and patient are now ready to logically progress to the next phase i.e. identification.

Identification

In this phase, the patient responds selectively to people who can meet his or her needs. Each patient responds differently in this phase. The patient identifies with those who can help him or her (relatedness) and might actively seek out the nurse or stoically wait until the nurse approaches. The response to the nurse is three fold:
- Participate with and be interdependent with the nurse
- Be autonomous and independent from the nurse, or
- Be passive and dependent on the nurse. (e.g. meal planning of diabetic patient).

Also the nurse permits explorations of feelings to aid the patient in undergoing illness as an experience that reorients feelings and strengthens positive forces in personality and provides needed satisfaction.

In the identification phase, all the time both patient and nurse clarify each other's perceptions and expectations. Past experiences of both the patient and the nurse will influence their expectations during this interpersonal process. Here, the perception and expectation of the patient and nurse are even more complex than in the orientation phase. The patient now responding to the helper selectivity. This requires a more intense therapeutic relationship while working through this phase the patient begins to have feelings of belonging and a capacity for dealing with the problem. These changes begin to decrease feeling of helplessness and hopelessness, creating an optimistic attitude from which inner strength ensues. In this phase, patient is prepared to move to next phase, i.e. exploitation.

Exploitation

During exploitation phase, patient attempts to derive full value from what is offered him through the relationship. New goals to be achieved through personal efforts can be projected and power shifts from the nurse to the patient as the patient delays gratification to achieve the newly formed goals. In this phase, the patient takes advantage of all services available. The degree to which these services are used based upon the needs and interests of the patient. The individual begins to feel as though he or she is integral part of the helping environments and begins to take control of the situation by extracting help from the services offered.

In exploitation, the nurse uses communication tools, such as clarifying, listening, accepting, teaching, and interpreting to offer services to the patient. The patient then takes advantages of the services offered based upon his or her needs and interests. Throughout this phase, the patient works collaboratively with the nurse to meet challenges and work towards maximum health. Thus in this phase, the nurse aids the patient in using services to help solve the problem. Progress is made towards the final stage, i.e., the resolution phase.

Resolution

In this phase, old goals are gradually put aside and new goals adopted. This is a process in which the patient frees himself from identification with the nurse. Because then patients needs have already been met by the collaborative efforts between the patient and nurse. The patient and nurse now need to terminate their therapeutic relationship and dissolve the links between them. Sometimes the nurse and patient have difficulty in dissolving these links. Dependency needs in a therapeutic relationship often continue psychologically after the physiological needs have been met. The patient may feel that it is just not time yet to end the relationship.

During successful resolution, the patient drifts away from identifying with the helping person, the nurse. The patient then becomes independent from the nurse as the nurse becomes independent from the patient. As a result of the process, both the patient and nurse becomes stronger maturing individuals. The patient needs are met and movement can be made toward new goals. Resolution occurs only with the successful completion of the previous phases. The focus of each phase is as follows:

Phases	Focus
1. Orientation	Problem defining phase.
2. Identification	Selection of appropriate professional assistance.
3. Exploitation	Use of professional assistance for problem solving alternatives.
4. Resolution	Termination of the professional relationships.

Nursing Roles

Peplau describes six different nursing rules that emerge in the various phases of the nurse-patient relationships. Different nursing roles are assumed during the various phases. These roles can be broadly described as follows:

Role of the Stranger

The first role is the role of the stranger. Peplau states that because the nurse and patient are strangers to each other, the patient should be treated with ordinary courtesy. In other words, the nurse not prejudge the patient, but accept him as he is. In the initial phase of orientation the nurse and patient meet as two strangers, during this non-personal phase, the nurse should treat the patients as emotionally able, unless evidence indicates otherwise. This coincides with the identification phase.

Role of Resource Person

Resource person is one who provides specific needed information that helps in understanding of a problem or a new situation. In the role of the resource person the nurse provides specific answers to questions, especially health information and interprets to the patient the treatment or medical plan of care. These questions often arise within the context of a larger problem. The nurse determines what type of response is appropriate for constructive learning, either straight forward factual answers, or providing counseling. While the patient and family talking to the nurse, a mutual decision needs to be made regarding what type of professional assistance the patient and family need. The nurse as a resource person may work with them. As an alternative, the nurse might wit the mutual agreement of all parties involved, refer the family to another source, such as psychologist, social worker or psychiatric or specialists, areas of medicine.

Teaching Role

Teacher refers to one who imparts knowledge concerning a need or interest. The teaching role as a combination of all roles, and always proceeds from what the patient knows and develops around his interest in wanting and ability to use information. Peplau separates teaching into two categories, i.e. instructional and experiential.
- Instructional, which consists largely of giving information and is the form explained in educational literature and
- Experiential, which is using the experience of the learner as the basis from which learning products are developed. The products of learning are generalizations and appraisal. The patient makes about his/her experiences. This concept of learning used in the teaching role overlaps with the nurse considers role, because the concept of learning is carried out through psychotherapeutic techniques.

Leadership Role

Leader is one who carries out the process of initiation and maintenance of group goals through interaction. The leadership role involves the democratic process. The nurse helps the patient meet the tasks at hand through a relationship of co-operation and active participation. As technical expert, nurse provides physical care by displaying clinical skills and operating equipments in their care.

Surrogate Role

Surrogate is one who takes place of another. The patient casts the nurse in the surrogate role. The nurse's attitude and behaviours create 'feeling tones' in the patient that reactivate feelings generated in a prior relationship. The nurses functions to assist the patient in recognizing similarities between herself or himself and the person recalled by the patient. She then helps the patient see the differences in her role and that of the recalled person. In this phase, both patient and nurse define areas of dependence independence and finally interdependence.

Counselling Role

Counsellor is one who, through the use of certain skills and attitudes, aids another in recognizing, facing, accepting, and resolving problems that are interfering with other persons, ability to live happily and effectively. Counselling functions in the nurse-patient relationship by the way nurse responds to patient demands. The purpose of interpersonal techniques is to help the patient remember to understand fully what is happening to him/her in the present situation, so that experience can be integrated rather than dissociated from other experience in life.

PARADIGM OF PEPLAU'S THEORY

Nursing's metaparadigm includes four concepts of human being, health, environment and nursing.

Human Being

Peplau defines person in terms of man. Man is an organism that lives in an unstable equilibrium and that strives in its own way to reduce tension generated by needs.

Health

Health is defined as "a word symbol that implies forward movement of personality and other ongoing human processes in the direction of creative, constructive, productive, personal and community living."

Environment

Peplau implicitly defines the environment in terms of "existing forces outside the organism and in the context of culture." From which mores, customs and beliefs are acquired." However, general conditions that are likely to lead to health always include the interpersonal process. Although Peplau does not directly address environment, she does encourage the nurse to consider the patient's culture and mores when the patient adjust to hospital routines.

Nursing

Peplau considers and describes nursing as "a significant therapeutic, interpersonal process." It functions co-operatively with other human processes that make health possible for individuals in communities. "When professional health team offers health services, nurses participate in the organization of conditions that facilitate natural ongoing tendencies in human organisms." Nursing is an educative instrument, a maturing force that aims to promote forward movement of personality in the direction of creative, constructive, productive, personal and community living.

Peplau defines nursing as a "human relationship between an individual who is sick or in need of health services and a nurse especially educated to recognize and to respond to the need for help." The nurse assists the patient in this interpersonal process. Major concepts within the process are nurse, patient, therapeutic relationship goals, human needs, anxiety, tension and frustration.

Interpersonal Process and Nursing Process

Peplau's phases and Interpersonal process can be compared to the nursing process. The nursing process is a deliberate intellectual activity whereby the practice of nursing is approached in an orderly, systematic manner. Both Peplau's phases and the nursing process are sequential and focus on therapeutic interaction. Both stress that the nurse and patient should use problem solving technique collaboratively with the end purpose of meeting the patient's needs. Both emphasize assist the patient to define general complaints more specifically so that the specific patient needs can be identified. Both use observation communication and recording as basic tools for nursing practice.

The similarities between the nursing process and Peplau's interpersonal phases are as follows:

Nursing process	*Peplau's phases*
1. Assessment • Data collection and analysis. • Need not necessarily be a "felt need," may be nurse initiated.	1. Orientation • Nurse and patient come together as strangers. • Meeting initiated by patient who expresses a "felt need" • Work together to recognize, clarify and define facts related to need (Data collection continual)
2. Nursing diagnosis • Summary statement based on nurse analysis.	2. Patient clarifies 'felt need'
3. Planning • Mutually set goals.	3. Identification • Interdependent goal setting. • Patient has feeling and belonging and selectively responds to those who can meet his or her needs. • Patient initiated.

4. Implementation
 - Plans initiated that move toward achievement of mutually set goals.
 - May be accomplished by patient health care professionals, or patient's family.

5. Evaluation
 - Based on mutually established expected behaviours.
 - May lead to termination of relationship or initiation of new plans.

4. Exploitation
Patient actively seeking and drawing on knowledge and expertise of those who can help. Patient-initiated.

5. Resolution
 - Occurs after other phases are successfully completed.
 - Leads to termination of relationships.

Assessment

Professional nursing today has more defined goals and more specialty areas of practice. Nursing has moved from the role of physician helper and toward consumer, advocates. Peplau's orientation phase parallels the beginning of the assessment phase in that both the nurse and patient come together as strangers. This meeting is initiated by the patient, who expresses problems with nurse understood. Conjointly, the nurse and patient begin to work through recognizing, changing, and gathering facts important to this need. Orientation and assessment are not synonymous and must not be confused, collecting data is continuous through the Peplau's phases.

Nursing Diagnosis

The nursing diagnosis evolves the health problem or deficits are identified. The nursing diagnosis is a summary statement of the data collected and analyzed. During the period of orientation, the patient clarifies his first, whole impression of his problem. Whereas the nursing process, the nurse's judgments form the diagnosis from the data collected.

In the planning, the nurse must specifically formulate how the patient is going to achieve mutually set goals. Here, the nurse considers the patients own skills for handling his or her problem. Planning can still be considered to be within the Peplau's identification phase, as the patient selectively responds to people who can meet his or her personal needs. The nurse incorporates the patient's individual strength and weakness into the plan.

As in Peplau's exploitation, implementation phase, the patient is finally reaping benefits from the therapeutic relationship by drawing on the nurses' knowledge and expertise. In both the phases, the individualized plans have already been formed, based on the patient's interests and needs.

Evaluation is the separate step in nursing process if the situation is clear-cut, the problem moves toward termination. Once needs have been met and resolution and termination are the end result. Resolution and evaluation both lead to termination.

Peplau's Work and Characteristics of Theory

Generally, Peplau's work is a theory of Nursing, on the basis characteristics of theory:
1. *Theories can interrelate concepts in such a way as to create a different way of looking at a particular phenomenon.*
The phases of orientation, identification, exploitation and resolution interrelationships create a different a different perspective from which to view the nurse-patient interaction and the transaction of health care. This interaction can apply the

concepts of human being health, society / environment and nursing. For example, in the phase of orientation, there are components of nurse, patient, stranger problem and anxiety.

2. *Theories must be logical in nature (Logical sequence)*

   Peplau's theory provides a logical systematic way of viewing nursing situations. The four progressive phases in the nurse-patient relationship are logical, i.e. orientation, identification, exploitation and resolution. Key concepts are clearly defined.

3. *Theories should be relatively simple yet generalizable. (Simplicity)*

   The phases provide simplicity regarding the natural progressing of the nurse-patient relationship. This simplicity leads to adaptability in any nurse patient interaction thus providing generalizability.

4. *Theories can be the bases for hypotheses that can be tested or for theory to be expanded.*

   Peplau's theory has generated testable hypotheses. Most of the research has centered on the concept of anxiety, not the nurse-patient relationship that is the case of her work. In 1989, Forchuk and Brown created an instrument to assess the Peplau's nurse-client relationships and tested the instrument on 132 clients. Burd SF (1963), Hay (1) (1961) also tested the aspects of Peplau's work.

5. *Theories contribute to and assist in general body of knowledge within the discipline through the research implementation to validate* Peplau's work has contributed greatly to nursing's body of knowledge such as her work on anxiety.

6. *Theories can be used by practitioners to guide and improve their practice.*

   Nursing is still defined as an interpersonal process built upon the progressive nurse patient phases. As Peplau proposed, communication and interviewing skills remain fundamental nursing tools. Also her anxiety continuum is still used for nursing intervention in working with anxious patients except unconscious patients.

7. *Theories must be consistent with other validated theories, laws, and principles but will leave open unanswered questions that need to be investigated.*

   In general, this theory is consistent with current theories and research. Interpersonal theories, including Sullivan's (1947), and Frommes (1947) are foundation on the theory. Peplau's concepts and phases are consistent with other theories such as Maslow's (1954) need theory and Selyed (1956) stress theory. General system theory can also be broadly applied to the four phases of the nurse-patient relationship (von Bertalanffy 1968). For example, the nurse and patient can each define on a system. Both nurse and patient systems interact with each other, processing input throughputs, and outputs so that a specific goal can be met.

   The impact and significance of Peplau's conceptual model can be best described by Suzanne Lego in a through discussion of the history, trends, patterns, and assessment of published research that notes the direction of the one-to-one nurse-patient relationship. she states that ambiguity about the nurse-patient relationship abruptly ended in the literature as a result of Peplau's *Interpersonal Relations in Nursing* (1952). As she would continue to do for the next 22 years, Dr. Peplau pulled together loose, ambiguous data and put them into systematic, scientific terms that could be tested, applied, and integrated into the practice of psychiatric nursing. It also stated that most of the published literature describing the one-to-one nurse-patient relationship is based on theoretical concepts inspired principally by Peplau. And also she makes a significant contribution to the nursing community through the research done to evaluate, validate, and make more precise the Theory of Interpersonal Relations.

As nursing broadens its scope, there appears to be a need for further development of Peplau's theory for use with the healthy patient, group, and community. Further development is also indicated for clients who are unable to use their communication skills effectively. Increased use of Peplau's theory in practice is needed. Continued research is needed to further refine the theory and to build on nursing's knowledge base.

Peplau herself continues to write about the expansion and development needed to test her theory of interpersonal relations as well as to offer explanations of such constructs as concepts, processes, patterns, problems, energy, and anxiety. Further, she suggests that the constructs of focal attention, dissociation, forbidding gestures, and personification deserve additional study.

EVALUATION OF THEORY

- The major focus of Peplau's theory, interpersonal relations between patient and nurse, is easily understood. The theory's basic assumptions and key concepts are defined. Of the assumptions Peplau listed, two are explicit and one is implicit. Peplau sequentially describes her four phases of the interpersonal process. The roles of the nurse and the four psychobiological experiences are clearly indicated. Her logic is based on inductive reasoning. Ideas are taken from observations of the specific and applied to the general. Peplau draws from other disciplines' theories. She is consistent with established theories and principles, such as those of Sullivan, Freud, and Maslow. Peplau deals with the relationships of the interpersonal process, nurse, patient, and psychobiological experiences. Each of these relationships is then developed, within the theory, in an understandable way. Thus Peplau's theory can be described as meeting the evaluative quality of simplicity.
- In meeting the criteria of generality, Peplau states, "While clinical situations are stressed, any nurse can apply principles that are presented in any other interpersonal relationship in any other area of living." The one drawback to the theory's generality is that an interpersonal relationship must exist. The theory is adaptable only to nursing settings where there can be communication between the patient and nurse. Its use is limited in working with the comatose, senile, or newborn patient. In such situations, the nurse-patient relationship is often one-sided. The nurse and patient cannot work together to become more knowledgeable, develop goals, and mature. Even Peplau admits, "Understanding of the meaning of the experience to the patient is required in order for nursing to function as an educative, therapeutic, maturing force." Since Peplau's theory cannot be applied to all patients, the quality of generality is not meet.

- Peplau provides us with a theory based on reality. The relationship between the theory and empirical data allows for validation and verification of the theory by other scientists. The definitions described by Peplau are in a middle range on a connotative-denotative continuum. Peplau operationally defines the four phases of the interpersonal process, the nurse with regard to her roles, and the patient with regard to his state of dependence. According to Duffey and Mullencamp, "Peplau relates behaviour to theory by naming and categorizing, operationalizing definitions of behaviour, thematic abstractions of interaction phenomena, and diagnosis of problems and principles guiding nursing interactions." Peplau's theory can be considered empirically precise. With further research and development, the degree of precision will increase.
- In historical perspective, Peplau is one of the first theorists since Nightingale to present a theory for nursing. Therefore her work can be considered pioneering in the nursing field. "She provided nursing with a meaningful method of self-directed practice at a time when medicine dominated the health care field.

Peplau's work, thoughts, and ideas have touched many nurses, from students to practitioners. Although her book was published in 1952, four decades ago, it continues to provide direction for nursing practice, education, and research. Peplau's work has provided a significant contribution to nursing's knowledge base. The evaluative criteria of derivable consequences are unquestionably met.

Chapter 9

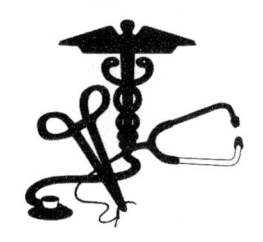

Orlando's Nursing Process Theory

Ida Jean Orlando was born August 12, 1926. In 1947 she received a diploma in nursing form New York Medical College, Flower Fifth Avenue Hospital School of Nursing in New York. She received a BS in Public Health Nursing from St. Johns University in Brooklyn, New York, in 1951, and an MA in Mental Health Consultation from Columbia University Teachers College in New York in 1954. While pursing her education, Orlando worked intermittently, and sometimes concurrently, as a staff nurse in obstetrical, medical, surgical, and emergency nursing services. She also worked as a supervisor in a general hospital. In addition, as an assistant director of nurses, she was responsible for a general hospital's nursing service and for teaching several courses in the hospital's nursing school.

After receiving her master's in 1954, Orlando went to the Yale School of Nursing in New Haven, Connecticut, for 8 years, where she was a research associate and principal project investigator on a federal project grant entitled "Integration of Mental Health Concepts in a Basic Curriculum" until 1958. The project focused on identifying factors influencing the integration of mental health principles in a basic nursing curriculum. Orlando carried out this project by observing and participating in student experiences with patients and medical, nursing, and instructional personnel through out the basic curriculum. She recorded her observations for 3 years and then spent a fourth year analysing the accumulated data. She reported her findings in 1958 in her first book, *The Dynamic Nurse-Patient Relationship; Function, Process and Principles of Professional Nursing Practice*. It was not published until 1961, but since then five foreign language editions have appeared. The formulations in this book provided the foundation for Orlando's nursing theory. During the next 4 years (1958-1961), as an associate professor and the director of the Graduate Program in Mental Health and Psychiatric Nursing, Orlando used her theory as the foundation of the program. She married Robert J. Pelletier and left Yale in 1961.

From 1962 through 1972, Orlando was Clinical Nursing Consultant at McLean

Hospital in Belmont, Massachusetts. From this position she studied the interactions of nurses with patients, other nurses, and other staff members and how these activities affected the process of the nurses help to patients. Orlando convinced the hospital director that a training program for nurses was needed, whereupon McLean Hospital initiated one based on her theory. The nursing service of the hospital was reorganized as a result of this program. Orlando subsequently applied for and received federal funding to evaluate training in the process discipline.

While at McLean Hospital, Orlando published "The Patient's Predicament and Nursing Function" in a 1967 issue of Psychiatric Opinion. In 1972 she reported the 10 years of work at the hospital in her second book, *The Discipline and Teaching of Nursing Process: An Evaluative Study*.

From 1972 to 1981 Orlando lectured, served as a consultant, and conducted about 60 workshops in her theory throughout the United States and Canada. She has served on the Board of the Harvard Community Health Plan in Boston, Massachusetts, from 1972 to 1984 and on the Hospital Committee of the board from 1979 to 1985. She has since served in various capacities such as on the membership, programme, and services committees.

In 1981 Orlando accepted a position as nurse educator for Metropolitan State Hospital in Waltham, Massachusetts. From 1984 until 1987 Orlando held various administrative nursing positions there. In September 1987, she became the assistant director of nursing for education and research as Metropolitan State Hospital.

In 1990 the National League for Nursing reprinted Orlando's 1961 publication. In the preface to the NLN edition Orlando states, "If I had been more courageous in 1961, when this book was first written, I would have proposed it as "nursing process theory" instead of as a "theory of effective nursing practice."

Orlando's nursing theory emphasizes the reciprocal relationship between patient and nurse. Both are affected by what the other says and does. Orlando may have facilitated the development of nurses as logical thinkers rather than conformers to the medical orders of a physician. She was one of the first nursing process and the critical importance of the patient's participation during the nursing process.

EVOLUTION OF THEORY

Orlando says that her search for facts in observing nursing situations influenced her most before the development of her theory and that she derived her theory from the conceptualisation of those facts. Her overall goal was to find an organizing principle for professional nursing, that is, a distinct function. Orlando has made a major contribution to nursing theory and practice. Her conceptualisations fulfil the criteria of theory because she presents interrelated concepts that present a systematic view of nursing phenomena; she specifies what happens during the nursing process and why; she prescribes how nursing phenomena can be controlled; and she explains how the control leads to prediction of outcome. Although nursing writers such as Fitzpatrick and Whall do not believe any current nursing model meets the level of specificity of theory described by Ellis, Orlando's theory has considerable merit in application to practice, education, and research.

The patient is an individual with a need that, if diminishes distress, increases adequacy; or enhances well being. Needs include requirements for implementing physicians' plans or other innate requirements. The nurse acts to meet needs and thus alleviate distress.

Patients with needs behave verbally and nonverbally in a given manner. The nurse reacts to patient behaviour by ascertaining both the meaning of the distress and what would alleviate the distress. Finally the nurse acts to alleviate the distress. Distress can be due to (i) physical limitation, either temporary or permanent; (ii) adverse reactions to the setting such as being misinterpreted or misinterpreting; and (iii) inability to communicate.

Three elements—patient behaviour, nurse reactions, and nurse actions—compose a nursing situation. Patient behaviour and nurse process and involve ongoing interaction with the nurse. Having clearly ascertained the need through assessment, the nurse act s automatically or deliberatively. Automatic actions are those carried out for reasons other than resolving an immediate need, where as deliberative actions seek to meet assessed needs. Automatic actions make problems by creating situational conflict that is evidenced through lack of resolution of needs and cooperation (i.e., distress is not alleviated).

Deliberative action yields solutions to problems and also prevents problems. Once the nursing action occurs, the nurse evaluates patient behaviour to determine if the need met and resultant distress has been alleviated. The overall goal is to meet needs and, in that way, to alleviate distress.

Orlando's Nursing Theory emphasizes the reciprocal relationship between patient and nurse. Both are affected by where the other says and does. She may have facilitated the development of nurses as logical thinkers rather than conformers to the medical orders of a physician. She was one of the first nursing leaders to emphasize the elements of nursing process and critical importance of the patient's participation during the nursing process. She describes a nursing process based on the interaction between a patient and nurse. Her nursing process discipline was developed through research and presented in two books titled as:

1. The dynamic nurse patient relationship: Functions, process and principles (1961, 1990).
2. The discipline and teaching of nursing process (1972).

Orlando's Educational background and the work lead to her publications provide insight into the contents of her theory. Her advanced nursing preparation and area of teaching responsibility and practice were in mental health and psychiatric nursing. The focus of her work is interactions.

CONCEPTS USED BY ORLANDO

Orlando describes her model as revolving around five major interrelated concepts:
1. The function of professional nursing.
2. The presenting behaviour or the client.
3. The immediate reactions or internal response of the nurse.
4. The nursing process discipline and
5. Improvement.

The details of concepts as given below:

Professional Function

Nurses often work with other professionals and are subject to the authority of the organization that employs them. It is inevitable, therefore, that at time, and conflicts will arise between the actions appropriate to the nurse's profession and those required by the job. Non-professional action can prevent the nurse from carrying out her professional function, and this can lead to inadequate potentate. A well-defined function of the profession can help to prevent and resolve the conflict. The purpose of nursing is supply the help a patient requires in order for his needs to be met. Need is situation ally defined as a requirement of the patient which, if supplied, relieves or diminishes his immediate distress or improves his immediate sense of adequacy or well being. Whatever help the patient may require for his needs to be met are the professional nurse's responsibility. Nurses must be constantly aware that their "activity professional only when it deliberately achieves the purpose of helping the patient.

Patient Behaviour

Orlando stresses in her first principle that the "presenting behaviour of the patient, regardless of the from in which it appears, may represent plea for help" patient behaviour may be very or non-verbal. Inconsistently between these two types of behaviour may be the factor that alerts the nurse that the patient needs help. *Verbal behaviour* encompasses all the patients' use of language. It may take the form of complaints, requests, questions, refusals, demands, and comments or statements. *Non-verbal behaviour* includes physiological manifestations such as heart rate, perspirations, oedema, and urinations and motor activity such as smiling, walking, and avoiding eye contacts. Non-verbal behaviour may also be vocal including such actions, as sobbing laughing, shouting and sighing. The patient behaviour reflects distress when a patient experiences a need that he cannot resolve a sense of helpless of helplessness occurs.

Some categories of patient distress which includes physical limitations, adverse reactions to the setting and experience which prevent the setting and experience which prevent the patient from communicating his needs. For example, feelings of helplessness caused by physical limitations that may result from incomplete developments, temporary or permanent disability or restrictions of the environment real or imagined.

Ineffective patient behaviour 'prevents the nurse from carrying out her concerns for the patient's care or from maintaining a satisfactory relationship to patient." Resolution of ineffective patient behaviour deserves high priority. For this behaviour, usually becomes worse over time if the need for help that it expresses remain unsolved. The nurse's reactions and actions are designed to resolve ineffectual patient behaviours as well as to meet the immediate need.

Nurse's Reaction

Nurse's reaction is comprised of three sequential parts. First, the nurse perceives the behaviour through any of her senses. Second, the perception leads to automatic thought. Finally the thought produces an automatic feeling. For example, the nurse sees a patient grimace, thinks he is in pain and feels concern. The nurse then shares her reactions with the patient to ascertain that she has corrected identified the need for help and identity the nursing antiphon appropriate to resolve it. Orlando offers a principle to guide the nurse in her reaction to patient behaviour, i.e. the nurse does not assume any aspect of her reaction to the patient is correct, helpful, or appropriate until she checks the validity of it in exploration with the patient. *Perception, Thought,* and *Feeling* occur automatically and almost simultaneously. Therefore the nurse must learn to identify each part of her action this helps her to analyze the reaction and for the purpose of helping to the patient.

Orlando (1972) offers a diagram depicting open sharing of the nurse reaction versus keeping the reaction secret the nurse's action that results from the reaction becomes a behaviour which stimulates a reaction by the patient. Only openness in sheering the nurse's reaction assures that the patient's needs will be effectively resolved. This sharing in the manner prescribed, differentiates professional nursing practice from automatic personal response (Figs. 9.1 and 9.2).

Nurse's Action

Orlando includes "only what she (the nurse) says or does with or for the benefit of the patient" as professional nursing actions. The nurse must be certain that her reaction is appropriate to meet the patient's need for help. Orlando's principle for guiding Nursing action states. I .The nurse initiates a process of exploration to ascertain how the patient is affected by what she says or does. The near can act in two ways: *automatic* or *deliberative actions* are those nursing actions decided upon farther ascertaining a need and then meeting this need. Carrying out the physician order is the purpose of the nursing action. For example, giving sedation to patient is the automatic action. Only deliberative action fulfills the nurse's professional function. The feeling list identifies the criteria for *deliberative actions*:

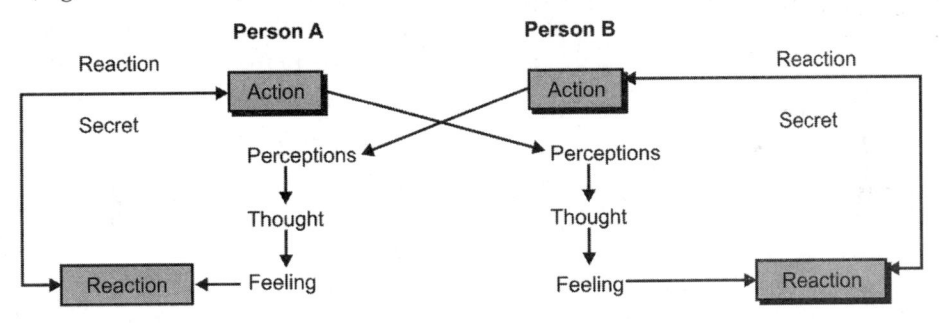

Figure 9.1: The action process in a person-to-person contact functioning in secret. The perception, thought, and feelings of individual are now directly available to the perceptions of the other through the observable action

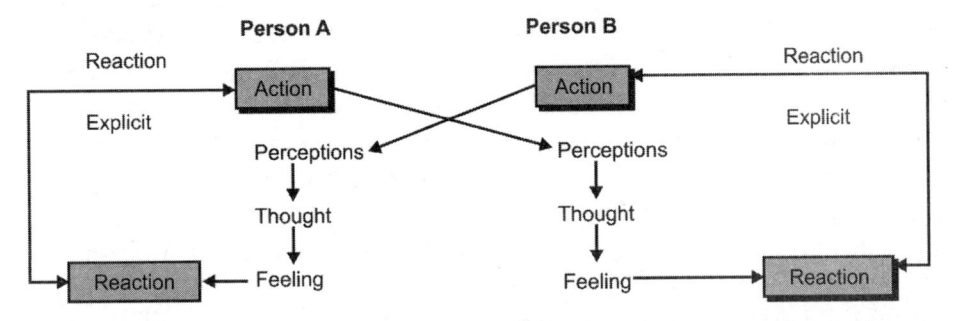

Figure 9.2: The action process in a person-to-person contact functioning by open disclosure. The perceptions, thoughts, feelings, of each individual are directly available to the perception of other individual through the observable action

1. Deliberative actions results from the correct identification of patient need by validation of the nurses reactions to patient behaviour.
2. The nurse explores the meaning of the action with the patient and its relevance to meeting his need.
3. The nurse validates the actions effectiveness immediately after completing it.
4. The nurse is free to stimuli unrelated to the patient's need when she acts.

Automatic action fails to meet this criterion. They are most lindy to be done by nurses permanently concerned with carrying out orders of physicians, routine patient car, or general principles of protecting health, etc. The purpose of nursing will be fulfilled when the criteria of deliberate action a followed and acted accordingly.

Improvement: Means to grow better to turn to profit to use of advantage.

PARADIGM OF ORLANDO

Orlando includes material specific to the major concepts like human, health, and nursing, but not included environment.

Human Being

She assumes that persons behave verbally non-verbally relationship. For her, human in need are the focus of nursing practice.

Health

She does not define health but assumes that freedom from mental or physical discomfort, feelings; of adequacy and well-being contribute to health. For example, the sense of helplessness replaces the concept of health of illness as the initiator of a need for nursing.

Nursing

Orlando assumed about nursing is that it should be distinct profession that functions autonomously. Although nursing has been historically aligned with medicine, and continues to have relationship with medicine, nursing and the practice of medicine are independent in its concern of an individual's need for help as carried it in an interactive situation and in a disciplined manner that requires proper training\education in the nursing.

Nursing Process and Orlando Process Discipline

Orlando's nursing process discipline may be compared with the present nursing process. Certain over all characteristics are similar in both processes. For example, both are interpersonal in nature and require interactions between patient and nurse. The patient is assessed for in put throughout the process. Both processes also view the patient on a total person. She does not use the term holistic but effectively described a holistic approach. Both process and used as method to provide nursing care and as a means to evaluate their care. Finally both are deliberate intellectual processes. The following figure shows comparison of nursing process and Orlando process. Both processes also view the patient on a total person. She does not use the term holistic but effectively describes a holistic approach. Both process and used as a method to provide nursing care and as a means to evaluate their care. Finally both are deliberate intellectual processes. Figure 9.3 shows comparison of *Nursing process* and *Orlando process*.

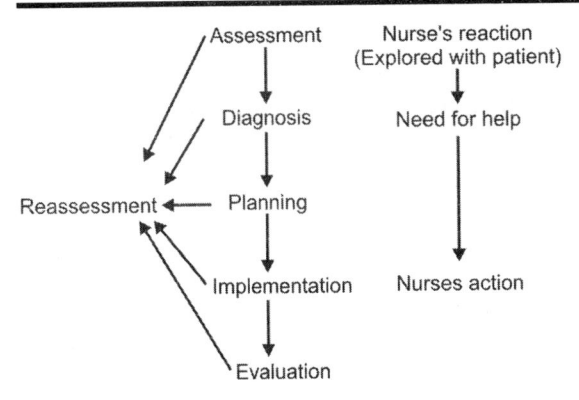

Figure 9.3: Nursing process and Orlando process comparison

The Assessment Phase

The assessment phase of nursing process corresponds to the sharing of nurse reaction to the patient's behaviour in Orlando's nursing process discipline. Patient behaviour initiates the assessment. Direct data are comprised of any perception; thought or feeling the nurse has from her own experience of the patient's behaviour at any or several moments in time. Indirect data comes from sources that the patient such as recorders other health team members, or patient's significant other the sharing of the nurses a reactions in Orlando's process discipline has components similar to the analysis in the nursing process. Although Nurses' action is automatic, her awareness of it and the ways the shares it is deliver intellectual activity.

Nursing Diagnosis

Nursing diagnosis the product of the analysis in the nursing process is the Nursing diagnosis. Exploration of the Nurse's reaction with the patient in the Orlando's process discipline leads to identification of his need for help.

- *The planning phase:* Of the nursing process involves writing goals and objectives and deciding upon appropriate nursing actions. This corresponds to the nurse's action phase of the Orlando's process discipline. Her goal is always relief of the patient's need for help; the objective relates to the improvement in the patient's need for help, the objective relates to the improvement in the patient's behaviour. Both the processes require patient participation in determining the appropriate action.
- *Implementation:* Involves the final selection and carrying out of the planned actions and is also part of the nurse's action phase of Orlando's process of discipline,. Both processes mandate that the action be appropriate for the patient's as a unique individual. The nursing process expects the nose to consider all possible effects of the action upon the patient; Orlando's process discipline is concerned only with the effectiveness of the action in resolving the immediate need for help.
- *Evaluation:* It is inherent in Orlando's action phase of her process Discipline. For an action to be deliberative, the nurse much evaluates its effectiveness when it is completed. Evaluation in both processes is based on objective criteria.

Both the nursing process and Orlando's prices of discipline are described as series of sequential steps.

Characteristics of Theory and Orlando's Work

1. Nursing is the focus of Orlando's work. Her theory views nursing as a unique discipline that interacts with an individual in an immediate situation to relieve a sense

of helplessness. She does relate concepts into new and meaningful whole.

2. Orlando's work does provide a reasonable and sequential process for nursing. Patient behaviour initiates the nurse reaction. Exploration of this reaction with the patient leads to identification of a need of and an action to resolve this need. The nurse must reach and in a carefully prescribed manner to certain she meets her goal of helping the patient. She must evaluate her actins to be certain of its effectiveness. Thus Orlando provides logical order.

3. Orlando's theory is simply in nature. It does generalize will be all nursing practice. The theory remains simply by revolving around the nurse-patient interactions, the basic of nursing. This simplicity makes the theory generalizable. This basic unit applicable regardless of the setting of nursing care of the type of patient receiving care.

4. Orlando did derive hypotheses from her theory and tested them. Although her initial study was observation, she tested her ideas in variety of setting. In her second study, she developed criteria for the nurse's reaction that were specific enough for the development of hypothesis and statistical testing.

5. In testing her theory, Orlando (1972) added to the general body of nursing knowledge.

6. Orlando has been quite successful in developing a theory useful to practice. Nurses can easily use her principles and process discipline in their interactions with patients and fellow workers.

7. Orlando's theory does not conflict with other validated theories. If it is viewed in the somewhat limited sense of a nurse-patient interaction theory. It is most consistent with interaction theory, but general system theory related to it with difficulty.

EVALUATION OF THEORY

- Orlando's first book, *The Dynamic Nurse Patient Relationship*, presented concepts clearly. The second book, *The Discipline and Teaching of Nursing Process*, redefined and renamed *deliberative nursing process as nursing process discipline*. Orlando's writing style involves defining concepts minimally at first and then developing them throughout the book. Because of the evolution of the theory the reader must be familiar with both books to evaluate her theory thoroughly.

- As Orlando deals with relatively few concepts and their relationships with each other, her theory would be considered simple. Her theory may also be viewed as simplistic because she is able to make some predictive statements as opposed to just description and explanation. The simplicity of Orlando's theory has benefited research application.

Walker and Avant use Orlando as an example of grand nursing theory. They state that grand nursing theories have provided a global perspective, but by virtue of their generality and abstractness, most grand theories are untestable in their current form. Although Orlando's theory has undergone testing, its global perspective would support labelling this work as grand theories. Orlando's theory has also been described as a practice theory. Practice theories provide a framework to specify when the guidelines

should be applied, describe the means to be used, and specify the goals to be used for outcome evaluation.
- Orlando discussed and illustrated nurse patient contacts in which the patient is conscious, able to communicate, and in need of help. Although she did not focus on unconscious patients and groups, application of her theory to groups or unconscious patients is feasible. Actually, any other person could make use of the process discipline if educated properly. Therefore, although Orlando's theory focuses on a limited number of situations, it could be adapted to other nursing of situations, it could be adapted to other nursing situations and other professional fields.
- Two thirds of Orlando's second book is a report of a research project designed to test the validity of her nursing formulations. A training programme based on her formulations had been in progress for 3 years before the project began. Nurses were trained to use the process discipline in nurse-patient contacts. Those nurses who became clinical nursing supervisors were trained to use the process discipline in their supervisory and other contacts as well. The following is a brief description of the research methodology.
- The purpose of the project was to evaluate the effectiveness of the process discipline in the nurse's contacts at work and the effectiveness of the training programme. But these evaluation could not take place before hypothetical measures for the process discipline were identified. A discipline variable was defined. Effectiveness of a *helpful outcome*, as judged by two reliable outcome coders. The outcome coders compared the beginning behaviour of the subject with the behaviour at the end of the record. Testing the relationship of the process discipline (in use) with the presence or absence of a helpful outcome in patient, staff, and supervisee contacts was also done. Evaluation of the training programme was done by testing whether nurses increased their use of the process discipline after being trained.

Chapter 10

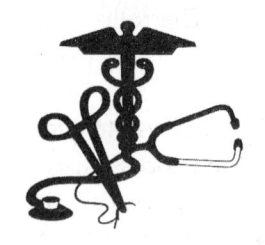

Wiedenbach's Helping Art of Clinical Nursing

Ernestine Wiedenbach's interest in nursing began with her childhood experiences with nurses. She greatly admired the private duty nurse who cared for her ailing grandmother and later enjoyed hearing accounts of nurses' roles in the hospital experiences of a young intern her sister was dating. Captivated by the role of the nurse, Wiedenbach enrolled in the Johns Hopkins Hospital School of Nursing after graduating from Wellesley College with a bachelor's degree in liberal arts. After completing her study at Johns Hopkins, she held a variety of positions in hospitals and public health nursing agencies in New York. She also continued her education by attending evening classes at Teachers College, Columbia University, from which she received a master's degree and a Certificate in Public Health Nursing. During this period Hazel Corbin, director of the Maternity Center Association of New York, persuaded Wiedenbach to enrol in the Association's School for Nurse-Midwives. After completing the program, Wiedenbach practiced as a nurse midwife in the home delivery service of the Maternity Center Association.

In addition to her practice, she also developed her academic career. She taught an evening course in advanced maternity nursing at Teachers College, wrote several articles for professional publications, and remained active in professional nursing organizations. Then in 1952 she moved from New York to Connecticut, where she was subsequently appointed to the faculty of the Yale University School of Nursing. She wrote *Family-Centered Maternity Nursing*, a text on clinical nursing which was published in 1958.

It was out of this vast practical experience and education that she developed her model, and after a long career at Yale, she retired and moved to Florida.

EVOLUTION OF THEORY

At Yale, Wiedenbach's theory development benefited from her contact with other faculty members. Ida Orlando Pelletier stimulated Wiedenbach's understanding of the use of self and the effect a nurse's thoughts and feelings has on the outcome of her actions. In addition, Patricia James and William Dickoff, who taught a course in nursing theory, reviewed the manuscript for Wiedenbach's book, *Clinical Nursing; A Helping Art*. In it they identified elements of a prescriptive theory, which Wiedenbach developed more fully in *Meeting the Realities in Clinical Teaching*.

The patient is an individual under treatment or care who experiences needs. Needs are requirements for maintenance or stability in a situation that may be perceived by the individual as a requirement for help and may be met by the person or others. Also, people may have needs and not seek help or may help themselves without recognizing a need. Needs for help are defined as "measures or actions required and desired, which potentially restore or extend ability to cope with situational demands." Nursing is concerned with patient's needs for help. What the nurse does and how she or he does it compose clinical nursing. Clinical has four components: (i) philosophy, (ii) purpose, (iii) practice, and (iv) art.

Philosophy is a personal stance of the nurse that embodies attitudes towards reality, and purpose is the overall goal. The purpose of clinical nursing is "to facilitate efforts of individuals to overcome obstacles which interfere with abilities to respond capably to demands made by the condition, environment, situations or time." This purpose is embodiment of meeting needs for help, which implies goal-directed, deliberate, patient-centred practice actions that require (i) knowledge (factual speculative and practical), (ii) judgement, and (iii) skills (procedural and communication). Practice includes four components; (i) identification of the perceived need for help, (ii) ministration of help need (iii) validation that help given was the help needed, and (iv) coordination of help and resources for help (i.e., reporting consulting and conferring). The art of clinical nursing requires individualised interpretation of behaviour in meeting needs for help.

The helping process is triggered by patient behaviour that the nurse perceives and interprets. In interpreting behaviour the nurse compares the perception to an expectation or hope. Nursing actions may be rational, reactionary, and deliberative. A rational response by the nurse is based on the immediate perception without going beyond to explore hidden meaning. A reactionary response is taken in reaction to strong feelings. Deliberative actions—the desirable mode—intelligibly, fulfil nursing's purpose. Identification of needs, for help involves (i) observing inconsistencies, acquiring information about how patients mean the cue given, or determining the basis for an observed inconsistency; (ii) determining the cause of the discomfort or need for help; and; (iii) determining whether the needs for help can be met by the patient or whether assistance required. Once needs for help are identified, ministration and validation that help was given follow.

The practice of clinical nursing is bounded by professional, local, legal, and personal constraints. Nursing administration, nursing education, nursing organizations, and nursing research support clinical nursing practice. The clinical goal is to meet for help, integrating the practice and process of nursing. Greater professional goals include conservation of life and promotion of health.

Wiedenbach started her career in the 1920s and first published *Family-centred Maternity Nursing* (1958). It is of interest that in this book, she recommended that babies be in hospital rooms with their mothers rather than in a central Nursing. In 1964, she wrote *Clinical Nursing–A Helping Art* in which she described her ideas about nursing art concept and philosophy" derived from her experience in the field of nursing. In collaboration with Dickoff and James, she presented the symposium and co-authored "Theory in a practice discipline"(1968). In 1970 she defined the essential of her prescriptive theory in "Nurse's Wisdom in Nursing theory."

Nursing is nurturing and caring for some one in a motherly fashion. That care is given in the immediate present and can be given by any caring person (1964). Nursing is a helping service that is rendered with compassive skill and understanding to those in need of care, counsels and confidence is the area of health (1977). Nursing wisdom is acquired through meaningful experience. Sensitivity alerts the nurse to an awareness of inconsistencies in one situation that might signify a problem. It is a key factor in assisting the nurses to identify the patient's need for help. The nurse's belief and values regarding reference for the gift of life, the worth of the individual and the aspirations of each human being determine the quality of the nursing care. The nurse's purposes in nursing represents a professional commitment

Concepts Used by Wiedenbach

Patients

Wiedenbach defines a patient as "any individual who is receiving help of some kind, be its care, instruction or advice, from a member of the health profession or from a worker in the field of health. Thus to be patient, one does not necessarily have to be sick. Someone receiving preventive health care teaching would qualify as a patient.

Need for Help

She believed every individual experience needs as a normal part of living. A need is anything that the individual may require "to maintain or sustain himself comfortably or capably in his situation. A need for help is any measure or action required and desired by the individual and which has potential for restoring or extending his ability to cope with the demands implicit in his situations. It is crucial to the nursing profession that a need-for-help be based on the individual perception of his own situation. If one does not perceive a need as a need for help, one may not take action to relieve or resolve it.

Nurse

The nurse is a functioning human being. As such, she, not only acts, but she thinks and feels as well. The thoughts she thinks and the feelings she feels as she gives about her nursing are important. They are intimately involved not only in what she does, but also in how she does it. They underlie every action she takes, be it the form of a spoken work, a written communication, a gesture, or a deed of any kind. For the nurse when action is directed toward achievement of a specific purpose, thoughts and feelings have a disciplined role.

Purpose

Purpose that which the nurse wants to accomplish, what she does, is the overall goal toward which she is striving, and so is constant. It is her reason for being and for doing, it is the why of clinical nursing and transcends the immediate intent of her assignment or tasks by specifically directing her activities toward the 'good' of her patient.

Philosophy

Philosophy is an attitude toward life and reality that involves from each nurse's beliefs and code of conduct, motivates nurses to act, guides her thinking about what she is to do and influence her decisions. It seems from both her culture and subculture, and is an integral part of her. It is personal in character, unique to each nurse, and expressed in her way of nursing. Philosophy underlies purpose, and purpose reflects philosophy.

Practice

Over action, directed by disciplined thoughts and feelings toward meeting the patient's need-for-help constitutes the practice of clinical nursing. It is goal-directed, deliberately carried out and patient-centered.

Knowledge, judgement and skills are three aspects necessary for effective practice. Identification, ministration and validation are three components of practice directly related to the patient's care. Co-ordination of resources is indirectly related to it.

Knowledge

Knowledge encompasses all that has been perceived and grasped by the human mind; its scope and range are infinite. Knowledge may be acquired by the nurse, apart from judgement and skills, in a so-called ivory-tower setting. When acquired in this way, it has potentially for use in directing, reaching, coordinating and planning care of the patient, but is not sufficient to meet his need-for-help. To be effective in meeting this need, such knowledge must be supplemented by opportunity for the nurse to function in a nurse-patient relationship with responsibility to exercise judgement and to implement skills for the benefit of the patient. Knowledge may be factual, speculative or practical.

Factual Knowledge

"Factual knowledge is something that may be accepted as existing or as being true."

Speculative Knowledge

Speculative knowledge on the other hand, encompasses theories, general principles offered to explain phenomena, beliefs or concepts, and the content of such special subject areas as the natural sciences, the social sciences and the humanities.

Practical Knowledge

"Practical knowledge is knowing how to apply factual or speculative knowledge to the situation at hand."

Judgement

Judgement represents the nurse's potentiality for making sound decisions, judgement flows out of a cognitive process, which involves weighing facts, both general and particular– against personal values derived from ideals, principles and convictions. It also involves differentiating facts from assumptions, and relating them to cause and effect. Judgement is personal in character, it will be exercised by the nurse according to how clearly she envisions the purpose to be served, how available relevant knowledge is to her at the time, and how she reacts to prevailing circumstances such as time, setting, and individuals. Decisions resulting from the exercise of judgement will be sound or unsound according to whether or not the nurse has disciplined the functioning of her emotions and of her mind. Uncontrollable emotions can blot out knowledge as well as purpose. Unfounded assumptions can distort facts. Although whatever decision the nurse may make represents her best judgement at the moment of making it, the broader her knowledge and the more available it is to her, and the greater her clarity of purpose, the firmer will be the foundation on which her decisions rest.

Skills

Skills represent the nurse's potentially for achieving desired results. Skills comprise numerous and varied acts, characterized by harmony of movement, expression and intent, by precision, and by adroit use of self. These acts are always carried out with deliberation to achieve a specific purpose and are not goals in themselves. Deliberation and purpose, therefore, differentiate skills from nurses' actions, which, although they may be carried out with proficiency, are performed with the execution of the act as the end to be attained rather than the means by which it is reached. Skills may be classified as procedural or communication.

Procedural Skills

"Procedural skills are potentialities for implementing procedures that the nurse may need to initiate and carry out in order to identify and meet her patient's need-for-help."

Communication Skills

"Communication skills are capacities for expression of thoughts and feelings that the nurse desires to convey to her patient and to others associated with his care. Both verbal and nonverbal expression may be used, singly or together, to deliver a message or to elicit a particular response.

Identification

Identification involves individualization of the patient, his experiences, and recognition of the patient's perception of his condition.

Activities in identification are directed toward ascertaining: (i) whether the patient has a need; (ii) whether he recognizes that he has a need; (iii) what is interfering with his ability to meet his need; and (iv) whether the need represents a need-for-help, in other words, a need that the patient is unable to met himself.

Ministration

Ministration is providing the needed help. It requires the identification of the need-for-help, the selection of a helping measure appropriate to that need, and the acceptability of the help to the patient.

Validation

Validation is evidence that the patient's functional ability was restored as a result of the help given.

Coordination

While striving for unity and continuity, the nurse coordinates all services provided to the patient so care will not be fragmented. Reporting, consulting and conferring are functional elements of coordination.

Reporting

Reporting is the act of presenting information or oral form and is important in keeping others informed not the patient's health and social history, but also about his current condition, progress, care and plan of care.

Consulting

Consulting, the act of seeking information or of asking advice, is a means of gaining, from others, an opinion or suggestion that may help the nurse to broaden her understanding before deciding on a course of actions.

Conferring

"Conferring, the act of exchanging and comparing ideas, is most often initiated to reviews the patient's response to the care he has so far received and to plan his future care.

Art

Art is the application of knowledge and skill to bring about desired results. Art is individualized action. Nursing art, then, is carried out by the nurse in a one-to-one relationship with the patient and constitutes the nurse's conscious responses to specifics in the patient's immediate situation. The art of clinical nursing is directed toward achievement of four main goals: (i) understanding of the patient, and his condition, situation and need; (ii) enhancement of the patient's capability; (iii) improvement of his condition or situation within the framework of the medical plan for his care; and (iv) prevention of the recurrence of his problem or development of a new one which may cause anxiety, disability or distress. Nursing art involves three initial operations, stimulus, preconception, and interpretation. The nurse reacts based on those operations. Her actions may be rational, reactionary, or deliberative.

Stimulus

The helping process is triggered by a stimulus that is the patient's presenting behaviour.

Preconception

Preconception is an expectation of what the patient may be like. The preconception is based on knowledge gained from a great variety of sources including the patient's chart, reports from other nurses, doctors or family members, what the nurse has read or heard of patients in similar condition, her own experiences with patients in similar condition, and, finally, her recollection of previous contacts with the patient.

Interpretation

Interpretation is comparison of perception with expectation or hope. Perception is an interpretation of the stimulus and may misinterpret the patient's behaviour.

Rational Action

Rational action is an over act taken in response solely or mainly to the doer's immediate perception, of another's action—verbal or nonverbal–or situation. In a nurse-patient relationship, the nurse's action would be called rational if she responds in a way guided by only her immediate perception of the patient's behaviour—what he says, what he does, or how he appears.

Reactionary Action

Reactionary action, in contrast with rational action, is an overt act taken spontaneously in response to strong feelings the doer experiences when he compares his perception of behaviour. In a nurse-patient relationship, the nurse's action is reactionary if it is taken solely or mainly in responses to her reaction to the feelings aroused in her comparing what she perceived as the patient's behaviour with what she hoped for or expected.

Deliberative Action

Deliberative action is in contract with both rational action and reactionary action. A deliberative action is an overt act which, although not failing to take account of the doer's immediate perceptions and feeling-reactions is, nonetheless, not based solely on these perceptions or feelings. Rather, deliberative action is interaction directed toward fulfilment of an explicit purpose and carried out with judgment and understanding of how the other means the behaviour which he is manifesting either verbally of non-verbally. In a nurse-patient relationship, the nurse's action is deliberative if her overt action is based on the application–in the fulfilment of her nursing purpose–of principles of helping to gain understanding of how the patient means the behaviour he is manifesting.

Wiedenbach concluded her consideration of the types of action by saying "My thesis is that nursing art is not comprised of rational nor reactionary actions but rather of deliberative action.

Framework of Clinical Nursing

Limits supports and research provide a broad framework in which clinical nursing functions. Limits or boundaries, in a professional service are the individual guidelines to follow in practicing that profession. Professional limits are set the profession's code: legal limits are those found in sate laws and licensing requirements local limits are set by the hospital, agency, or individual the nurse herself.

Supportive facilities for the practicing nurse are nursing administration, nursing education, and nursing organisation. Although these are rarely found at the patient's bedside or in the one-to-one relationship between the nurse and patient, they are nevertheless important to the nurse by maintaining standards of quality of nursing care for the profusion.

Wiedenbach recognised that nursing research had not received a great deal of emphasis from the profession in the past, although more nursing research was beginning to occur. She acknowledged that such activity was essential to the growth of nursing and might even "prove to be crucial to the conservation of life and the promotion of health."

Wiedenbach has following assumptions:

Nurses describe to an explicit philosophy. Basic to this philosophy of nursing are "(i) reverence for the gift of life; (ii) respect for the dignity, worth, autonomy and individuality of each human being; (iii) Resolution to act dynamically in relation to one's beliefs. "The rationale for nursing is stated in" the reason she has come into being is that there is a patient who needs her help. Wiedenbach identifies five essential attributes of a professional person. These characteristics are:

1. Clarity of purpose.
2. Mastery of skill and knowledge essential for fulfilling the purpose.
3. Ability to establish and sustain purposeful working relationships with them, both

professional and nonprofessional individuals.
4. Interest in advancing knowledge in the area of interest and in creating new knowledge.
5. Dedication to furthering the goal of mankind rather than to self-aggrandisement.

Nurses describe to an explicit philosophy. Basic to this philosophy of nursing are:
1. Reverence for the fit life.
2. Respect for the dignity, worth, autonomy, and individuality of each human being
3. Resolution to act dynamically in relations to one's belief. Wiedenbach (1964) stated that the characteristics of a professional person that are essential for the professional nurse includes the following:
   - *Clarity* of purpose.
   - *Mastery* of skills and knowledge essential for fulfilling the purpose.
   - *Ability* to establish and sustain purposeful working in relationships with others, both professional and non-professional.
   - *Interest* in advancing knowledge in the area of interest and in creating new knowledge.
   - *Dedication* to furthering the good of mankind rather than to self-agreement.

The practice of nursing comprises a wide variety of services each directed toward the attainment of one of its three components.
1. Identification of the patient's need-for-help.
2. Ministration of the help needed; and
3. Validation that help provided was indeed helpful to the patient.

Wiedenbach presents three principles in identification of the patient's need-for-help, the principles and their brief description are as follows:

1. The principles of inconsistency/consistency refers to the assessments of the patient to determine some action, word or appearance that is different from that expected, that is, something out of the ordinary for this patient. It is important for the nurse to observe the patient astutely and then critically analyse her observations.
2. The principle of purposeful perseverance is based on the nurse's sincere desire to help the patient. The nurse needs to strive to continue her helping efforts in spite of difficulties she encounters while seeking to use her resources and capabilities effectively.
3. The principle of self-extension recognizes that each nurse has limitations that are both personal and situational. It is important that she recognizes when these limitations arte reached and that she seeks help from others

PRESCRIPTIVE THEORY

Theory may be described as a system of conceptualization invented to some purpose. This prescription theory is a situation-producing, which may be described as one that conceptualizes both a desired situation and the prescription by which it is to be brought about. Thus, this theory directs action toward an explicit goal.

Wiedenbach's (1969) prescription theory (Fig. 10.1) is made up of three factors or concepts as follows:
1. The central purpose which the practitioner recognizes as essential to the particular discipline.

2. The prescription for the fulfilment of the central purpose.
3. The realities in the immediate situation that influence the fulfilment of the central purpose.

The diagrammatic representation of prescriptive theory is as follows:

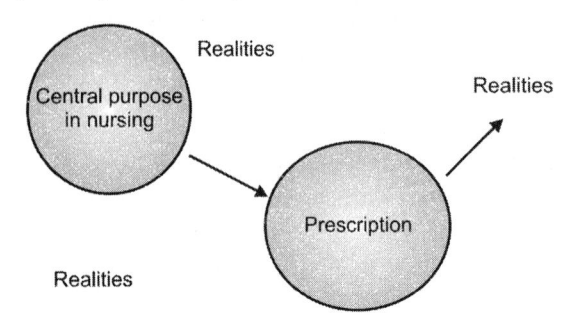

Figure 10.1: Prescriptive theory (Wiedenbach)

Central Purpose

The nurses' central purpose defines that quality of health she desires to effect or sustain in her patients and specifies what she recognizes to be her special responsibility in caring for the patient. This central purpose or commitment is based on individual nurses philosophy. Wiedenbach identifies three essential components for a nursing philosophy.
   i. A reverence for the gift of life.
   ii. A respect for dignity, worth, autonomy and individuality of each human being.
   iii. A resolution to act dynamically in relation to one's belief.

She emphasized human beings in her work, formulating following beliefs about the individual.
- Each human being is endowed with unique potential to develop within himself/themselves the resources that enable them to maintain and sustain themselves.
- Human beings are basically strived toward self-direction and relative independence, and desire not only to make the best use of their capabilities and potentialities but also to fulfil their responsibilities.
- Human beings need stimulation in order to make the best use of their capabilities and realize their self-worth.
- Whatever individuals do represent their best judgement at the moment of doing it.
- Self-awareness and self-acceptance are essential to the individual's sense of integrity and self-worth.

This central purpose is a concept the nurse has thought through one she has put into words, believes in, and accepts as standard against which to measure the value of her action to the patient. It is based on her philosophy and suggests the nurse's reason for being, the mission she believes is here to accomplish.

Prescription

Once the nurse identified her own philosophy and recognizes that the patient has autonomy and individuality, she can work with the individual to develop a prescription or plan of his or her care.

A prescription is directive to a directive to activity which specifies both the *nature of the action* that will most likely lead to fulfilment of the nurse's central purpose and the *thinking* process that determines it. A prescription may indicate the broad general action appropriate to implementation of the basic concept as well as suggest the kind of behaviour needed to carry out these actions in accordance with the central purpose. These actions may be voluntary or involuntary.

Voluntary action is an intended response, whereas involuntary action is an unintended response.

A prescription is a directive to at least three kinds of voluntary actions.
   i. Mutually understood and agreed upon action (recipient and practitioner).
   ii. Recipient-directed action and (ways in which to be carried out).
   iii. Practitioner-directed actions (practitioner carried action).

Realities

When the nurse has determined her central purpose and has developed the prescription, she must consider the *realities* of the situation in which she is to provide nursing care. Realities consists of all factors—physical, physiological, psychological, emotional and spiritual that are at a play in a situation in which nursing actions occur at a given moment. Wiedenbach defines five realities as: the *agent*, the *recipient*, the *goal*, the means and the framework.

Agent

The agent who is the practising nurse or her delegate is characterized by the personal attributes, capacities, capabilities, and most importantly commitment and competencies in nursing. as the agent the nurse is the propelling force that moves her practice towards its goal. In the course of goal directed movement, she may engage in innumerable acts called forth by the encounter with actual or discrepant factors and situations within the realities of which she herself (nurse) is a part. The agent or nurse has the following four basic responsibilities:

1. To reconcile her assumptions about the realities with her central purpose.
2. To specify the objectives of her practice in terms of behavioural outcomes that are realistically attainable.
3. To practice nursing in accordance with her objectives.
4. To engage in related activities which contribute to her self-realization and to the improvement of nursing practice.

Recipient

1967: The recipient, the patient is characterized by personal attributes, problems, capacities, aspirations and most important the ability to cope with the concerns or problems being experienced. The patient is the recipient of the nurse's actions or the one on whose behalf the action is taken.

1970: The patient is vulnerable, depending on others for help and risk in losing individuality, dignity worth and autonomy.

Goal

The goal is the desired outcome the nurse wishes to achieve. The goal is the end result to be attained by the nursing action. The stipulation of an activity's goal gives focus to the nurse's action and implies her reason for taking it.

Mean

The means comprise the activities and devices through which the practitioner is enabled to attain her goal. The means include skills, techniques, procedures, and devices that may be used to facilitate nursing practice. The nurse's way of giving treatment of expressing concerns of using the means available is individual and is determined by her central purpose and the prescription.

Framework

The framework consists of human, environmental, professional and organizational facilities that not only make up the context within which nursing is practiced but also constitute its currently existing limits. The framework is composed of all the extraneous factors and facilities in the situation that affect the nurse's ability to obtain the desired results. It is a conglomerate of object, existing or missing, such as policies setting, atmosphere time of day, humans and happenings that may be current, past or anticipated.

The realities offer uniqueness to every situation. The success of professional nursing practice is dependant on them. Unless the realities are recognized and dealt with, they may prevent the achievement of the goal. The nurse develops a prescription of care that is based on her central purpose, which is implemented in the realities of the situation.

Nursing Practice and Process

Nursing practice is an art in which the nursing action is based on the principles of helping. Nursing action may be thought of as consisting of the following four distinct kinds of action (Wiedenbach, 1967).
- Reflex (spontaneous)
- Conditioned (automatic)
- Impulsive (impulsive)
- Deliberate (responsible).

Nursing practice as a discipline is goal-directed. The nature of the nursing act is based on thought. The nurse thinks through the kind of results she wants, fears her actions to obtain those results, then accepts responsibility for the acts and the outcome of those acts. Since nursing requires thought, it can be considered a deliberate responsible action.

Nursing practice has three components which as already stated earlier will include:
1. Identification of the patient's need for help.
2. Ministration of the help needed, and
3. Validation that the action taken was helpful to patient.

Identification

Within the identification, there are four distinct steps, first the nurse observes the patient, looking for an inconsistency between the expected behaviour of the patient and the apparent behaviour. Second she attempts to clarify what inconsistency means. Third she determines the cause of the inconsistency. Finally she validates with the patient that her help is needed (Fig. 10.2).

Ministration

In ministering to her patient, the nurse may give advice or information, make referral, apply a comfort measure, or carry out therapeutic procedure. During this, she makes an adjustment in the plan of action if necessary (Fig. 10.3).

Validation

After help has been ministered the nurse validates that the actions were indeed helpful. Evidence must come from the patient that the purpose of the nursing actions has been fulfilled (Fig. 10.4).

Wiedenbach (1977) views the nursing process essentially as an internal personalized

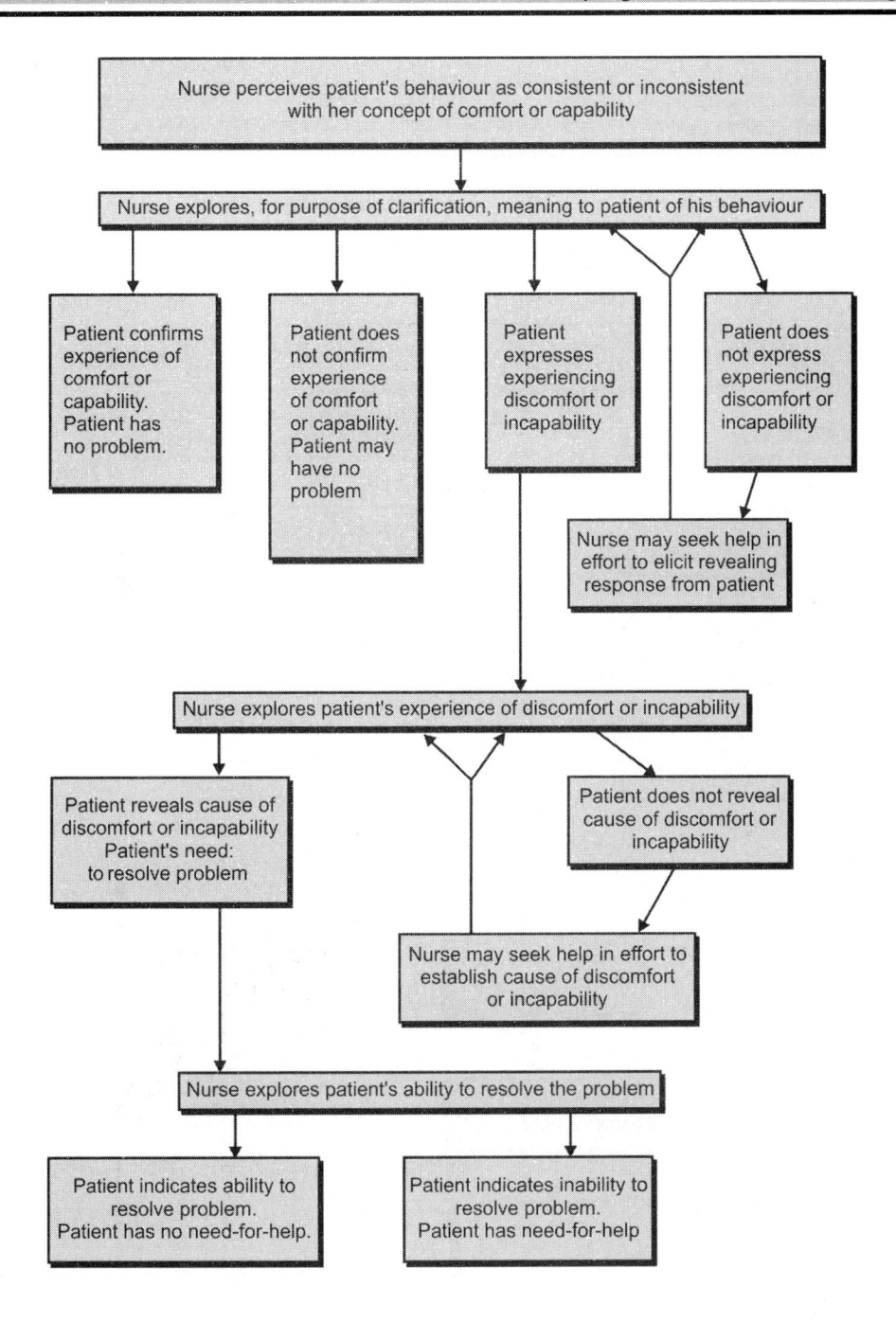

Wiedenbach's Helping Art of Clinical Nursing 141

```
                Nurse perceives patient's behaviour as consistent or inconsistent
                           with her concept of comfort or capability
                                              ↓
              Nurse explores, for purpose of clarification, meaning to patient of his behaviour
               ↓             ↓                      ↓                      ↓
    ┌──────────────┐  ┌──────────────┐  ┌──────────────┐  ┌──────────────┐
    │ Patient confirms │ Patient does │ Patient        │ Patient does     │
    │ experience of    │ not confirm  │ expresses      │ not express      │
    │ comfort or       │ experience   │ experiencing   │ experiencing     │
    │ capability.      │ of comfort   │ discomfort or  │ discomfort or    │
    │ Patient has      │ or capability│ incapability   │ incapability     │
    │ no problem.      │ Patient may  │                │                  │
    │                  │ have no      │                │                  │
    │                  │ problem      │                │                  │
    └──────────────┘  └──────────────┘  └──────────────┘  └──────────────┘
                                              ↓                  ↓
                                      Nurse may seek help in
                                      effort to elicit revealing
                                      response from patient

              Nurse explores patient's experience of discomfort or incapability
               ↓                                                    ↓
    ┌────────────────────────┐                         ┌────────────────────────┐
    │ Patient reveals cause of│                         │ Patient does not reveal│
    │ discomfort or incapability                        │ cause of discomfort or │
    │ Patient's need:         │                         │ incapability           │
    │ to resolve problem      │                         │                        │
    └────────────────────────┘                         └────────────────────────┘
                                    Nurse may seek help in effort to
                                    establish cause of discomfort
                                    or incapability

              Nurse explores patient's ability to resolve the problem
               ↓                                         ↓
    ┌────────────────────────┐              ┌────────────────────────┐
    │ Patient indicates ability to           │ Patient indicates inability to │
    │ resolve problem.        │              │ resolve problem.        │
    │ Patient has no need-for-help.          │ Patient has need-for-help │
    └────────────────────────┘              └────────────────────────┘
```

Figure 10.2: Identification of patient's need for help

142 Nursing Theories

```
┌─────────────────────────────────────────────────────────────────────┐
│ Nurse formulates plan for meeting patient's need-for-help based on  │
│ available resources: what patient thinks, knows, can do, has done + │
│ what nurse thinks, knows, can do, has done. Nurse presents plan to  │
│ patient. Patient responds to presentation of plan                   │
└─────────────────────────────────────────────────────────────────────┘
                                    ↓
┌─────────────────────────────────────────────────────────────────────┐
│ Nurse perceives patient's behaviour as consistent or inconsistent   │
│ with her concept of acceptance of the plan                          │
└─────────────────────────────────────────────────────────────────────┘
                                    ↓
┌─────────────────────────────────────────────────────────────────────┐
│ Nurse explores, for purpose of clarification, meaning to patient of │
│ perceived behaviour following presentation of plan                  │
└─────────────────────────────────────────────────────────────────────┘
            ↓                                           ↓
┌──────────────────────────┐              ┌──────────────────────────┐
│ Patient concurs with plan│              │Patient does not concur   │
│                          │              │with plan                 │
└──────────────────────────┘              └──────────────────────────┘
            ↓                                           ↓
┌──────────────────────────┐              ┌──────────────────────────┐
│ Nurse suggests to patient│              │ Nurse may seek help in   │
│ way of implementing plan │              │ effort to elicit         │
│                          │              │ definitive response      │
└──────────────────────────┘              └──────────────────────────┘
      ↓              ↓
┌───────────┐  ┌──────────────┐
│ Patient   │  │ Patient does │
│ accepts   │  │ not accept   │
│ suggestion│  │ suggestion   │
└───────────┘  └──────────────┘
      ↓              ↓
┌───────────────┐ ┌──────────────────────────────┐
│ Nurse         │ │ Nurse explores for cause of  │
│ implements    │ │ patient's nonacceptance      │
│ plan:         │ │                              │
│ Ministration  │ │                              │
│ of help needed│ │                              │
└───────────────┘ └──────────────────────────────┘
                        ↓                    ↓
              ┌──────────────────┐  ┌──────────────────┐
              │ Patient reveals  │  │ Patient does not │
              │ cause of         │  │ reveal cause of  │
              │ nonacceptance    │  │ nonacceptance    │
              │ interfering      │  │                  │
              │ problem.         │  └──────────────────┘
              │ Patient's        │           ↓
              │ immediate need:  │  ┌──────────────────┐
              │ to resolve       │  │ Nurse may seek   │
              │ problem          │  │ help in effort to│
              └──────────────────┘  │ establish cause  │
                        ↓           │ of patient's     │
              ┌──────────────────┐  │ nonacceptance    │
              │ Nurse explores   │  └──────────────────┘
              │ patient's ability│  ┌──────────────────┐
              │ to resolve       │  │ Nurse formulates │
              │ problem          │  │ plan for meeting │
              └──────────────────┘  │ this need-for-   │
                   ↓        ↓      │ help based on    │
         ┌──────────┐ ┌──────────┐ │ newly recognized │
         │ Patient  │ │ Patient  │ │ resources;       │
         │ indicates│ │ indicates│ │ presents this    │
         │ ability  │ │ inability│ │ plan to patient; │
         │ to       │ │ to       │ │ and explores     │
         │ resolve  │ │ resolve  │ │ meaning to       │
         │ problem  │ │ problem  │ │ patient of his   │
         │ patient  │ │ patient  │ │ behaviour in     │
         │ has no   │ │ has      │ │ response to the  │
         │ need-for-│ │ need-for-│ │ new plan         │
         │ help     │ │ help     │ │ according to the │
         └──────────┘ └──────────┘ │ outline on this  │
                                   │ chart            │
                                   └──────────────────┘
```

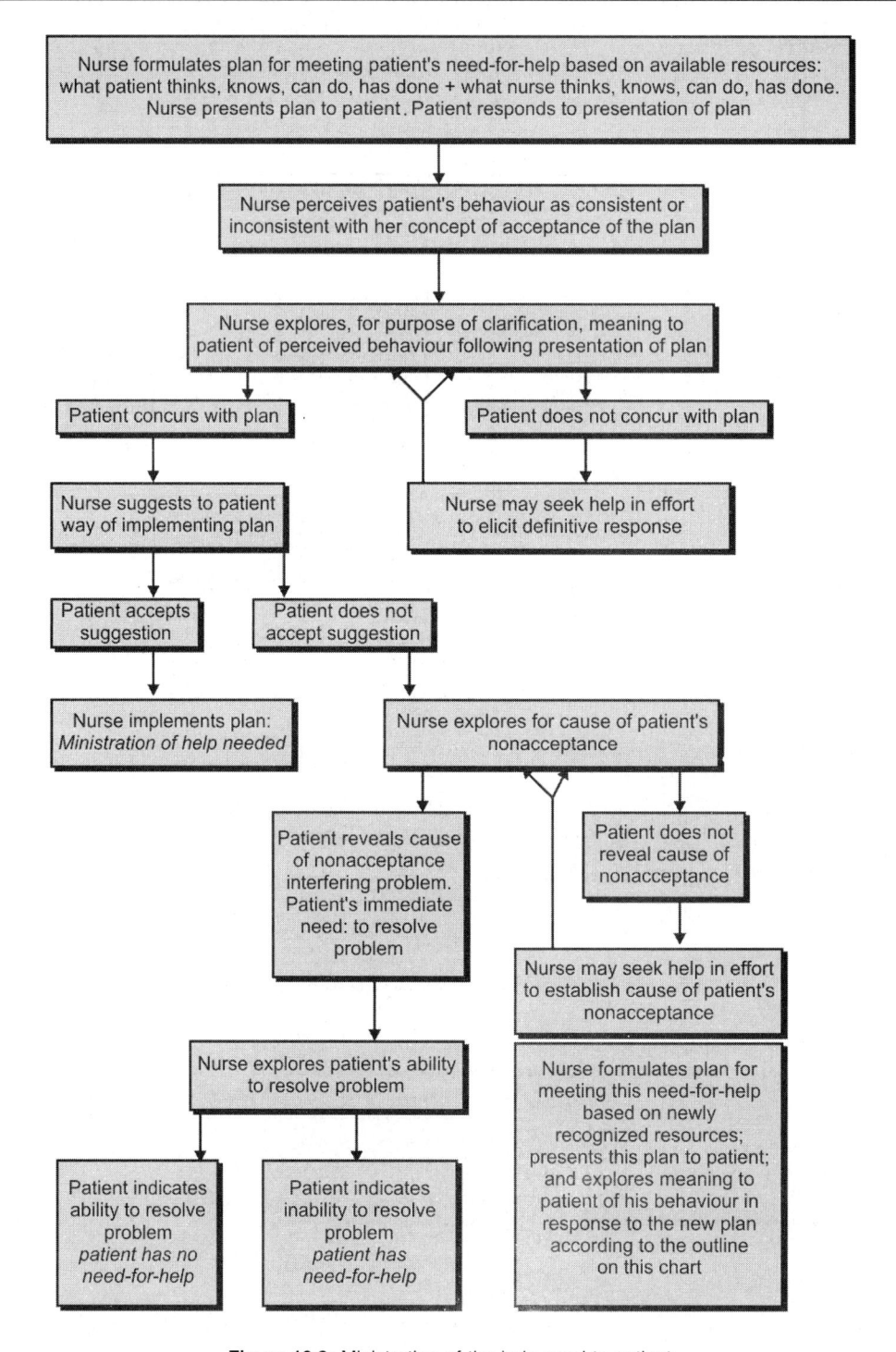

Figure 10.3: Ministration of the help need to patient

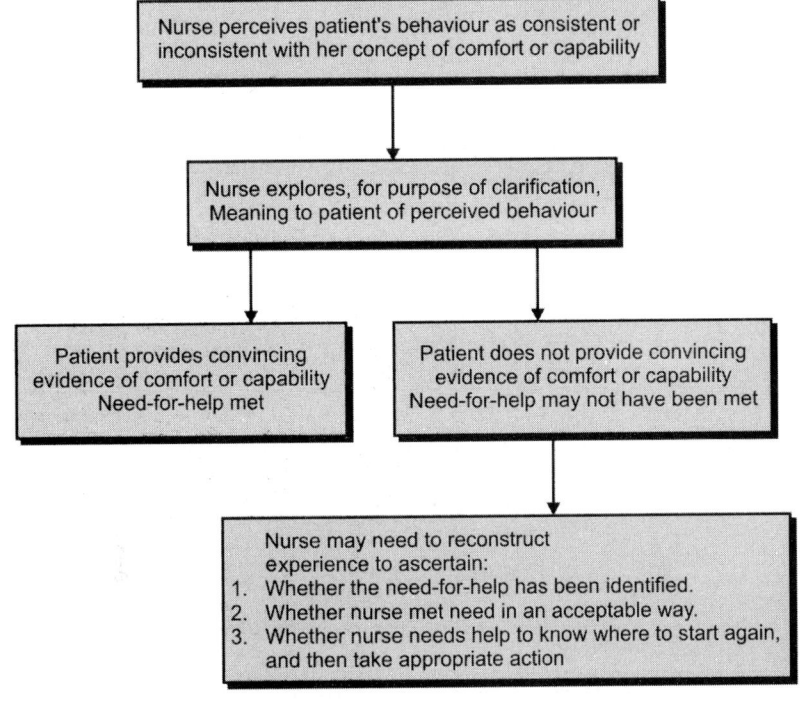

```
┌─────────────────────────────────────────────┐
│ Nurse perceives patient's behaviour as consistent or │
│ inconsistent with her concept of comfort or capability │
└─────────────────────────────────────────────┘
                       │
                       ▼
┌─────────────────────────────────────────────┐
│ Nurse explores, for purpose of clarification, │
│ Meaning to patient of perceived behaviour    │
└─────────────────────────────────────────────┘
           │                         │
           ▼                         ▼
┌──────────────────────┐   ┌──────────────────────┐
│ Patient provides     │   │ Patient does not provide │
│ convincing evidence  │   │ convincing evidence of │
│ of comfort or        │   │ comfort or capability │
│ capability           │   │ Need-for-help may not │
│ Need-for-help met    │   │ have been met        │
└──────────────────────┘   └──────────────────────┘
                                     │
                                     ▼
┌─────────────────────────────────────────────┐
│ Nurse may need to reconstruct               │
│ experience to ascertain:                    │
│ 1. Whether the need-for-help has been identified. │
│ 2. Whether nurse met need in an acceptable way. │
│ 3. Whether nurse needs help to know where to start again, │
│    and then take appropriate action         │
└─────────────────────────────────────────────┘
```

Figure 10.4: Validation that need for help was met

mechanism. As such, influenced by the nurses culture, purpose in nursing, knowledge, wisdom, sensitivity and concern. In nursing process, she identifies severe level of awareness: sensation, perception, assumption, realization, insight, design and decision.

Sensation   Experienced sensory impression.

Perception   The interpretation of a sensory impression.

Assumption   The meaning the nurse attaches to the nurse's attention on the stimulus.

Realization   In which nurse begins to validate the assumptions previously made about the patient.

Insight   Which includes joint planning and additional knowledge about the cause of the problem.

Design   The plan of action decided upon by nurse and confirmed by patient.

Decision   The nurse's performance of a responsible action.

Paradigm or Wiedenbach

Human Being

She emphasized that human or individual possesses unique potential, strives towards self-direction, and needy stimulation. Whatever the individual does, represents his or her best judgment at the moment. Self-awareness and self-acceptance are essential to individuals sense of integrity and self-worth. These circumstances require respect from the nurse.

Health

She does not define health, however, she supports the WHO's definition of health.

144 Nursing Theories

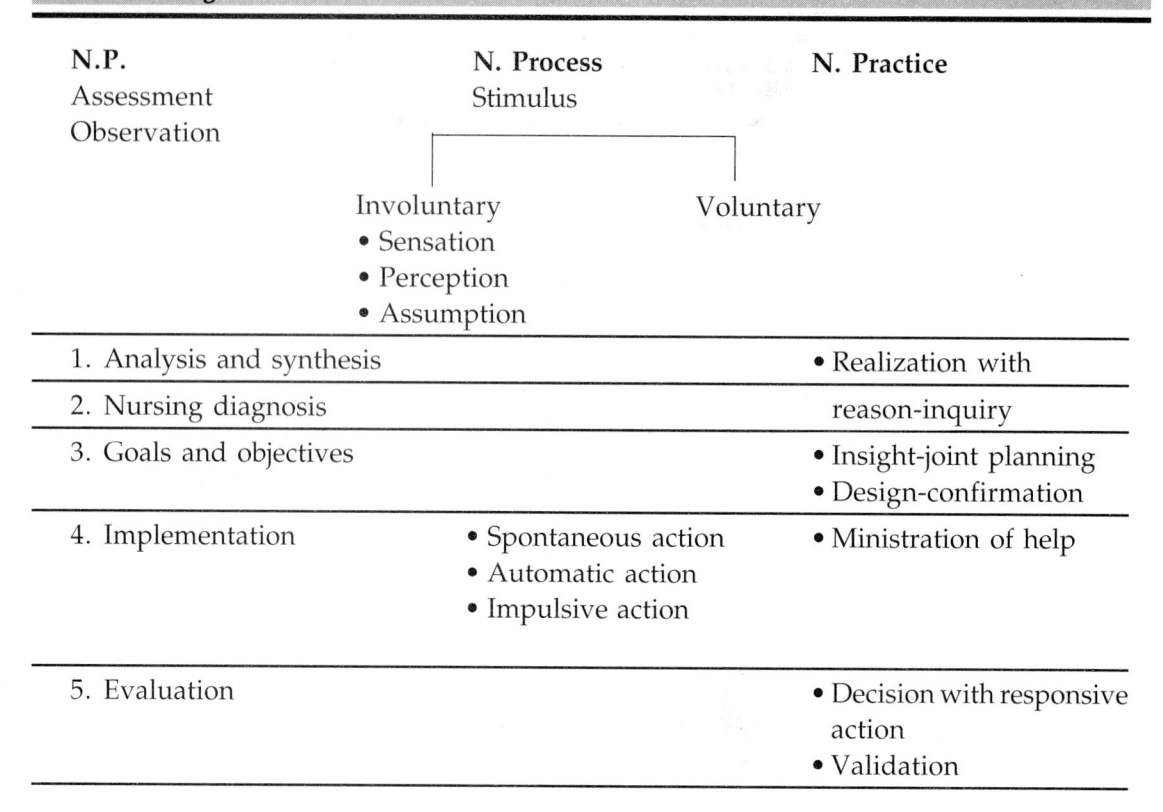

N.P.	N. Process		N. Practice
Assessment	Stimulus		
Observation	Involuntary	Voluntary	
	• Sensation		
	• Perception		
	• Assumption		
1. Analysis and synthesis			• Realization with
2. Nursing diagnosis			reason-inquiry
3. Goals and objectives			• Insight-joint planning
			• Design-confirmation
4. Implementation	• Spontaneous action		• Ministration of help
	• Automatic action		
	• Impulsive action		
5. Evaluation			• Decision with responsive action
			• Validation

Environment

Wiedenbach incorporating the environments within the realities–a major component of her theory. One element of the realities in frame work which is a complex of extraneous factors and circumstances, that are present in every nursing situation. Framework includes objects such as policies, setting, atmosphere, time of day, humans and happenings.

Nursing

Nursing, a clinical discipline, is a practice discipline designed to produce explicit desired results. The art of nursing is goal directed activity requiring the application of knowledge and skill towards meeting a need for help experienced by a patient. Nursing is helping process that extends or restores the patient's ability to cope with demands implicit in the situation.

In Wiedenbach's nursing practice, the steps of observation ministration of help and validation are comparable to the nursing process phase of assessment, implementation and evaluation as follows:

Characteristics of Theory and Wiedenbach's Work

1. Wiedenbach's work does interrelate concepts in such a way as to create a different way of looking at particular phenomenon. She defines and interrelate that concept of realities and central purpose to devise a prescription of nursing care.

2. Wiedenbach stated that she was presenting prescription rather than a predictive theory. When using her theory, it is difficult, if not impossible, to follow a logical thought process and predict the outcome of nursing care, because the prescription and desired outcome will vary from one nurse to another on each nurse's central purpose.
3. This theory is simple yet generalizable to all nursing. Although theory is situation producing, it is not situation specific. The situation is produced by the nurse's central purpose and prescription within the existing realities. The situation is not site oriented, so it can be anywhere house, school.
4. Wiedenbach theory presents a philosophical approach that has not been tested, hypotheses can be formed.
5. Wiedenbach theory can be used to support, guide and assist the nurse to fulfil her commitments to nursing. The nurses commitment to nursing is her central purpose that will influence prescription within the situational realities. Thus, the nurse whose central purse is the holisting support of the optimal development of the individual will develop the prescription that deal with multitude of aspects of the individual rather than focussing solely on the problem that led to initial contact.
6. Wiedenbach does not use theories or support her theory from other disciplines. However, her work is consistent with interaction and communication theory and principles.

Wiedenbach displayed in a graph all the constituent parts of her clinical nursing model at the end of her 1964 treatise (Fig. 10.5).

Wiedenbach is a pioneer in the writing of nursing theory. Her model of clinical nursing is one of the early attempts to systematically describe what it is that nurses do and what nursing is all about. It needs to be further developed by more clearly defining the concepts of health and environment. In addition, the component of nursing art needs to be identified in an operational way.

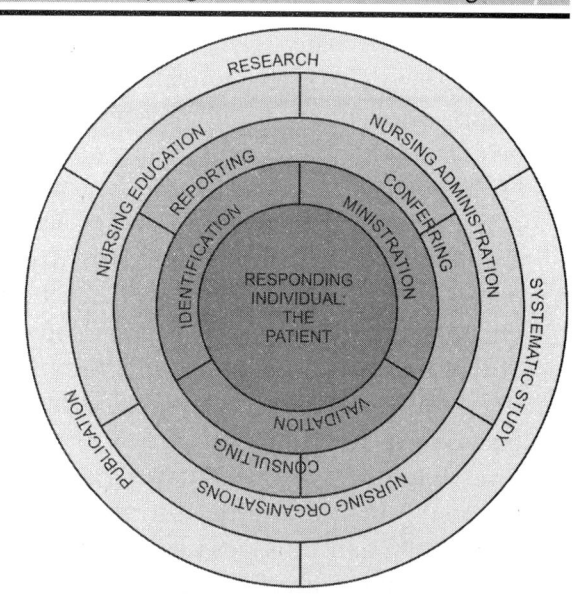

Figure 10.5: Clinical nursing—the relationship between its focus and its constituents

EVALUATION OF THEORY

- Wiedenbach's model evolved out of a desire to describe the practice of professional nursing. Her theory was influenced by Ida Orlando Pelletier and the philosophy of Dickoff and James, her colleagues at Yale University. Hers was one of the earlier nursing theories developed.
- Wiedenbach's model meets the criterion of clarity in that the concepts and definitions are clear, consistent, and intelligible.

- There are too many relational statements for the theory to be classified as a simple theory. The concepts include the need-for-help, nursing practice, and nursing art. All of these concepts are interrelated, equal in importance, and have no meaning aside from their interaction. Relationships between the major components can be linked, but it is difficult to diagram some of the concepts in the model. In addition, the concepts describe or explain phenomena but do not predict.
- The scope of the concepts of patient (person), nursing, and need-for-help are very broad and thus possess generality. However, the concept of need-for-help is based on the patient's recognition of his or her need for help. This concept is not applicable to the infant, comatose patient, or many other physiologically or psychologically incompetent persons. Also, the assumption that all nurses do not share a similar philosophy of nursing lessens the generality of the model.
- Substantiation of a theory is accomplished through research, and thus the usefulness of the theory is determined. In Wiedenbach's model, the criterion is only partially met. The concepts of nursing practice and need-for-help are operationally defined and measurable. However, the concept of need-for-help is not always applicable. Also, within this theory there is little attempt to operationally define nursing art. Therefore it would be difficult to test this theory.

  However, the potential exists for research to be done with this model. J. Fawcett believes three steps must be taken before the model can be tested. "First, the model must be formulated; second, a theory must be derived from the model; and third, operational definitions must be given to the concepts, and hypothesis derived."
- Derivable consequences refer to the overall effect of the theory and its importance to nursing research, practice, and education. Wiedenbach's model fulfils the purpose for which it was developed and that is to describe professional practice. The theory focuses on nurse patient interactions and regards the patient from a holistic point' of view. Wiedenbach's work influenced the work of other early scholars, including Orlando and Peplau.

As one of the early nursing theorists, Wiedenbach made an important contribution to the nursing profession.

Chapter 11

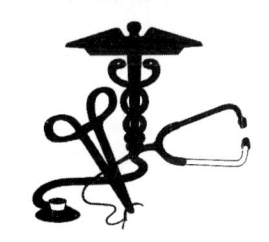

King's Theory of Goal Attainment

Imogene King earned a diploma in nursing from St. John's Hospital of Nursing in St. Louis in 1945. She then worked as an office nurse, school nurse, staff nurse, and private duty nurse to support herself while studying for a baccalaureate degree. In 1948 she received a Bachelor of Science in Nursing Education from St. Louis University. From 1947 to 1958 King worked as an instructor in medical-surgical nursing and then as an assistant director at St. John's Hospital School of Nursing. She went on to earn an MSN in 1957 from St. Louis University and a Doctor of Education degree from Teachers College, Columbia University, New York, in 1961. King was awarded an honorary PhD from Southern Illinois University in 1980.

From 1961 to 1966, King was an associate professor of nursing at Loyola University in Chicago, where she developed a master's degree program in nursing using a conceptual framework. During this time her book, Toward a Theory for Nursing; General Concepts of Human Behaviour, was conceptualised, the literature reviewed, and a contract from a publishing company signed.

Between 1966 and 1968, king served as Assistant Chief of Research Grants Branch, Division of Nursing in the Department of Health, Education, and Welfare. While she was in Washington, DC, her article "A Conceptual Framework for Nursing" was published in Nursing Research. From 1968 to 1972 King was the director of the School of Nursing at The Ohio State University in Columbus. The manuscript for her book had been submitted to the publisher by the time she accepted this administrative position, and it was subsequently published in 1971. In Toward a Theory for Nursing King concludes, "A systematic representation of nursing is required ultimately for developing a science to accompany a century or more of art in the everyday world of nursing."

King returned to Chicago in 1972 as a professor in the Loyola University graduate program. Form 1978 to 1980 she also served as the Coordinator of Research in Clinical Nursing at the Loyola Medical Center, Department of Nursing. From 1972 to 1975 she was a member of the Defense Advisory Committee on Women in the services for the

Department of Defense. In 1980 King moved to Tampa, Florida, where she is currently a professor at the University of South Florida College of Nursing. The manuscript for her second book, *A Theory for Nursing Systems, Concepts, Process*, was published in 1981 (Fig. 11.1)

King has been a member of the American Nurses Association, the Florida Nurses Association, National League for Nursing, and several honorary and professional societies. In addition to her books, she has authored several book chapters and multiple articles in professional journals. A third book, *Curriculum and Instruction in Nursing*, was published in 1986. King retired in 1990. She continues to provide community service by teaching and helping plan care with her theory at Tampa General. She keynoted two Sigma Theta Tau theory conferences in 1992.

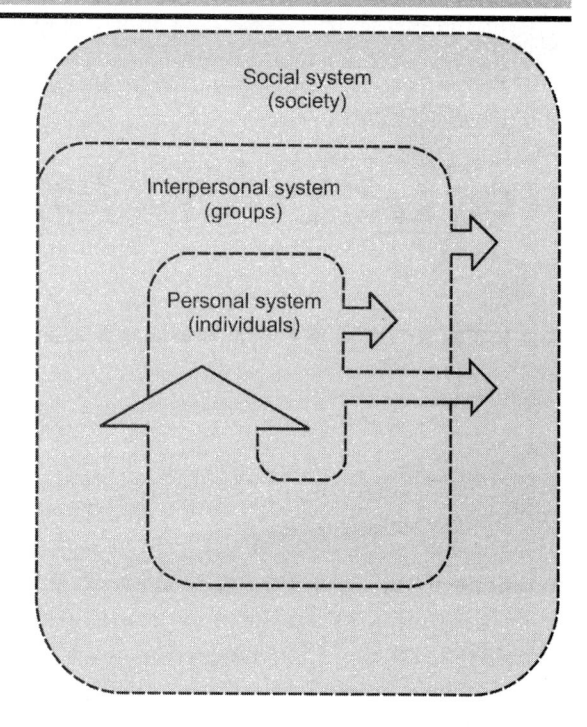

Figure 11.1: Dynamic interacting systems

EVOLUTION OF THEORY

King states in the preface of Toward a Theory for Nursing that the book's purpose "is to propose a conceptual frame of reference for nursing to be utilized by students and teachers, and also by researchers and practitioners to identify and analyze events in specific nursing situations. The framework suggests that the essential characteristics of nursing are those properties that have persisted in spite of environmental changes." King proposed that her first book was "a way of thinking about the real world of nursing." that it suggested "an approach for selecting concepts perceived to be fundamental for the practice of professional nursing," and that it showed "a process for developing concepts that symbolize experiences within the physical, psychological, and social environment in nursing." "A search of the literature in nursing and other behavioural science fields, discussion with colleagues, attendance at numerous conferences, inductive and deductive reasoning, and some critical thinking about the information gathered, lead me to formulate my own theoretical framework." King wrote in 1971 that although nurses were individuals and professionals, nursing was "not yet a science."

During a telephone interview, King was asked who influenced her work. She said the sources were "too numerous to mention." However, at a conference of nursing theorists she stated the general systems theory from the behavioural sciences led to the development of her "dynamic interacting systems." She identified in this system three distinct levels of functions: (i) individuals, (ii) groups, and (iii) society. King states in her second book that "if the goal of nursing is concern for the health of individuals and the health care of groups, and if one accepts the premise that human beings are open systems interacting with the environment, then a conceptual framework for nursing must be organized to incorporate these ideas. King's concepts and definitions of those concepts were derived from theories and research."

King defines theory as "a set of concepts, which, when defined, are interrelated and observable in the world of nursing practice."

Concepts are abstract ideas that give meaning to our sense perceptions...mental images formed by generalizations from these particular impressions." For King, theory serves to "build scientific knowledge for nursing," and she has identified two methods for cultivating theory. First, a theory can be developed and then tested with research. But the procedure can also be reversed and enable research to initiate the development of theory, King states, "It is my opinion that in today's world of building knowledge for a complex profession such as nursing, one must consider a composite of these two strategies."

Many research studies are cited in King's books, especially with regard to the development of the concepts relating to her theory, but only a few of those studies are briefly mentioned here. With regard to "perception" King examined studies by F.H. Allport, K.J. Kelley and K.R. Hammon, W.H. lttleson and H. Cantril, and others. In her development of definitions for "space," R. Sommer and R. Ardrey's studies were used and B.B. Minkley's research was noted. For "time", J.E. Orme's work was acknowledged. In the examination of communication, theories and models were presented and the studies of P. Watzlawick, J.H. Beavin, and D.D. Jackson; and D. Krieger were noted. Studies by J.F. Whiting, I. Orlando, and J. Bruner were examined for information on "interaction" and "transaction." J. Dewey's theory of knowledge, which deals with self-action, interaction, and transaction in knowing and the known, and A. Kuhn's work on transactions were also used.

With regard to research, in 1975 King noted, "Most studies have centered on technical aspects of patient care and of the health care systems rather than on patient aspects directly....Few problems have been stated that begin with what the patient's condition demands or what the patient wants." In her 1981 book king states, "Several theoretical formulations about interpersonal relations and nursing process have been described in nursing situations," citing studies by H. Peplau, I. Orlando, H. Yuro and M. Walsh, and herself. However, "Few nursing studies have provided empirical data about nursing process phenomena related to human interaction."

King notes that Orlando's study "supports the idea that nursing process is reciprocal" because goal identifications exists for nurses and patients. She adds that this study varies from others in that it "described the nurse-patient interaction process that leads to goal attainment." King also discusses her own descriptive study, which tested goal attainment and operationally defined a concept of transaction as an integral component of the theory. A method of nonparticipant observation was used to collect information on nurse-patient interactions in a patient care hospital setting. Volunteer patients and graduate nursing students participated, and the students is open to permit feedback, because perception is potentially influenced by each phase of the activity.

As previously noted, King's descriptive study relating to the **theory of goal attainment** resulted in a means for analysing interactions, as presented in Figure 11.2.

King derived the following seven hypotheses from Goal Attainment Theory.
1. Perceptual congruence in nurse-patient interactions increases mutual goal setting.
2. Communication increases mutual goal setting between nurses and patients and leads to satisfactions.
3. Satisfactions in nurses and patients increase goal attainment.
4. Goal attainment decreases stress and anxiety in nursing situations.
5. Goal attainment increases patient learning and coping ability in nursing situations.
6. Role conflict experienced by patients, nurses, or both decreases transactions in nurse-patient interactions.
7. Congruence in role expectations and role performance increases transactions in nurse-patient interactions.

Classification system of nurse-patient interactions that lead to transactions, which includes the elements in interactions:
- Action
- Reaction
- Disturbance
- Mutual goal setting
- Explore means to achieve goal
- Agree on means to achieve goal
- Transaction
- Goal(s) achieved.

Figure 11.2 combines some factors from the classification system and the process of human interaction. Both client and nurse perceive throughout the process; they communicate, thus creating action. Actions result in reactions, and, if there is a disturbance, goals may be set. At this point, means for goal achievement are explored and agreed upon, transactions are made, and goal attainment results.

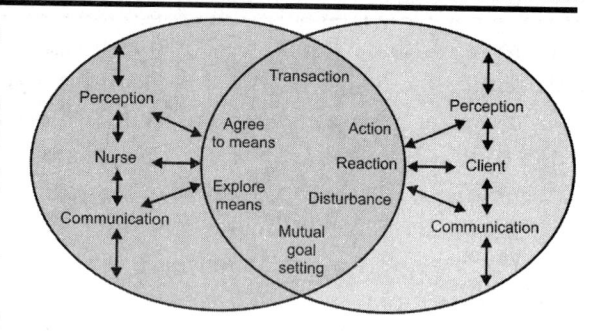

Figure 11.2: Schematic diagram of a theory of goal attainment

The patient is a personal system within the environment who coexists with other personal systems. Individuals form groups that comprise interpersonal systems, and interpersonal systems contribute to social systems. Thus patient and nurse are composed of personal systems as subsystems within interpersonal and social systems. The nurse must understand given aspects of all three systems. Concepts identified for each system affect total system function. There are three comprehensive concepts: perception for the personal system, organization for the social system, and interaction for the interpersonal system. Personal system concepts related to perception include self, body image, growth and development, time, space, and learning. The nurse also must have knowledge of role, communication, transaction, and stress to understand interactions central to interpersonal system function. Because interaction occurs within social systems—including family, belief, educational, and work systems—nurses require knowledge or organizational concepts of power, authority, control, status, and decision making to function adequately.

The focus for nursing is the human being in the system context. The goal is health. Health implies helping people in groups attain, maintain, and restore health; live with chronic illness or disability; or die with dignity. Interactions of the individual with the environment are significant in influencing life and health. Nurse and patient meet in a health care organization—a patient who needs help and a nurse who offers help. Nurse and patient perceive one another, act and react, interact, and transact. In this process, presenting conditions are recognized, goal-related decisions are made, and motivation to exert control over events to achieve goals occurs. Transactions are basic to goal attainment and include social exchange, bargaining and negotiating, and sharing a frame of reference towards mutual goal setting. Transactions require perceptual accuracy in nurse-client interactions and congruence between role performance and role expectation for nurse and client. Transactions lead to goal attainment, satisfaction, effective care, and enhanced growth and development. The goal of nursing process interaction is transaction, which leads to attainment of goals set in relation to health promotion, maintenance, and recovery from illness.

During 1960s, rapidity of scientific and technological advances has had great impact on the profession of Nursing as on other components of society. As emerging professionals, nurses were identifying the knowledge base specific to nursing practice and to an expanding role for nurses. In this period, of environment, Imogene M. King (1971) published *Towards a Theory of Nursing: General Concepts of Human Behaviour* and *A Theory for Nursing; systems, Concepts, Process in 1981*. These publications grew from King's thoughts about the vast amount of knowledge available to nurses and the difficulty this presents to the individual nurse in choosing the facts and concepts relevant to a given situation. She identifies the conceptual framework as an open system frame work and the theory as one of goal attainment. As her extensive documentation indicates, she has drawn from a wide variety of sources in developing the framework and deriving the theory from that framework.

Open System Framework

The purposes of the conceptual work are to organize concepts that represent essential knowledge that ought to be used by many disciplines and to construct theories from the framework and test them from the prospective of nursing as discipline. The concepts and knowledge may be similar across disciplines. But the way each profession uses them will differ. The framework represents knowledge essential for nursing and has an additional purpose of allowing the construction and testing of theories from the perspective of nursing. The conceptual framework includes goal, structure, function, resources and decision making, which are essential elements.

The framework has health as the *goal* for nursing. *Structure* is represented by the three open systems. *Function* is demonstrated in reciprocal relations of individuals in interaction.

Resources include both people (health professional and their clients) and money, goods and services for items needed to carry out specific activities. *Decision making* occurs when choices are made in research allocation to support obtaining system goals.

In her conceptual framework, King (1989) presents several assumptions which include the assumptions that human beings are open systems in constant interaction with their environment, that nursing focus is human being, interacting with their environment, and that nursing's goal is to help individuals and groups maintain health. Her framework is composed of three interacting systems which include, "personal system, the interpersonal system and the social systems. About her conceptual framework she states that the

"Nursing phenomena are organised within three dynamic interacting systems (i) *Personal systems* (individuals; (ii) *Interpersonal systems* (friends, small and large groups) and (iii) *Social system* (family, school, industry, social organizations and health care delivery system) (Fig. 11.1).

She identifies several concepts as relevant for each of these systems and also states that the placement of concepts with each system is arbitrary because all the concepts are interrelated in the human-environment interaction. For each system of a comprehensive or major concepts with additional sub-concepts is identified.

Personal Systems

She conceives each individual is a personal system. For a personal system, the relevant concepts are perception, self, growth and development, body image, space, learning and time.

Perceptions

Refer to each person's representation of reality. According to King, it includes the import and transformation of energy, and processing, storing, and exporting information. Perceptions are related to past experiences, concept of self, socio-economic group, biological inheritance, and educational background. Perception influences all behaviours or to which all other concepts are related. The characteristics of perceptions are that is universal or experienced by all; subjective or personal; and selective for each person, meaning that any given situation will be experienced in a unique manner by each individual involved.

Perception is action oriented in the present and based on the information that is available. Perception is transactions; that is, individuals are active participants in situation and their identities are affected by their participation. Further, perception is a process in which data obtained through the senses and from memory are organized, interpreted and transformed. This process of human interactions with the environment influences behaviour, provides meaning to experience and represents the individual image of reality.

Self

The self is a composite of thought and feelings which constitutes a person's awareness of his individual existence, his conception of who and what he is. A person's self is the sum total of all he can call his. The self includes, among other things, a system of ideas, attitudes, values, and commitments. The self is a person's total subjective environment. It is a distinctive centre of experience and significance. The self constitutes a person's inner world as distinguished from the outer world consisting of all other people and things. The self is the individual as known to the individual. It is that to which we refer when we say 'I'.

King accepted this definition. The characteristics are *self* as dynamic individual, an open system and goal orientation.

Growth and Development

It is defined as a continual changes in individuals at the cellular, molecular and behavioural levels of activities, conducive to helping individuals move towards maturity. The growth and development is the process in people, lives through which they move from a potential for achievement to actualization of self. The characteristics of growth and development include cellular, molecular and behavioural changes in human beings. These changes usually occur in an orderly manner. One that is predictable but has individual variation and is a function of genetic endowment, of meaningful and satisfying experiences, and of an environment conducive to helping individuals move towards maturity.

Body Image

It is characterized as very personal and subjective, acquired or learned, dynamic and changing as the person redefines self. Body image is part of each stage of growth and development. King defines body image as the way one perceives both one's body and other's reactions to one's appearance.

Space

It is defined operationally "as existing in all directions and is the same everywhere and it is this immediate environment in which nurse and client interact." It is also defined by the physical area known as "territory" and by the behaviours of those who occupy it. Space is characterized as universal because all people have some concept of it. It may be personal or subjective; individual, situational and dependent on the relationships in the situation; dimensional as a function of voluntary area, distance and time, and transactional or based on individual perception of situation.

Time

It is defined as a sequence of events moving onwards to the future. It is a duration between one event and another as uniquely experienced by each human being; it is the relation of one event to another event. Time is characterized as universal or inherent in life process, relational or dependent on distance and the amount of information occurring, unidirectional or irreversible as it moves from past to future with a continuous flow of events; measurable; and subjective because it is based on perception.

Learning

It is a subject concept in the personal system. King did not define it operationally.

Perception, self, growth and development, body image, space and time are concepts of the personal system. In this, the focus of nursing is the person. When personal systems come in contact with one another, they for interpersonal system.

Interpersonal System

Interpersonal system are formed by human beings interacting. Two interacting individuals form a dyad, three form a triad, and four or more form small or large groups. As the number of interacting individuals increases, so does the complexity of interactions. The relevant concepts for interpersonal systems are interactions, communications, transactions role and stress. The concepts from the personal system are also used in understanding interaction.

Interaction

King, defines interaction as "a process of perception and communication between person and environment and between person and person, represented by verbal or nonverbal behaviours that are goal directed." Each individual is interaction (nurse and client) "brings different knowledge, needs, goals, past experiences, and perceptions which influence the interactions."

Interaction is a major or comprehensive concept and is characterized by values; mechanisms for establishing human relationship, being universally experienced, being influenced by perceptions; reciprocity; being mutual or interdependent; containing verbal and nonverbal communication; Learning occurring when communication is effective, unidirectionality, irreversibility, dynamism, and having temporal-spatial dimensions. Interactions are defined as the observable behaviour of two or more persons in mutual presence.

Communication

King, defines communication as "a process whereby information is given from one person to another either directly in face to face meeting or indirectly through telephone, television or the written word. Communication is fundamental social process develops and maintains human relations and facilitates the ordered functioning of human groups and societies. As the information components of human interactions communication occurs in all behaviours.

The characters of communication are then, it is verbal, nonverbal, situational, perceptual, transactional, irreversible; or moving forward in time, personal and dynamic. Symbols of verbal communications are provided by language, for such communication includes the spoken and written language that transmits the ideas from one person to another. An important aspect of non-verbal behaviour is touch, other aspects of nonverbal behaviour are distance, posture, facial expression, physical appearance, and body movements.

Transactions

Transactions, are defined as purposeful interactions that lead to goal attainment. King goes on subsequently expand this definition of transaction to include "observable behaviour of human beings interacting with their environment... the valuation components of human beings communicated with the environment to achieve goals that are valued... goal directed human behaviour.

Transactions for this conceptual framework are derived from cognitions and perceptions and not from transaction or analysis. The characteristics of transactions are that they are unique because each individual has a personal world of reality based on that individual's perceptions; they have temporal and spatial dimensions, and they experience a series of events in time.

Role

It is defined as "a set of behaviour expected and persons occupying a position in a social system; rules that define rights and obligations in a position." Expectations of a role different than role conflict and confusion exists. This may lead to decreased effectiveness of nursing care provided.

The characteristics of *role* include reciprocity in that person may be a giver at one time and a taker at another time, with a relationship between two or more individuals who are functioning in two or more roles that are learned, social, complex and situation. There are three major elements of role as follows:

1. The role consists of a set of expected behaviours of those who occupy a position in a social system.
2. The role consists of a set of procedures or rules that define the obligations and rights associated with a position in an organization.
3. The role is a relationship of two or more persons who are interacting for a purpose in a particular situation.

The nurse's role can be defined as interacting with one or more others in a nursing situation in which, the nurse as a professional uses those skills, knowledge and values identified as belonging to nursing to identify goals and help others achieve the goals.

Stress

Stress is a "dynamic state, whereby a human being interacting with environment. It involves an exchange of energy and information between the person and the environment for regulation and control of stressors ... an energy response of an individual persons, objects and events." An increase in the stress of individuals interacting can narrow the perceptual field and decrease rationality. An increase in stress may also affect nursing care.

The characteristics of stress are that it is dynamic as a result of open systems being in continuous exchange with the environment; the intensity varies; there is a temporal-spatial dimension that is influenced by past experiences: it is individual, personal and subjective–a response to life events that is uniquely personal.

King (1981) derives a definition of stress to be a "dynamic state whereby a human being interacts with the environment to maintain balance of growth, development, and performance, which involves an exchange of energy and information between the persons and the environment for regulation and control of stressors. In addition, stress involves objects, persons and events as stressors that evoke an energy response from the person. Stress may be positive or negative, and may simultaneously help an individual to a peak of achievement and wear the individual down.

The concepts of interpersonal system are interaction, communication, transaction, role and stress. The focus of nursing in the interpersonal system is the environment. Interpersonal system join together to form larger system known as social system.

Social System

A social system is defined as "an organized boundary system of social roles, behaviours, and practices developed to maintain values and the mechanisms to regulate the practice and rules". An example of social system includes families, religious groups, educational systems work systems, and peer groups. The concept, relevant to social systems are *organization, authority, power, status, decision making and control* plus all the concepts from the personal and interpersonal systems.

Organization

King defines organization as being made up of human beings who have prescribed roles and positions and who make use of resources to meet both personal and organizational goal. She proposes four parameters for organization:
1. Human values, behaviour patterns, needs, goals and expectations.
2. A natural environment in which material and human resources are essential for achieving goals.
3. Employers and employees, or parents and children, who form groups that collectively interact to achieve goals, and
4. Technology that facilitates goal attainment.

Organization is characterized by a structure that orders positions and activities and relates formal and informal arrangement of individuals and groups to achieve personal and organizational goals; functions that describe the roles, positions, and activities to be performed; goals or outcomes to be achieved; and resources.

Authority

Authority is an active, reciprocal process of transaction in which the actors, background, perception, and values influence the definition. Validation and acceptance of those in organizational positions associated with authority.

The characteristics of authority include that it is observable through provisions of order, guidance and responsibility of actions; universal; essential in formal organization; reciprocal because it requires co-operation, resides in a holder who must be perceived as legitimate, situational, essential to goal achievement and associated with power. Assumptions about authority include that it can be:
- Perceived by individuals and be legitimate.
- Associated with a position in which the position holder distributes rewards and sanctions.
- Help by professional through their competence in using special knowledge and skills, and
- Exercised through group leadership by those with human relation skills.

Power

King defines power in a variety of ways.
- Power is the capacity to use resources in organizations to achieve goals.
- Power is the process whereby one or more persons influence other person in a situation.
- Power is the capacity or ability of person or a group to achieve goals.
- Power occurs in all aspects of life and each person has potential power determined by individual resources and the environmental forces encountered.
- Power is social force that organizes and maintaining society.
- Power is the ability to use and mobilize resources to achieve goals.

Status

Status refers to the position of an individual in a group or groups in relation to other groups in an organization and identifies that status is accompanied by privileges, duties and obligations. Status is characterized as situational, position dependent and reversible.

Decision-making

Decision-making in organization is defined as "a dynamic and systematic process by which goal-directed choice of perceived alternatives is made and acted upon by individuals or groups to answer a question and attain a goal" (King, 1981). It is characterized as necessary to regulate each person's life and work, universal individual, personal, subjective, situational, a continuous process and goal-directed.

Control

It is not defined by King, and control is added as a subconcept in the social system.

As in personal and interpersonal system, King identified a nursing in this system and nursing focus on health.

The major thesis of King's conceptual framework are:
1. That "each human being perceives the world as a total person in making transactions with individuals and things in the environment", and
2. That transactions represent a life situation in which perceiver and thing perceived are encountered and in which each person entered the situation as an active participant and each is changed in the process of these experiences.

Theory of Goal Attainment

The major components of the theory of goal attainment are stated in her (King's) interpersonal systems in which two people who are usually strangers come together in a health care organization to help and be helped to maintain a state of health that permits functioning in roles. The theory's focus on interpersonal systems reflect her beliefs that the practice of nursing is differentiated from that of other health professions by what nurses do with and for individuals. The concept of the theory are interaction, perception, communication, transactions, self, role, stress, growth and development, time and personal space. Their concepts are interrelated in every nursing situation. Although these terms have already been defined as concepts in the conceptual framework, they are defined again here as a part of the theory of goal attainment.

Interaction

It is defined as "a process of perception and communicated between person and environment and between person and person represented by verbal and non-verbal behaviours that are goal-directed. King's diagram of interaction is as given below (Fig. 11.3).

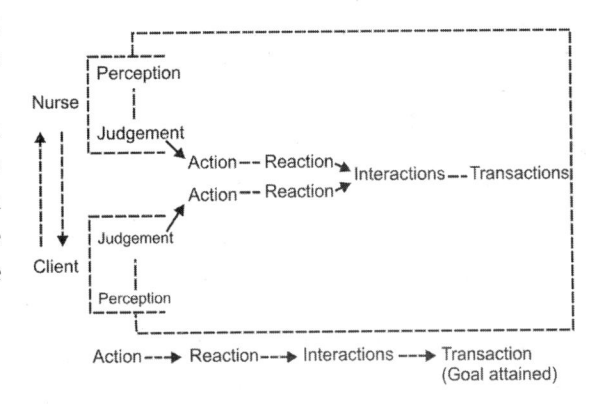

```
                    ┌─────────────┐
                    │ Perception  │
              Nurse │      ↓      │
                    │ Judgement   │
                    └─────────────┘
                         Action-- Reaction↘
                                            Interactions -- Transactions
                         Action-- Reaction↗
                    ┌─────────────┐
                    │ Judgement   │
             Client │      ↑      │
                    │ Perception  │
                    └─────────────┘

       Action ---> Reaction ---> Interactions ---> Transaction
                                                   (Goal attained)
```

Figure 11.3: A human interaction process

Hence, each individual involved in an interaction brings different ideas, attitudes and perceptions to exchange. The individuals come together for a purpose and perceive each other; each makes a judgment and takes mental action or decides to act. The neach reacts to the other and the situation (perception, judgment, action and reaction). King indicates that only the interaction and transactions are observable.

Perception is "each person's representation of reality". The elements of perception are the importing of energy from the environment and organizing it by information, transforming, energy, processing, information, storing information and exploring information in the form of overt behaviours.

Communication is defined as a process whereby information is given from one person to another either directly in face-to-face meetings or indirectly through telephone, television or written word. Communication represents, and is involved in, the information component of interaction.

Transaction is defined as observable behaviours of human beings interacting with that environment. Transactions represent the valuation component of human interactions and involve bargaining, negotiating and social exchange. When transactions occur between nurses and clients goals are attained.

Role is defined as 'set of behaviours expected of persons occupying a position in a social system; rules that defines rights and obligations in a position; a relationship with one or more individuals interacting in specific situation for a purpose.' It is important that roles be understood and interpreted clearly to avoid conflict and confusion.

Stress is a dynamic state whereby a human being interacts with the environment to maintain balance for growth, development and performance... an energy response of an individual to persons, objects, and events called stressors. Although stress may be positive or negative, too high level of stress may decrease an individual ability to interact and to attain goals.

Growth and development can defined as the 'continuous changes in individuals at the cellular, molecular and behavioural levels of activities—the process that takes place in the life of individuals that help them move from potential capacity for achievement of self-actualization.

Time is a sequence of events moving onward to the future a continuous flow of events in successive order that implies a change, a past and a future... a duration between one event and another as uniquely experienced by each human being... the relation of one event to another.

Space exists in every direction and in the same in all directions. Space includes that physical area named territory. Space is defined by the behaviours of those individuals, who occupy it.

Health is not stated as a concept in King's theory, but is identified as an outcome variable. She indicates the outcome is an individual's state of health or ability to function in social roles.

Here the operational definition of transactions has been used to identify the elements in interactions at other times called a model of transactions. These elements in interactions, and other times called a model of transactions. These elements are *action, reaction, disturbance* (problem), *mutual goal setting,* explorations of meaning to achieve the goal, agreement or means to achieve goal, transactions and goal attainment. The model essentially described as interpersonal dyad, (nurse and client) in interactions using mutual goal setting or decision making as a process that leads to goal attainment.

King developed predictive proposition from her theory of goal attainment, which includes:
- Perceptual accuracy, role congruence, and communication in a nurse-client interaction leads to transactions.
- Transaction leads to goal attainment and growth and development.
- Goal attainment leads to satisfaction and to effective nursing care.

She suggested that additional propositions may be generated.

In addition, she specifies internal and external boundary determining criteria as follows:
1. Internal boundary criteria are derived from the characteristics of the concepts of theory and speak to the theory itself. The internal boundary criteria for King's theory of goal attainment are the following:
   - Nurse and client do not know each other.
   - Nurse is licensed to practice professional nursing.
   - Client is in need of the services provided by the nurse.
   - Nurse and client are in a reciprocal relationship in that the nurse has special knowledge and skills to communicate appropriate information about self and perceptions of problems or concerns that when communicated to nurse will help in mutual goal setting.
   - Nurse and client are in mutual presence, purposefully interacting to achieve goals.
2. The external boundary criteria speaks to the area in which the theory is applicable. The external boundary criteria for King's theory of goal attainment is the following:
   - Interaction in a two-person group.
   - Interaction limited to licensed professional nurse and to client in need of nursing care.
   - Interactions taking place in natural environments.

Further, King (1987) added the boundary for client locus of control and states that it is difficult to achieve mutual goal setting with a client who has an external locus of control.

Thus, King states that 'a professional nurse, with special knowledge and skills, a client in need of nursing. With knowledge of self and perceptions of personal problems, meet as strangers in a natural environment. They interact mutually to identify problems and to establish and achieve goals. The personal system of the nurse and the personal system for the client meet in interactions with interpersonal systems that surround them as well as by each of their personal system.

PARADIGM OF KING'S THEORY

In King's theory of goal attainment, she discussed the four major concepts of human beings, health, environmental society, and nursing and defined.

Human Being

King's personal philosophy about human beings and life influenced her assumptions. Her conceptual framework and theory of goal attainment "are based on overall assumption that the focus of nursing is human beings interacting with their environment leading to a state of health for individuals, which are ability to function in social roles."

King identifies several assumptions about human beings. She describes human being as social beings, sentiment, rational reacting, perceiving, controlling, purposeful, action-oriented and time oriented. From these beliefs, about human beings, she has derived the following assumptions that are specific to nurse-client interactions:

- Perceptions of nurse and of client influence the interaction process.
- Goals, needs, and values of nurse and client influence the interaction process.
- Individuals have a right to knowledge about themselves.
- Individuals have a right to participate in decision that influence their life, their health, and community services.
- Health professionals have, a responsibility to share information that helps individuals make informed decisions about their health care.
- Individuals have a right to accept or reject health care.
- Goals of health professionals and goals of recipients of health care may be incongruent.

Further, King states that "nurses are concerned with human beings interacting with their environment in ways that lead to self-fulfillment and to maintenance of health." Human beings have three fundamental health needs.

i. The need for health information that is usable at the time when it is needed and can be used.
ii. The need for care that seeks to prevent illness, and
iii. The need for care when human beings are unable to help themselves.

She states, "nurses are in a position to assess what people know about the health, what they think about their health, what they think about their health, how they feel about it and how they act to maintain it.

Health

King defines health as "dynamic life experience of human being, which implies continuous adjustment to stressors in the internal and external environment through optimum use of one's resources to achieve maximum potential for daily living. "and" as a dynamic state of an individual in which change is constant and ongoing and may be viewed as the individuals ability to function in his or her usual roles.

She affirms that health is not a continuum but a holistic state. The characteristics of health are "genetic, subjective, relative, dynamic, environmental, functional, cultural, and perceptual. King discusses health as a functional state and illness is an interference with that functional state. She then defines illness as "a deviation from normal, that is an imbalance in a personal biological structure or in an imbalance in a person's biological structure or in his psychological make up, or a conflict in a person's social relationship.

Health is viewed as a dynamic state in the life cycle, illness is an interference in the life cycle. Health implies continuous adaptation to stress" in the internal and external environment through optimum use of one's resources to achieve maximum potential for daily living. Health is the function of nurse, patient, physicians, family and other interactions.

Environment

King's framework does not specifically define environment, but views as the social system, portion of her open system framework. She extended the ability to interact in goal setting and selection of means to achieve the goal to include mutual goal setting with family members in relation to client and families. An understanding of the ways that human beings interact with their environment to maintain health is essential for nurses.

Although her definition of health mentions both internal and external environment, she stated, "environment is a function of balance between internal and external interactions," the usual implication of the use of environment in a "Theory for Nursing" in that of external environment. Open system, imply interactions occur between the system and its environment, interfering that the environment is constantly changing "Adjustment to life and health are influenced by an individual's interaction with environment. Each human being perceives the world as a total person in making transactions with individuals and things in the environment. It is understood that definition of external environment drawn for general systems theory. She does say that three systems form the environment that influence individuals.

Nursing

Nursing is an observable behaviour found in the health care system in society. The goal of nursing is to help individuals maintain their health so they can function in their roles. Nursing is viewed as "interpersonal process of *action, reaction, interaction and transaction,* whereby nurse and client share information about their perceptions in the nursing situation" and as a process of human interaction, between nurse and client whereby each perceives the other and the situation, and through communications, they set goals explore means and agree on means to achieve goals.

- *Action* is defined as a sequence of behaviour, involving mental and physical action. The sequence is first mental action to recognize the presenting conditions; and physical action to begin activities related to those conditions; and finally, mental action in effort to exert control over the situation, combined with physical action seeking to achieve goals.
- *Reaction* is not specifically defined, but might be considered to be included in the sequence of behaviours described in action.
- *Interaction* has been discussed.

Further, King discussed the definition of nursing's goal, domain, and function of the professional nurse.

- The *goal* of the nurse is to "help individuals maintain their health so they can function in their roles."
- Nursing *domain* includes promoting, maintaining, and restoring health, and caring for the sick, injured and dying.
- The *function* of the professional nurse is to interpret information in what is known as the nursing process to plan, implement, and evaluate nursing care.

Theory of Goal Attainment and the Nursing Process

The basic assumption of the theory of goal attainment—that nurses and clients communicate information, set goals mutually, and then act to attain those goals—is also the basic assumption of the nursing process. King describes the steps of the nursing process as a system of interrelated actions and identifies concepts from her work that provide the theoretical basis for the nursing process as method.

According to King, *Assessment* occurs during the interaction of the nurse and client, who are likely to meet as strangers. Assessment may be viewed as paralleling action and reaction. The concepts King identifies are the perception, communication, and interaction of nurse and client. The nurse brings knowledge of self and perceptions of the problems that are of concern. Assessment, interviewing and communication skills are needed by the nurse as is the ability to integrate knowledge of natural and behavioural sciences for application to a concrete situation.

All concepts of the theory apply to assessment, growth and development, knowledge of self and role, and the amount of stress influence perception and in turn influence communication, interaction, and transaction. In assessment, the nurse needs to collect data about the client's level of growth and development, view of self, perception of current health status, communication patterns, and role socialization, among other things. Factors influencing the client's perception include the functioning of the client's sensory system, age, development, sex, education, drug and diet history, and understanding of why contact with the health care system is occurring. The perceptions of the nurse are influenced by the cultural and socio-economic background and age of the nurse and the diagnosis of the client. Perception is the basis for gathering and interpreting data, thus the basis for assessment. Communication is necessary to verify the accuracy of perceptions, without communication, interaction and transaction cannot occur.

The information shared during assessment is used to derive a *Nursing Diagnosis*, defined by King as a statement that "identifies the disturbances, problems, or concerns about which patients seek help". The implication is that the nurse makes the nursing diagnosis as a result of the mutual sharing with the client during assessment. Stress may be a particularly important concept in relation to nursing diagnosis because stress, disturbance, and problem or concern may be closely connected.

After the nursing diagnosis is made, *Planning* occurs. King says that the concepts involved are *decision-making* about goals and *exploring means* and *identifying means* to attain goals. King describes planning as setting goals and making decisions about how to achieve these goals. This is part of transaction and again involves mutual exchange with the client. She specifies that clients are requested to participate in decision making about how the goals are to be met. Although King assumes that in nurse-client interactions clients have the right to participate in decisions about their care, she does not say they have the responsibility. Thus, clients are requested to participate, not expected to do so.

Implementation occurs in the activities that seek to meet the goals. Implementation is a continuation of transaction in King's theory. She states that the concept involved is the making of *transactions*.

Evaluation involves descriptions of how the outcomes identified as goals are attained. In King's (1981/1990a) description, evaluation not only speaks to the attainment of the client's goals but also to the effectiveness of nursing care. She also indicates that the involved concept is goal attainment or, if not, why not.

Although all the theory concepts apply throughout the nursing process, communication with perception, interaction, and transaction are vital for goal attainment and need to be apparent in each phase. King emphasizes the importance of mutual participation in interaction that focuses on the needs and welfare of the client and of verifying perceptions while planning and activities to achieve goals are carried out together. Although King emphasizes mutuality, she does not limit it to verbal communication, nor does she require the client's active participation in actions to achieve goal attainment.

In a *Theory of Nursing*, King presents an application of her theory of goal attainment that she identifies as the use of a goal-oriented nursing record. Her description of this goal-oriented nursing record closely parallels the steps of the nursing process.

King's Work and the Characteristics of a Theory

King has stated that she has derived a theory of goal attainment from her open system framework of personal, interpersonal, and social systems. How her work compares with the characteristics of a theory presented and discussed below.

1. Theories can interrelate concepts in such a way as to create a different way of looking at a particular phenomenon. King has interrelated the concepts of interaction, perception, communication, transaction, self, role, stress, growth and development, time, and space into a theory of goal attainment. Her theory deals with a nurse-client dyad, a relationship to which each person brings personal perceptions of self, role, and personal levels of growth and development. The nurse and client communicate, first in interaction and then in transaction, to attain mutually set goals. The relationship takes place in space identified by their behaviours and occurs in forward-moving time. In particular, the specification of transaction as dealing with mutual goal attainment is a different way of looking at the phenomenon of nurse-client relationships.

2. Theories must be logical in nature. King's theory of goal attainment does describe a logical sequence of events. For the most part, concepts are clearly defined. However, a major inconsistency within her writing is the lack of a clear definition of environment, which is identified as a basic concept for the framework from which she derives her theory. In addition, she indicates that nurses are concerned about the health care of groups but concentrates her discussion on nursing as occurring in a dyadic relationship. Thus, the theory essentially draws on only two of the three systems described in the conceptual framework. The social systems portion of the framework is less clearly connected to the theory of goal attainment than the personal and interpersonal systems. The definition of stress always implies that it is both negative and positive, but discussion of stress always implies that it is negative. Finally, King says that the nurse and client are strangers, yet she speaks of their working together for goal attainment and of the importance of health maintenance. Attainment of long-term goals, such as those concerning health maintenance is not consistent with not knowing each other.

3. Theories should be relatively simple yet generalizable. Although the presentation appears to be complex, King's theory of

goal attainment is relatively simple. Ten concepts are identified, defined, and their relationships considered; two concepts are identified only. Even though King indicates that many of the concepts are situation-dependent, they are not situation specific; that is, they are influenced by the situation but may occur in many different situations. The theory of goal attainment is limited in setting only in regard to "natural environment" and, with growth and development as a major concept, is certainly not limited in age. They theory of goal attainment is generalizable to any dyadic nursing situation with a possible limitation relating to difficulties associated with seeking mutual goal setting with a client who has an external locus of control. The emphasis on mutuality would initially appear to limit the theory to dealing with those clients who can verbally interact with the nurse and physically participate in implementations to meet goals. However, King points to observable behaviours and to both verbal and nonverbal communication. Indeed, even the comatose individual has observable behaviours in the form of vital signs and does communicate nonverbally. The major limitation in relation to the characteristic is the effort required of the reader to sift through the presentation of a conceptual framework and a theory with repeated definitions to find the basic concepts. Another limitation relates to the lack of development of application of the theory in provided nursing care to groups, families or communities.

4. Theories can be the basis for hypotheses that can be treated or for theory to be expanded. King (1990) presents the following hypotheses that she states are being tested:

- Mutual goal setting will increase ability to perform activities of daily living.
- Mutual goal setting by nurse and patient leads to goal attainment.
- Goal attainment will be greater in patients who participate in goal setting than those who do not participate in goal setting.
- Mutual goal setting will increase elderly patients' morale.
- Perceptual congruence in nurse-patient interactions increases mutual goal setting.
- Goal attainment decreases stress and anxiety in nursing situations.
- Congruence in role expectations and role performance increases transactions in nurse-patient interactions.

These and other hypotheses could be used to test the theory.

5. Theories contribute to and assist in increasing the general body of knowledge within the discipline through the research implemented to validate them. King reports the results of a descriptive study conducted to test the theory of goal attainment. The study resulted in a classification system to analyze nurse-patient interactions and found that goal attainment is facilitated when the nurse and patient have accurate perceptions, adequate communication, and set goals mutually. She also states that data about interactions from two separate studies have confirmed the presence of transactions. Studies reported in the literature include using King's conceptual framework and/or theory of goal attainment to investigate nurse's attitude

towards the elderly, attending behaviour and mental status measurements promoting postoperative participation in self-care (used in conjunction with Orem's theories), and parenting; These are examples of contributions to the general body of knowledge. The theory of goal attainment needs to be tested further. Such testing will expand the theory's contribution to the discipline.

6. Theories can be used by practitioners to guide and improve their practice. As demonstrated in the discussion of nursing process, King's theory of goal attainment can be used as a guide to practice, King has also developed the goal-oriented nursing record in an effort to assist the practice of nursing. She presents the goal-oriented nursing record as an application of the theory of goal attainment in nursing. She has also developed a criterion-referenced tool for measuring attainment of health goals. Others have reported the use of King's work in nursing curricula.

7. Theories must be consistent with other validated theories, laws, and principles but will leave open unanswered questions that need to be investigated. King's theory of goal attainment is not in apparent conflict with other validated theories, laws and principles. She has clearly documented the sources on which she has based her characteristics and definitions of concepts, and she states that "the major technique used in developing concepts... has been a review of the literature in nursing and related fields to identify characteristics of the concept. From this information, an operational definition of the concept is formulated. Using the review of the literature as a base has helped to avoid being in conflict with others. King shares many similarities with other nursing theorists. As does Peplau, King indicates that the nurse and client usually enter the relationship as strangers when the client has a need. King's basic assumptions about human beings as thinking, sentient decision makers who have a right to information and to participation in decisions about themselves has a humanistic base similar to that of Paterson and Zderad (1975). The emphasis on the right to participate in decisions is similar to that of Orlando among others.

Throughout *A Theory of Nursing*, King identifies those theories from other fields that support what she is saying. Although there is no apparent conflict, many questions are open for exploration. A few of these are discussed in the hypotheses presented earlier in this chapter.

King derived the Goal Oriented Nursing Record (GONR), based on L.L. Weed's problem Oriented Medical Record (POMR), from Goal Attainment Theory. A method of collecting data, identifying care, it has been used effectively in patient settings. King states, "Nurses who have knowledge of the concepts of this theory of goal attainment are able to accurately perceive what is happening to patients and family members and are able to suggest approaches for coping with the situations." "The theory and the GONR are useful in practice as nurses have the ability to provide individualized plans of care while encouraging active participation from clients in the decision making phase." The GONR is one approach to document effectiveness of nursing care.

King's conceptual framework was recently used at Ohio State University for curriculum design in the nursing program, and presently the graduate program at the University of Texas at Houston is doing the same. The Department of Medical-Surgical Nursing at Loyola University in Chicago was using portions of King's steps of nursing process at the graduate level. In 1980, Brown and Lee noted that King's concepts were useful in developing a framework "for use in nursing education, nursing practice, and for generating hypotheses for research... It provides a systematic means of viewing the nursing profession, organizing a body of knowledge for nursing, and clarifying nursing as a discipline." Shirley Steel used King's framework as the framework for her book, Child Health and the Family.

"Research can be designed and conducted to implement this system in a hospital unit, in ambulatory care, in community nursing and home care. This information system can be designed for any patient population and for current and future computerization of records in health care systems." In a telephone interview King provided more examples of how her conceptual framework and her GONR are presently being or will soon be used in nursing practice and research. King has said that she would be happy to assist students in testing her theory and working with faculty developing curriculum from her conceptual framework. Polit and Hunger cite her theory in giving examples and discussing different aspects of the research process.

Because this theory was published only in 1981, there has been little time for digesting, testing, and evaluating. King is coinvestigator with a colleague, Dr. Ross, in a study of goal attainment related to functional abilities in residents in two nursing homes.

While maintaining her position as a professor at the University of South Florida, King serves as a consultant and continues to expand her GONR in diverse situations. She states, "Any profession that has its primary mission in the delivery of social services requires continuous research to discover new knowledge that can be applied to improve practice... The basis for the practice of nursing is knowledge; its activity is guided by the intellect, and applied in the practical realm."

EVALUATION OF THEORY

- King's theory presents nine major concepts, thus making the theory complex. The concepts are easily understood because they are defined to show interrelations in nursing practice.

  Some of the definitions of the basic concepts are derived from research literature. King's definition of stress states that stress has positive consequences. She gives examples of the negative effects of stress on patients with sensory deprivation and sensory overload.

  King maintains that her definitions are clear and conceptually derived from the identified characteristics.

- King's theory has been criticized for having limited application in areas of nursing where patients are unable to interact competently with the nurse. However, King maintains that she has made transactions with comatose patients; nurse midwives have made transactions with newborns; and psychiatric nurses have applied the knowledge of her theory to make transactions with psychiatric patients. Its use with groups has not been clarified.

King responds that 80 per cent of communication is nonverbal. She says, "Try observing a really good nurse interact with a baby or a child who has not yet learned the language. If you systematically recorded your observations, you would be able to analyze the behaviours and find many transactions at a nonverbal level. I have a beautiful example of that when I was working side by side with a graduate student in a neuro unit with a comatose patient. I was talking to the patient, explaining everything that was happening and showing the graduate student what I believe to be important in nursing care. When the patient regained consciousness a few days later, she asked the nurse in the unit to find that wonderful nurse who was the only one who explained what was happening to her. She wanted to thank her. I made transactions. I could observe her muscle movement. She was trying to help us as a physician poked a tube down her throat. A nurse midwife reports observing transactions between mothers and newborns. Psychiatric nurses have reported to me the value of my theory in their practice. So the need in nursing is to broaden nurses' Knowledge of communication and that is what my theory is all about.

King believes critics are assuming that a theory will address every person, event, and situation, which is impossible. She reminds critics that even Einstein's theory of relativity could not be tested completely until space travel made testing possible.

- King has gathered empirical data on the nurse-patient interaction process that leads to goal attainment. A descriptive study was conducted to test the goal attainment theory. From a sample of 17 patients, goals were attained in 12 cases (70% of the sample). If nursing students were taught the goal attainment theory, and if it were used in nursing practice, goal attainment could be measured along with the effectiveness of nursing care.

Because King's theory is relatively new, empirical testing is in the beginning stages, and it remains to be seen if relationships exist between the concepts. The Twenty-Seventh Annual Research Conference at the University of South Florida College of Nursing in February of 1988 was titled "Building knowledge for Nursing: Testing king's Theory." This was truly an international conference with presentations by nurses from Canada, Sweden, the United States, and Japan.

King is presently acting as a consultant to researchers testing hypotheses derived from her theory, in addition to conducting her research to test her theory. She hopes researchers will continue to do more testing of the theory.

- For theory to be useful in nursing practice, it should focus on at least one aspect of the nursing process. King's theory focusses on the planning and implementation phases of the nursing process. The nurse-patient dyad interact, devise mutually agreed-on goals, explore means to achieve goals, transact, and attain goals.

King maintains that her theory focusses on all aspects of the nursing process (assess, plan, implement, evaluate [APIE]), but her process is the theoretical basis for the Yura and Walsh process as method. King compares her process model, the Yura and Walsh nursing process model, and the scientific method by identifying the elements of each of the four processes and their similarities. She believes one must assess to set mutual goals, plan to provide alternate means to achieve goals, and evaluate to determine if the goal was attained. King says she is "the only one who has provided a theory that deals with choices, alternatives, participation of all individuals in decision making and specifically deals with outcomes of nursing care." Her theory is being used to implement theory based practice in several areas of nursing practice in Canada and the United States. King is presently working with a colleague to derive a theory of administration for nursing from her conceptual systems model.

Chapter 12

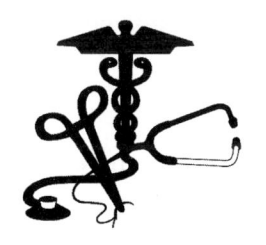

Paterson and Zderad Theory of Humanistic Nursing

The person is unique being, extant in all nursing situations, who innately struggles– to know. Humanistic nursing is an existential experience of being and doing so that nurturance with another occurs. Fundamentally, nursing is a response to human need that can be described to build a humanistic nursing science.

Humanistic nursing requires that the participants be aware of their uniqueness, as well as their commonality with others. Authenticity is required an in-touchness with self that comes in part with experiencing. Humanistic nursing also presupposes responsible choices. The ability of an individual to make choices based on authentic awareness and knowledge of such choices is a concern of humanistic nursing and cultivates moreness. Also, a commitment to the value of humanistic nursing must be present.

A nurse with the foregoing attitudes and qualities can offer genuine presence to another. Humanistic nursing concerns the basic nursing act: the response of one human in need to another. At this level nursing is related to the health-illness quality of the human condition: nurturance toward more being.

Josephine G. Paterson and Lorett T. Zderad began theorizing about the nature of nursing admist the clamor within the profession to develop a scientific basis of nursing practice. They have described what they call a "humanistic nursing practice" theory in several publications and presentations. The development of this theory won response to a call from within themselves to search for and articulate the meaning and value of their own nursing practices. Nursing "undescribed and unappreciated" is nursing inadequately conceptualised and uncommunicated to others. This, their personal call resonated with the call within the profession of nursing to explicate the nature and significance of nursing as professional discipline. Both (Paterson and Zderad) were among the pioneers in nursing who readily understood the value and nature of theory in practice discipline and responded by developing a method of theorizing that is congruent with the practice of nursing.

EVOLUTION OF THEORY

Theory is the articulated vision of experience (R.D. Laing) Zderad stresses the meaning of each key word in Laing's definition of theory.
- Articulated means that theory is expressed in an enduring form, so that it can be shared with others and also means that the connectedness among the concepts in the theory is evident.
- *Vision* refers to the heuristic nature of theory, it calls us forth to enact the possibilities as envisioned by the theory and goes beyond merely summarizing past concrete experience.
- *Experience* refers to the nurses lived acts as a nurse in the health illness community from multiple vantage points.

This means that nursing practice is the basis for what we believe about nursing. Our experience in the world of health care in the foundation for understanding the nature of nursing and what it means to be a nurse. These theorist maintain that nursing theory is valued resource for nurses as education, practitioners and researchers and for the humanity in general.

Paterson and Zderad convey their vision of nursing expressed as "humanistic nursing practice theory and general theory of nursing. In addition, they provide a rich metatheoretical landscape from which other theories can be sculpted. Paterson defined "metatheory" as a systematized body of knowledge formulated for the purpose of making something else possible." The most general forms of nursing phenomena of concern have been asserted by some nursing scholars to form the metaparadigm of nursing. Flaskerad and Hallman (1980) have termed the four elements, of nurse, person, health and environment areas of agreement in nursing theory.

Humanistic nursing is nursing's response to the humanistic movement and psychology which was seen as an alternative to the two dominant psychologic view of the time. **Freudian** psychology was seen on being too limited in its orientation towards the sick personality, and **behavioural** psychology was seen as being too mechanistically oriented. The humanistic orientation tries to take a broader view of the potential of human beings, trying to understand them from the context of their experience of living in the world.

It is not so easy to define the essence of humanistic nursing, because it is concerned with the phenomenological experiences of individuals, the exploration of human experience. It requires that who enters the nursing situation should be fully aware of the lenses, that they wear. They need to know what values, biases, myths and expectations they bring to the nursing experiences. And they need to fully appreciate what values, biases, myths and expectation to others bring to the nursing experience. The combination of these perspectives brings uniqueness to nursing.

The practice of nursing is rooted in existential thought. Existentialism is philosophical approach to understanding life. Individuals are faced with possibilities when making choices. These choices determine the direction and meaning of one's life. Like humanistic psychology, existentialism was a response to the dominant philosophies of the positivism and determinism. The early writings of existentialisms provided a basis for viewing human existence in individually meaningful terms. By having the opportunity for choice, each act we choose is significant and gives meaning to our lives. One of the criticism levelled against existentialism has been that it presents a despairing view of life. Since individuals are faced with freedom of choice, there is always the possibility for making errors. For example, imagine the experience of being an adolescent making career and personal choices while facing developmental needs of autonomy, identity, body image, and peer acceptance. Intimacy, sexual activity, success, independence, contraception, fear of failure, risk taking, and needs for intimacy all play a part in the daily experience of middle to late adolescent and influence the eventual outcome of this time of life. Consequently, individuals experience dread as well as hope, in the possible consequences of their actions.

Several propositions can be drawn from existential thought that have relevance for helping professions. Existentialism identified individual as:
- Having the capacity for self-awareness.
- Having freedom and responsibility.
- Striving to find their own identity while being in relation with others.
- Being involved in a search for meaning in life.
- Having to experience anxiety or dread if they are going to assume responsibility for their own lives, and
- Being aware of the reality of death in order to experience the significant of living.

Consequently when living in the world, there are many possibilities and the responsibility for making the most out of the existence, rests within each; as a philosophy, existentialism is particularly applicable to nursing within the framework of holistic health, because of the emphasis on self determination, free choice and self responsibility.

Phenomenology, the study of the meaning of a phenomenon to a particular individual, is often thought to have had a significant influence on the development of existentialism because, existentialism requires an analysis of the human situation from the perspective of the individual's own experience. When combined with humanism into an existential-phenomenological-humanistic approach, which refer to reverence for life that values the need for human interaction in order to determine the meaning that comes from the individual's unique way of experiencing the world. Although we are ultimately alone in choosing the pathis, our lives will take, we can find meaning in sharing our experiences with others who are also facing the uncertain choices of daily living. This means that we as nurses must acknowledge our own struggle and needs as a part of the process of living. Simultaneously, we must acknowledge the importance of the struggles and needs of others only by the interaction of sharing with others, of recognizing the human experience, that is unique for each of us but also shared, can we really enter into a humanistic nursing practice.

While developing humanistic nursing theory, Paterson and Zderad have been influenced by the writings of existentialists, humanistic psychologists and on the basis of their years of experience, in clinical nursing, reflection and exploration of these experiences as they have been lived with psychiatric clients, students, nurses, and others helping professionals.

Paradigm and Theory on Humanistic Nursing

- **Human Being** Paterson and Zdedard's view of persons is meant to apply to both the Nurse and the Patient and can be thought of as flashing out their implicit assumptions.
- Human beings viewed from an existential framework of becoming through choices. (Freedom).
- Man is an individual being necessary related to other men in time and space.
- As every man is beholden to other men for his birth and development, interdependent is inherent in the human situations (adequacy).
- Human existence is coexistence.
- Human beings are characterized as being capable, open to option, persons with values and unique manifestations of their past, present and future (uniqueness).
- It is through relationship with others that human beings become, which in turn allows for each person's unique individuality to become actualised (Relatedness).

Implications for nursing practice are clear. People need information. They need options. Individuals and groups need opportunities to make their own choices.

Health

Paterson and Zderad (1978) viewed health as a matter of personal survival, as a quality of living and dying. It is described as being more than the absence of disease. Individuals have the potential for well-being but also for more being. Well-being implies a steady state, whereas more-being refers to being in the process of becoming all that is humanly possible.

This conceptualization of health implies that disease, medical diagnosis or any form of labelling does little to determine a person's capacity for health. Health can be found in a person's willingness to open to the experiences of life regardless of his or her physical, social, spiritual, cognitive or emotional status. Implications for nursing practice include being open to wide range of definition of Health Diagnostic categories are useful only if agreed to by the person to whom they refer. The relationship is very essential that the nurse has with the person receiving care, is critical, but even more essential is the need for an appreciation of relationship that exist in daily living. By understanding the existential premise of humanistic theory, it become apparent that health is a process of finding meaning in life, as it is experienced in the process of living, of being involved in each movement.

Nursing

Nurse as a person means one who responds to the call of human beings, with needs within health-illness quality of life. The nursing act is an always related to the health-illness quality of the human condition, or fundamentally to man's sick personal survival that nothing related to health and illness is evident. Nursing then, is seen within the human context. It is a nurturing responses of one person to another in a time of need that aims towards the development of well-being and more-being. Nursing works towards the aim by helping to increase the possibility of making responsible choices, since this is how human beings are able to become.

The nursing situation is a particular kind of human situation in which the inter human relating is purposely directed towards nurturing the well-being of person with perceived needs related to health-illness quality of living. Nursing is concerned with the individual's unique being and striving toward becoming... Nursing focusses on the whole and looks beyond the categorization of the parts. For example, when person changes influence the person's world and the experiences of being in the world. The client's prospective of the world is a vital consideration in nursing.

Nursing is described as a unique blend of art and science. Science and arts both play critical roles in humanistic nursing practice. If one thinks, when nurses performing activities related to thermoregulations maintaining fluid and electrolytic balance, stages of grieving and growth of development, they follow principles or rules based on science, which will guide to their practice. Here the application of scientific principles laws effectually in the nursing situation is an art. Nursing is an art is being able to use theories within the context of life as people struggle to become all that they are capable of becoming.

ELEMENTS OF HUMANISTIC NURSING

The elements of the framework for humanistic nursing as stated by Paterson and Zderad may be described as follows:

"Incarnate men (patient and nurse) meeting (being and becoming) is a goal directed (nurturing well-being and more being), intersubjective transaction (being with and doing with) occurring in time and space (as measured and as lived by patient and nurse) in a world of men and things.

To use this framework for a nursing practice theory, it has been suggested three concepts together provide the basis or components of nursing, which includes—dialogue, community, and phenomonologic nursology.

Nursing as Dialogue

The notion of nursing as a dialogue conveys the back and forth ebb and flow of nursing. Nursing cannot take place without the nursed (patient). Within this image of nursing, the nursing lived as a "purposeful call and response." So, nursing is a lived dialogue. It is the nurse-nurses relating creatively. Humans need nursing. Nurses need to nurse. Nursing is an intersubjective experience in which there is real sharing. Involved in this dialogue are meeting, relating, presence, call and response.

Relating

The process of nurse-nursed 'doing with each other' is relating. There are two ways of relating which includes subject-object relating. *Subject-object* relating refers to how human beings are objects and know others through abstractions, conceptualisation, categorizing, labelling and so on. *Subject-subject* relating occurs when two persons are open to each other as fully human. Through the scientific objective approach, that is subject object relating, it is possible to gain certain knowledge about a person; through intersubjective approach, it is possible to know a person in his unique individuality. Thus, both relationships are essential to clinical nursing process. Both are the integral elements of humanistic nursing.

Presence

It refers to the quality of being open, receptive, ready and available to another person, in a reciprocal manner. Presence necessitates being open to the whole of the nursing experience, behaviour that is difficult to achieve when the nurse at times is required to focus on specific details of the client's body and/or behaviour. Man is an embodied being and the nurse is nurturing the patients well being and more being, must relate to him and his body, in them mysterious interrelatedness.

Call and Response

The complex nature of the lived dialogue is seen in call and response. Call and response are transactional, sequential and simultaneous. Nurses and clients call and respond to each other both verbally and non-verbally and there is the potential to be "all-at-once." All-at-once means, as nurses being able to relate simultaneously to the subjective and objective aspects of the lived situation.

Thus it is understood that it is through nursing acts that the dialogue of nursing is lived. The meaning of those acts to the nurse and the client may differ and may act as a potential catalysts, for effecting change in the dialogue. When considering nursing as dialogue, it is necessary to take into account the situation in which it occurs in the real world of others, human beings and things, within a framework of time and space.

Community

The nurse-patient relationship defined as a form of community. It is two or more persons struggling toward a common centre, i.e., struggling together, living-dying all at once. To understand community is to recognize and value uniqueness. Humanistic nursing leads to community. It occurs within the community and is affected by community. It is through inter-subjective sharing of meaning in community that human beings are comforted and nurtured. Community is experience of persons and it is through community, persons relating to others that it is possible to become. Community is considered "We", that occurs with clients, families, professional colleagues, and other health care providers.

Phenomenologic Nursology

Nursology is the name given to a process of scientific inquiry in nursing, that was first introduced by Paterson in 1971. She defined it as "the study of nursing aimed towards the development of nursing theory." Further, it has been viewed as a form of phenomenology. So named, it as "Phenomenologic nursology". There are five phases in this approach as follows:

- *Phase 1. Preparation of the knower:* It is the preparation of the nurse knower for coming to know. The nurse is ever prepared and striving to be open and caring. This involve learning to take risks, being open to experience, to one's own view of the world, and to another's perceptual framework. To achieve this, the nurse needs to be exposed to a wide range of experiences. Nurses can be prepared for this by immersing themselves in studies in the humanities, where varying views about the nature of being are expressed.
- *Phase 2. Knowing other intuitively:* It is the nurse knowing other intuitively, refers to the intuitive aspects of knowing in which the knower grasps the whole of the other through an imaginative process of getting

in touch with the others "rhythm and mobility." This phase on the merging of the self with the rhythmic spirit of the other. Intuitive knowing of the other requires getting "inside" the other into the rhythm of the other's experience, which results in a special, difficult to express, knowledge of the other. Intuitive knowing presumes the I-thou relationship (Buber, 1958) of nursing situation, several steps to be taken to facilitate openness.

- *Phase 3. Knowing the other scientifically:* It is the nurse, knowing the other scientifically. This phase highlights the kind of knowing that is a "look at." It implies a separateness from which is known. It requires taking the all-at-once phenomena that are known intuitively and looking at them, mulling them over, analysing, sorting, comparing, contrasting, relating, interpreting, giving a name to and categorizing them. This is taking the *I-thou* and reflecting it as an *I-It*. The challenge of communicating a lived nursing reality demands authenticity with the self and rigorous efforts in relation of words, phrases and precise grammar. To achieve this goal, the nurse must be adequately prepared in the liberal arts and sciences. Nurses need to be able to reflect critically on the experience at the same time that they are immersed in the experience communication skills are critical as the nurse seeks clarification and verification from the client.

- *Phase 4. Complimentary synthesis:* It is the nurse complementing synthesizing known others. This phase involves relating, comparing and contrasting what occurs in nursing situations to enlarge one's understanding of nursing. The nurse compares and synthesizes multiple known realities and arrives at an expanded view.

The nurse allows a dialogue between realities and permits differences. Here the nurse uses not only personal experiences but also the right theoretical foundation of education and practice in order to put the clinical situation in perspectives.

- *Phase 5. Succession from the "we" by "the many" to the "paradoxical one":* This is succession with the nurse from the many to the paradoxical one. This phase evolves from the descriptive process of a lived phenomenon. It is the articulated vision of experience that becomes expressed in a coherent whole. This phase is the process of refining the intuitive grasp achieved before, struggling with the known realities, and making an intuitive leap towards truth, thus forming a new hypothetical construct. Since the multiple realities and known truths are part of the nurse, the new truth is part of the nurse, the new truth is really an expression of the knower in abstract or conceptual terms beyond the individual data. It is a truth beyond the synthesis of whole. So, the paradox rests in the fact, that the nurse starts with a general notion, an intuitive grasp; then studies it, compares, contrasts and synthesizes it in order to arrive at truth, that is uniquely personal, but has meaning for all; a descriptive theoretical construct of nursing.

The last three phases can be termed as analysis, synthesis and description, phases involve many of the same techniques.

Nursing Process and Phenomenologic Nursology

Nursing Process and Nursology are similar and many aspects. Both use a systematic approach to client interactions.

Assessments

The first phase of nursology differs from nursing process. But assessment requires preparation of the Knower (Nurse). Almost all nurses are educated in the nurses are educated in the humanities and sciences prior to starting nursing practice in the clinical situation, and nurse has a sensitivity to and knowledge of human condition as well as self-knowledge.

The second phase "knowing the other intuitively, needed is prior to traditional assessment phase of nursing process. This phase is characterized by a "taking in" of the client in the human situation, the empathetic encounter, the beginning of the I-thou relationship, wherein the nurse understands the other's experience all-at-once. The use of intuition is vital to assessment.

The third phase, knowing other scientifically is comparable to the assessment and early analysis phase of the nursing process. This phase of nursology includes the more familiar method of looking at phenomenon from many aspects: comparing, clarifying and looking for themes in relationships and among parts, by dividing person into biological, psychological, social and spiritual.

The later state of analysis in the nursing process are quite similar to the phase of nursology called "complementary synthesis." Here, nurse compares the data with other known realities such as developmental stages, Maslow's hierarchy of needs, and physiological principles. In other words, the nurse examines the data and experience of the client in light of scientific and subjective knowledge and then compares, contrasts and ultimately synthesizes to an expanded view, which helps to identify the problems.

Nursing Diagnosis

Diagnosis refers to the step of nursing process in which the nurse makes a problem statement. The nurse stating the problem after careful collection of data, analysis and comparing and coming to a conclusions on basis of her education and experience after synthesizing the ideas, data and experience.

Planning and Implementation

The planning and implementation phases of the nursing process describes goal or outcome to be reached by the client with step (objectives) to be accomplished toward goal. Nursology does not describe the goal-directed nursing care plan. Humanistic nursing is concerned with being with another who is in need. The goal of more-being or well-being is accomplished through dialogue. In the dialogue between nurse and nursed, there is meeting in the presence of the nurse for other and the call and response between the nurse and the nursed. The I-thou relationship. This is the repeated relationship. This relationship takes place in the nursing situation in the real world; however they do not elaborate on incorporating the "doing" aspects of nursing into the dialogue.

Evaluation

The evaluation phase is deciding whether client's behaviour has changed as measured by the goals and objectives. The behaviour changes result from the action of the nurse and client. By nature of being humanistic, the concern is now with the resultant behaviour but with the meaning of the experience for the client. The humanistic nurse might see a change in the client. Perspective of his or her experience, a client who is able to make choices about health care activities and assume responsibilities for those choices would be able to find meaning in life. by doing this with a nurse, the client would have the opportunity to affirm the humanness of the situation from his or her own perspective, resulting in personal growth, more being or health.

Paterson and Zderad's Work and the Characteristics of a Theory

1. Theories can interrelate concepts in such a way as to create a different way of looking at a particular phenomenon. Paterson and Zderad say, that nursing is a lived dialogue between the nurse and the nursed directed toward, the goal of nurturing well-being and more-being in the everyday world of men and things. The authors have interrelated the four concepts of human beings, health, nursing, and society, so that a different way of looking at the phenomenon of nursing has been created for using existential philosophy and phenomenological methodology within a humanistic framework. Nursing is described as an intersubjective transaction that has a new and different description of nursing although it is similar in concept to other nursing theories. Theories describe, explain, or predict phenomena. Humanistic nursing theory is descriptive; the phenomenological approach is a descriptive method.

2. Theories must be logical in nature. Humanistic nursing theory is logical because Paterson and Zderad provide a framework and methodology for nursing in practice. also, the ideas and concepts fit together in a meaningful way.

3. Theories should be relatively simple yet generalizable. Humanistic nursing theory is not simple; indeed it is somewhat difficult to grasp unless the nurse is familiar with existential philosophy and phenomenology. The theory focuses on the dialogue between the nurse and the nursed as a unique encounter between two people. Knowledge gained by repeated study of this encounter provides a generalizable concept. In fact, the final step of nursology is the expression of a concept. Thus the theory is generalizable.

4. Theories can be the bases for hypotheses that can be tested or for theory to be generated, and

5. Theories contribute to and assist in increasing the general body of knowledge within the discipline through the research implemented to validate them. Paterson and Zderad's theory provides a basis for hypotheses that can be tested. The authors describe several replications of the methodology and present numerous concepts that could be examined. Since it is testable, phenomenologic nursology is an excellent medium for concept and theory development.

6. Theories can be used by practitioners to guide and improve their practice. Humanistic nursing theory, including phenomenologic nursology, can certainly be used by nurses to guide and improve

practice. Although nurses may find the concepts new at first, a study of humanistic psychology and existential philosophy facilities an understanding of the concepts and an appreciation of human potential.

7. Theories must be consistent with other validated theories, laws and principles but will leave open unanswered questions that need to be investigated. Humanistic nursing theory is consistent with existentialism, humanistic psychology, and phenomology upon which it is based. Because the theory is descriptive and generalizable, it can be applied in any nursing situation always open for examination.

Chapter 13

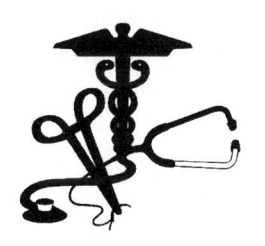

Erikson, Tomlin, Mary Ann's Theory of Modelling and Role Modelling

Helen C. Erikson, Evelyn M. Tomlin and **Mary Ann P. Swain** were instrumental in developing the theory of "Modelling and Role Modelling. The combination of talents of the three authors who collaborates at the university of Michigan in the mid-1970s was advantageous for the development of a nursing theory that was useful and related to practice, education and research. All three authors have been involved in nursing education. Two are expert nursing clinicians and remain actually involved in clinical practice and two remain active in research and scholarly pursuits.

THE THEORY OF MODELLING AND ROLE MODELLING

The theory of modelling and role modelling used psychological, cognitive, and biological theories on the theoretical base for the observation the theorists make regarding similarities and differences among individuals. The works of Abraham Maslow, Helen C. Erikson, Milton H. Erikson, Jean Pigget, George Engel and Hans Selye are salient on the development of the theory.

Modelling and role modelling is an interpersonal and interactive theory of nursing that requires the nurse to assess (model), plan (role model) and intervene (five aims of intervention) on the basis of client world. The nurse always acknowledges that uniqueness and individuality of the client and appreciates that individuals, at some level, know what makes them ill and which makes them well (self-care knowledge). Two additional concepts important in the theory are affiliated-individuation and adaptive potential.

Modelling

Modelling is the process used by the nurse to develop and understanding of the clients world as the client perceives at the way and perceives life and all of its aspects and components; the way an individual thinks, communicates, feels, believes and behaves;

and the underlying motivations and rationale for beliefs and behaviours—all these comprises the individuals model of the world. Modelling is both an art and science. The **art of modelling** is the empathetic development of an understanding of the present situation within the clients context of the world i.e., the development of "model" of the situation from the clients perspective. The **science of modelling** is the analysis of the information collected about the clients world. To truly understand the clients model of the world, the nurse must have a strong theoretical base in the physical and social science. The clients perspective is analysed on the basis of knowledge and theory regarding human behaviour, development, cultural diversity, interaction, pathophysiology, human needs and so forth.

Role Modelling

Role-modelling also both an art and science. The **art of role modelling** occurs when the nurse plans and implements interventions that are unique for the clients. It involves the individualization of care based on the clients model of world. The **science of role modelling** is the use of theoretical bases when planning and implementing nursing care. Role modelling is the facilitation of the individual in attaining, maintaining, or promoting health through purposeful interventions based on the individuals personal perceptions as well as the theoretical base for the practice of nursing.

Five Aims of Intervention

The aims of intervention based on five principles pertaining to similarities among human, which include the following:
1. The nursing process requires that a trusting and functional relationship exist between nurse and client (Building trust).
2. Affiliated-individuation is dependent on the individuals perceiving that he or she is an acceptable, respectable and worthwhile human being (Promote clients positive orientation).
3. Human development is dependent on the individuals perceiving that she or he has some control over her or his life, while concurrently sensing a state of affiliation (Promote clients control).
4. There is an innate drive towards holistic health that is facilitated by constitute and systemic nurturance (Affirm and promote clients strength).
5. Human growth is dependent on ratification of basic needs and facilitated by growth-need ratification (Set mutual goals that are health directed).

Individualized intervention are based on the clients model of the world and guided by the five aims of interventions defined as follows:
1. *Build trust:* Nursing requires a trusting relationship. This relationship involves honesty, acceptance, respect, empathy and belief in the clients model of the world. Therapeutic communication skills are essential in building trust. Trust is basic to any interpersonal relationship and is easily threatened if clients perceive that nurses lack respect for their view of world or fact that nurse consider the clients concerns or beliefs to be invalid, unwarranted, erroneous, or inappropriate.
2. *Promote positive orientation:* Nursing intervention need to promote clients self-worth as well as hope for the future. Reframing can be used to assist clients in changing their perceptions of a situations from one of threat to one of challenge from

one of hopelessness to one of hope, and from something negative to something positive.
3. *Promote perceived control:* Human development depends on individuals perceiving than they have some control over their lives. Nurses may understand that clients have control over what happens to them and may understand that clients are required to give informed consent for any procedure done to them. Generally patients will not perceive that they have any control. The responsibility of the nurses is not enough to promote control, but also must promote the clients perception of control.
4. *Promote strengths:* Identifications of strengths is a means of assisting clients to mobilize research. In the face of stressors, individual may become overwhelmed with their perceived weakness and not able to identify or use strengths.
5. *Set mutual goals that are health directed:* Nurses must use the individuals innate drive to be as healthy as he or she can be. The nurses and clients goals are the same to meet the clients basic needs. When the nurses and clients goals appear to differ, the nurse has most likely not fully modelled the clients world. Incomplete modelling can be the result of inadequate data gathering and empathy or a lack of knowledge for analysis and interpretation of the data collected.

Self-care

There are three aspects of self-care on the theory of modelling and re-modelling: self-care knowledge, self-care resources and self-care action.

Self-care Knowledge

Self-care is knowledge one has about "what has made him or her sick, lessened his or her effectiveness, or interfered with his or her growth. The person also known that will make him or her well, optimise his or her effectiveness or fulfilment (given circumstances), or promote his or her growth." Erickson (1990) found following four themes that relate to the nature of self-care knowledge includes:

1. An individuals perception of factors associated with his or her personal health problems are rarely obvious to the health care provider.
2. The individuals perceptions of what is needed to help him or her can best be defined by that person.
3. The nurses role is to facilitate clients to articulate what they perceive to be associated with their problem and what can be done to help them feel better.
4. Another nursing role is to assist the clients to resolve these problems in ways that meets personal needs and are health and growth directed.

Self-care Resources

All individual have internal and external resources (strengths and support) that will help gain, maintain, and promote an optimum level of holistic health. It is important for the nurse to assess these resources to assist the client in self-care action.

Self-care Action

Self-care action is the development and use of self-care knowledge and self-care resources. The basis of nursing is assisting clients in self-care actions related to health.

The self-care used in modelling and remodelling deficient of Orem's self-care theory. Orem's focuses on self-care in a universal needs met the ranging the ability of the care of ones self, nurses assists client and meeting self-care needs. When there is defect in the clients ability to meet the self-care needs. Modelling and remodelling theory focus on the individual personal knowledge about what makes him or her well or ill. All clients have self-care knowledge and nurse facilitates the clients identification and use of their knowledge.

Affiliated-individuation

Individuals have an instrumental need for affiliated-individuation. They need to be able to be dependent on support system while simultaneously maintaining independence from their support system. All individuals are seen as having simultaneous needs to be attached to other individuals and to be separate from them. This concept described in modelling and remodelling as "affiliated-individuation" are considered to be a motivation for human behaviour. Affiliated-individuation occurs where a person perceives himself or herself as simultaneously close to and separate from significant other.

Adaptive Potential

Adaptive potential refers to the individuals ability to mobilize resources to cope with stressors. The Adaptive Potential Assessment Model (APAM) 13.1 has the three categories. Equilibrium, arousal and impoverishment. Equilibrium has two possibilities: adaptive and maladaptive equilibrium. Arousal and impoverishment are both interstates. They differ in that those in impoverishment must seek to deal with stress with diminished, if not depleted, resources. Adaptive potentials in dynamic, and individuals can move from any of the three states to any other of the states. Movement among the states is influenced by the individual ability to cope. The APAM identifies states (not truth) of coping that can assist the nurse in planning interventions for the client. Adaptive potential has been well documented.

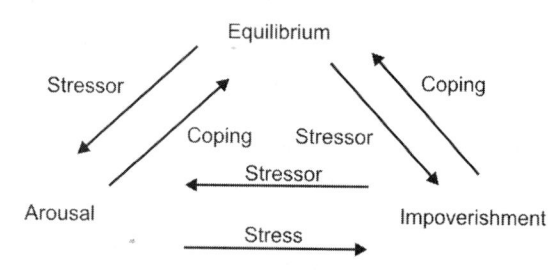

Figure 13.1: APAM model

Paradigm of Theory

Human Beings

Human beings are holistic persons with interacting subsystems (biophysical, psychological, social and cognitive) and inherent genetic bases and spiritual drive. Permeating all subsystems are the inherent bases. These include genetic makeup and spiritual drive. Body, mind, emotion and spirit are a total unit and they act together. They affect and control one another interactively. The intervention of the multiple subsystems, and the interests bases creates holism: Holism implies that the whole is greater than the some of the grats. People are seen on also in they are all holistic beings who wants to develop their potential. All individual have basic needs that motivate behaviour, including drive called affiliated-individuation. Although human beings are share these commonalities, each individual is unique. People differ from one another as a result of these individual inherited endowment, these situational ability to mobility these resources to respond to life stressors, and these models of the world. People are alike because of their holism, life stress growth and development and these need for affiliated-individuation. They are different because of their inherited endowment, adaptation and self-care knowledge.

Environment

Environment is not identified in the theory as an entity of its own. The theorist, seen environment in the social subsystems on the interaction between self and other, both cultural and individual. Biophysical stressors are seen as part of the environment. Environment on internal and external and include both stressors and resources for adopting to stressors. Stressors exist in life at all times and are necessary for overall growth and life enhancement. All individuals have both external and internal resources for dealing with stressors. Potential resources exist and individuals may need assistance in becoming aware of and constructively mobilizing them.

Health

Theorists consistence with that of WHO definition: "Health is a state of physical, mental and social well-being not merely the essence of disease or infirmity." The authors of this theory also writes that health connotes a state of dynamic equilibrium among the various subsystems. This dynamic equilibrium among the various subsystems. This dynamic equilibrium implies on adaptive equilibrium whereby individual learns to cope constructively with life stressors by mobilizing internal and external coping resources and leaving no subsystem in jeopardy when adaptation occurs.

Nursing

Nursing in the holistic helping of persons with that self-care activities in relation to their health. Nursing is a process between nurse and the client and requires an interpersonal and interactive nurse-client relationship. Three characteristics of the nurse in this theory are facilitation, nurturance and unconditional acceptance.

- Facilitation implies that the nurse help the individual to identify, mobilize and develop his or her own strengths.
- Nurturance is the fusing and integrating of cognitive, psychological and affective process with the action of assisting a client toward holistic health.
- Unconditional acceptance in the acceptance of each individual as unique, worthwhile, and important with no strings attached.

These theorists defined nursing as follows:

"Nursing is the holistic helping of persons with them self-care activities in relation to their health. This is an interactive, interpersonal process that nurses strength, to enable development, release and channelling of resources for coping with one's circumstances and environment. The goal is to achieve a state of perceived optimum health and consentment."

Additional statements to define nursing are the following:

- Nursing is the nurtherance of holistic self-care.
- Nursing in assisting persons holistically to use their adaptive strengths, to attain and maintain optimum biopsycho-socio-spiritual functioning.
- Nursing in helping with self-care to gain optimum health.
- Nursing is an integrated and integrative helping of persons to take better care for themselves.

Evaluation of Modelling and Role Modelling

There are two distinct meaning of nursing process acknowledge in the authors of this theory of Modelling and Re-modelling. The **first** is the formalized, step-by-step problem-solving process that includes gathering and analysing path, planning and implementing interventional and evaluating outcomes. The **second** is more basic use of the term and refers to an interactive process—the exchange between nurse and patient in which the nurse has purpose of the nurturing and supporting the clients self-care.

The theory of modelling and remodelling, emphasise the primary of the interaction interpersonal definition. Nursing involves an ongoing exchange of information feelings, and behaviours; the nursing process describes this exchange. Thus nursing process begins with the first interaction between nurse and patient. This theory accepts the view that nursing care begins with the first encounter because the nurses immediate contribution to care include the nurse himself or herself—the presence, the unconditional acceptance, and the support and comfort that are offered from one human being to another.

Since the theory directs the nurse to begin where the client is in modelling the clients world a comprehensive assessment in rarely done to initiate nursing care. The client will always be asked to express his or her questions, concerns, and needs. Client concerns have utmost priority because a person whose immediate needs are unattended will not progress in other ways. Thus, the theory directs the nurses priorities of care quite simply, beginning where the client requests care to begin, knowing that as one need is met, other unmet need will emerge to direct care. At any point, assumes as dictated by clients needs, and the nurse will gather whatever information required to understand and care of client expressed concerns. The interactive nursing process includes, formal, logical thinking.

When using the this theory there are no preset steps in applying the nursing process. Nurses provide care at the first moment of contact, they **assess** while they **implement**, that **analyze** while **evaluating**. Theorists write "when we view the nursing process predominating as an ongoing, interactive, interpersonal relationship that includes use of the formal scientific mode of thought, we can regard documentation of the nursing process primarily as a valuable way to communicate with others and keep records."

In providing care client data are gathered to model the clients world. An evaluation of the clients stress and adaptation is essential, as well as information on self-care knowledge, resources and actions. Diagnoses include adaptive potential, that is, the clients potential for mobilizing resources needed to contact with stressors. Theorists of the theory did not address the use of nursing diagnoses taxonomy developed by NANDA with Modelling and Remodelling.

While carrying out nursing care, the nurse must "role model", that is help client in attaining, maintaining, promoting health through purposeful interventions. Care is based on five aims of interventions and is consistent with the clients adaptive potential. The nurses role is to facilitate, nurture, and provide unconditional acceptance while assisting the client to achieve health. Evaluation and nursing care is directed towards goals mutually determined between patient and client.

Chapter 14

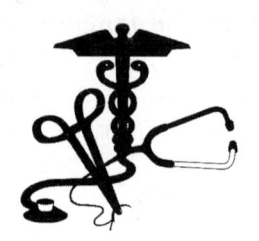

Boykin and Schoenhofer Theory of Nursing as Caring

Anne Boykin and Savina Schoenhofer (1993) write that work on their theory of "Nursing as caring" begin as 1983 as they worked together on curriculum development (a general new) and progressed overtime to an identification of the level of detail that led them to the label of a general theory of nursing. Major influences on the development of the theory are Maycroffs (1971) genetic discussion of caring and Roachs (1984) discussion of caring persons and caring in nursing. Roachs view of caring as process, rather than Maycroffs view of caring as end, is incorporated in the theory of 'Nursing as caring.'

Maycroffs caring ingredients are drawn in the theory of nursing caring, those ingredients are summarized by the these authors of nursing in caring includes the following:

- *Knowing:* Explicitly and implicitly, knowing that and knowing how, knowing directly and knowing indirectly.
- *Alternating rhythm:* Moving back and forth between narrower and wider framework, between action and reflection.
- *Patience:* Not a passive waiting but participating with the other giving fully of ourselves.
- *Honesty:* Positive concept that implies openness, genuineness and seeing truly.
- *Trust:* Trusting the other to grow his or her own time and own way.
- *Humility:* Ready and willing to learn more about other and self and what caring involves.
- *Hope:* An expression of plenitude of the present, alive with a sense of a possible.
- *Courage:* Taking risks, going into the unknown, trusting.

Theorists of this nursing as caring presents two major perspectives for theory are: (i) perception of persons as caring, and (ii) a conception of nursing as a discipline and profession.

Perception of Persons as Caring

The basic presence of nursing as caring in that all persons are caring. Seven major assumptions underlie the theory, as follows:

- Persons are caring by virtue of their humanisers.
- Persons are caring, moment to moment.
- Persons are whole or complete in the moment.
- Personhood is a process of living grounded in caring.
- Personhood is enhanced through participating in nurturing relationships with caring others.
- Nursing is both a discipline and a profession and
- Persons are viewed as already complete and continuously growing on completeness, fully caring and unfolding caring possibilities moment-to-moment.

The capacity for caring grows throughout ones life. Although the human is innately caring, not every human act is caring. Knowing oneself is caring person leads to a continuing commitment to know self and other as caring. This in turn leads to a moral obligation the quality of which is a "measure of being 'in place' on the world." The degree of authentic awareness of self as caring person influences how one is with others. It requires the coverage to let go of the present to discover new meaning about self and other.

Personhood, a process of living grounded in caring, recognizing the possibilities for caring in every moments and is enhanced through caring relationships with others. Caring-living in the context of relational responsibilities–responsibilities for self and other. the heat of the caring relationship is the importance of person-as-person. Viewing the person as a whole, as caring and complete, is intentional and does not provide for doidery, the other into parts or segments, such as mind, body, or spirit, at any time. The person, both self and other, is at all times whole. Unless the person is encountered as a whole, there is only a factual encounter. The person can be fully known as whole.

To understand the person as caring, one needs of focus on valuing to celebrate the wholeness of humans, to view humans as both living and growing in caring, and to actively seek engagements on personal level with others. The caring perspectives of human is basic to a view of nursing as an undertaking that focuses on humans, provides service from person to person, exerts because of a social need, and as a human science.

Conception of Nursing as a Discipline and Profession

The theory of nursing as caring is derived from a belief that nursing is both a discipline and a profession.

The discipline of nursing originates in the unique social call to which nursing is a response and involves being, knowing, living and valuing all at once. As a discipline, nursing is a unity of science, art and ethic. Discipline relates to all aspects of the development of nursing knowledge.

The profession of nursing is based on understanding the social need from which the call for nursing originates and the body of knowledge which is used in creating the response known on nursing. Professions are based in everyday human experiences and responses to one another.

Theory of Nursing as Caring

Theorists viewing nursing as "nurturing persons living, caring, growing and caring." Nursing is the response to the unique human need to be recognized as and supported in being, caring person. The nurse must know the person on caring person and take those nursing actions that seek to nurture the person in living and growing in caring.

The focus on nurturing persons living caring and growing is caring in broad in statement but specific to the individual situation in practice. As the nurse seeks to know the nurses who is having and growing in caring, the individuals unique ways of living caring become known. Although it is easy to identify instances of non-caring, it is the nurses commitment to discover the unique caring individual hopelessness, fear and anger and recognize these emotions as personal expressions of the caring value.

The nurse enters the world of the nursed with the intention and commitment to know the other as caring person. It is in knowing the other in this way than calls for nursing are heard. Knowing how other is living caring and expressing aspirations for growing in caring is as importance as knowing the other as caring person. The call for nursing is a call for a acknowledgement and affirmation of the person living caring in specific ways in this immediate situation. The nursing response to this call is a caring nurturance evidenced by specific caring responses to sustain and enhance the nursed is having caring and growing in caring in immediate situation. Theorists of this theory likes stress being in relationship to a **dance of caring** persons. The circle represents relating with respect for and valuing of the other in the basic dance to know self and other as caring person. Each dancer in the circle makes a contribution and moves within the dance as the nursing situation evolves. There is always room for more on the circle and dancers may move in or out as the nursed calls for services.

The nursing situations defined by the authors as and shared lived experience in which the caring between nurse and nursed enhances parenthood. The nursing situation is composed whenever a nurse engages in a situation from a nursing focus. It is the intention with which the situations, as approached and caring is expressed that creates the nursing situation and demonstrates nursing as caring.

The call for nursing comes from persons who are living caring and aspiring to grow in caring. The call is for nurturance through personal expression of caring. The nurse responds to the call of caring person, not to a lack of caring or to noncaring. The nurse brings to this response a deliberately developed, or expert, knowledge of which it means to be humane and to be caring, the nurse has made a commitment to recognize and nurture caring in all situations. Every nursing situation is original and differs from all others because each a lived experience that involves two individuals who do not have duplicates. The native of this lived experience is one of reciprocity with personal investment from both the nurse and nursed. Boykin and Schoenhofer identify the phenomenon that develops through the encountering of the nurse and the nursed as "caring between" when caring between occurs, personhood is nurtured.

It is important that in the theory of Nursing as Caring, the call for nursing is based on neither need or deficit. In this theory does not seek to report or wrong, solve a problem, meet a need to alleviate deficit. Rather nursing as caring in an egalitarian model of helping that celebrates the human and the fullness of being. Nursing responses areas varied as the calls for nursing.

or less automatic adjustments and adaptations to the "natural" focus impinging upon him.

It means that the individual is continuously presented with situations in everyday life, that require adaptation and adjustment. These adjustments are so natural that they occur without conscious effort by the individual.

3. That a behavioural system, which require and results in some degree of regularity and constancy in behaviour, is essential to man that is to say, it is fundamentally significant in that it serves a useful purpose both in social life and for the individual.

It means that the pattern of behaviour characteristics of the individual have purpose in the maintenance of homeostasis by the individual. The development of behavioural patterns that are acceptable to both society in the individual foster individual ability to adapt to minor changes in the environment.

4. The system balance reflects adjustments and adaptations that are successful in some way and to some degree. Achievement of this balance may and will vary from individual to individual. Most of individuals are flexible enough. However, to be on some state of balance that is "functional efficient and effective" for them.

The integration of these assumptions by the individual provides the behavioural system with the patterns of action to form "an organized, and integrated functional unit that determines and limits the interaction between the person and his environment and establishes the relationship of the person to the objects, events, and situations in his environment." The function of the behavioural system, that is to regulate the individual response to input from the environment so that the balance of the system can be maintained.

There are four assumptions made about the structure and function of each subsystem, which are the 'structural elements' common to each seven subsystems.

1. Each subsystem is "from the form the behaviour takes and the consequences it achieves can be inferred what **drive** has been stimulated or what **goal** is being sought." The ultimate goal for each subsystem is expected to be the same for all individuals. However, the way of achieving the goal may vary depending on culture and other individual variations.

2. Each individual has a "predisposition to act, with reference to the goal, in certain ways, rather than in other ways." Johnson labelled by predisposition to act as "Set" the concept of 'set' implies that despite having only a few alternatively from which to select a behavioural response, the individual will rank those options and choose the option considered most desirable.

3. Each system has available, a repertoire of choices or "scope of action" alternatives from which choices can be made." As life experience occurs, individuals add to the number of alternative actions available to them. However, **at same point**, the acquisition of new alternatives of behaviour decreases on the individual becomes comfortable with the available repertoire but which point individual loses desire or acquire alternative not mentioned

4. Each subsystem produces observable outcomes, i.e. the individual behaviour.

The observable behaviours allow an outsider–in the case ofcourse–to note the actions the individual is taking to reach a goal related to a specified subsystem. The nurse can then evaluate the effectiveness and efficiency of these behaviours in assisting the individual in reaching one of these goals.

In addition, each subsystem has three functional requirements as given below.

1. Each subsystem must be "**protected** from noxious influences which the system cannot cope."
2. Each subsystem must be "**nurtured** through the input of appropriate supplies from the environment" and
3. Each subsystem must be "**stimulated** for use to enhance growth and prevent stagnation."

As long as the subsystem are meeting their fundamental requirements, the system and subsystem are viewed as self-maintaining and self-perpetuating. The internal and external environments of the system need to remain orderly and predictable, for system to maintain homeostasis or remain in balance. The interrelationships of the structural elements of the subsystem are critical for each subsystem to function at a maximum state. The interaction of the structural elements allows the subsystem to maintain a balance that is adaptive to that individual's needs. Any imbalance in a behavioural subsystem produces tension, which results in disequilibrium. The presence of tension resulting in an unbalanced behavioural system requires the system the increase energy use to return the system to a state of balance. Nursing is viewed as a part of external environment that can assist the client to return to a state of equilibrium or balance.

BEHAVIOURAL SYSTEM MODEL

It has been believed by Johnson that each individual has patterned purposeful, repetitive ways of acting that comprise a behavioural system specific to that individual. These actions or behaviours form an "organized and integrated functional unit that determines and limits the interaction between the person and his environment and establishes the relationship of the person to the objects, events, and situations in his environment. These behaviours are "orderly, purposeful, predictable and sufficiently stable and recurrent to be amenable to description and explanations." (Johnson 1980)

Johnson identifies seven subsystem within the behavioural system model, which are considered to be inter related and changes in one subsystem affect all the subsystems. The schematic representation of Johnson model (Figs. 15.1 and 15.2).

Brief description of Johnson's seven behavioural subsystems are as follows:

1. The attachment or affiliative subsystem is identified as a first response system to develop in the individual. The optimal functioning of the affiliative subsystem allows "social inclusions, intimacy, and the formation and maintenance of a strong social bond." Attachment is significant, caregiver has been found to be critical for survival of an infant. As the individual matures, the attachment to other significant individuals as they enter both the child's and adults network. These 'significant others' provide the individual with a sense of security.
2. *The dependency subsystem* is distinguished from the affiliative or attachment subsystem. Dependency behaviours are

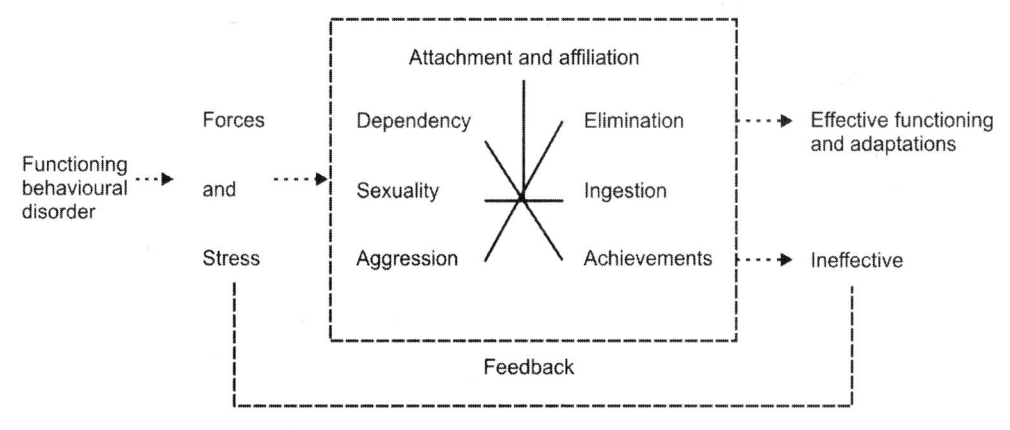

```
                    ┌─────────────────────────────────────┐
                    │     Attachment and affiliation      │
                    │                                      │
              Forces│  Dependency        Elimination       │····▶ Effective functioning
                    │                \  /                  │       and adaptations
Functioning    ···▶ │               \/                     │
behavioural ···▶ and│  Sexuality    /\  Ingestion          │
disorder            │              /  \                    │
                    │                                      │
              Stress│  Aggression        Achievements      │····▶ Ineffective
                    │                                      │
                    └─────────────────────────────────────┘
                                   Feedback
```

Figure 15.1: Johnson behavioural system model

"succouring" behaviours that precipitate nurturing behaviours from other individuals in environment. The results of dependency behaviour is "approval, attention, or recognition, and physical assistance." It is difficult to separate dependency subsystem from the affiliative or attachment subsystem because without someone invested in or attached to the individual to respond to that individual's dependency, behaviours, and the dependency subsystem has no animate environment in which to function.

3. The ingestive subsystem relates to the behaviours surrounding the intake of food. It is related to the biological system. Further nursing point of view, it emphasis the meanings and structures of the socio-events surrounding occasion when food is eaten. Behaviours related to the ingestion of food may relate more to what is society acceptable in a given culture than to the biological needs of the individual.

4. The elimination subsystem relates to behaviours surrounding the excretion of waste products from the body. It is difficult to separate from biological system perspective. However, as with behaviour surrounding the ingestion of food, there is socially acceptable behaviour for the time and place for humans to excrete waste human cultures to cultures have defined different socially acceptable behaviour for excretion to culture. Individuals who have gained physical control over the eliminative subsystem control those subsystems rather then behave in a socially unacceptable manner. For example, biological cues are often ignored if the social situation dictates that it is objectionable to eliminate wastes at a given time.

5. *The sexual subsystem* related to procreation. Both biological and social factors affects behaviours in the sexual subsystem. Again, the behaviours are related to culture and vary from culture to culture. Behaviour also vary according to the gender of the individual. The key is that the goal in all societies has the same outcome—behaviours acceptable to society at large.

6. *The aggressive subsystem* relates to behaviours concerned with protection and self preservations. It is the system that generates defensive responses from the individual when life or territory is

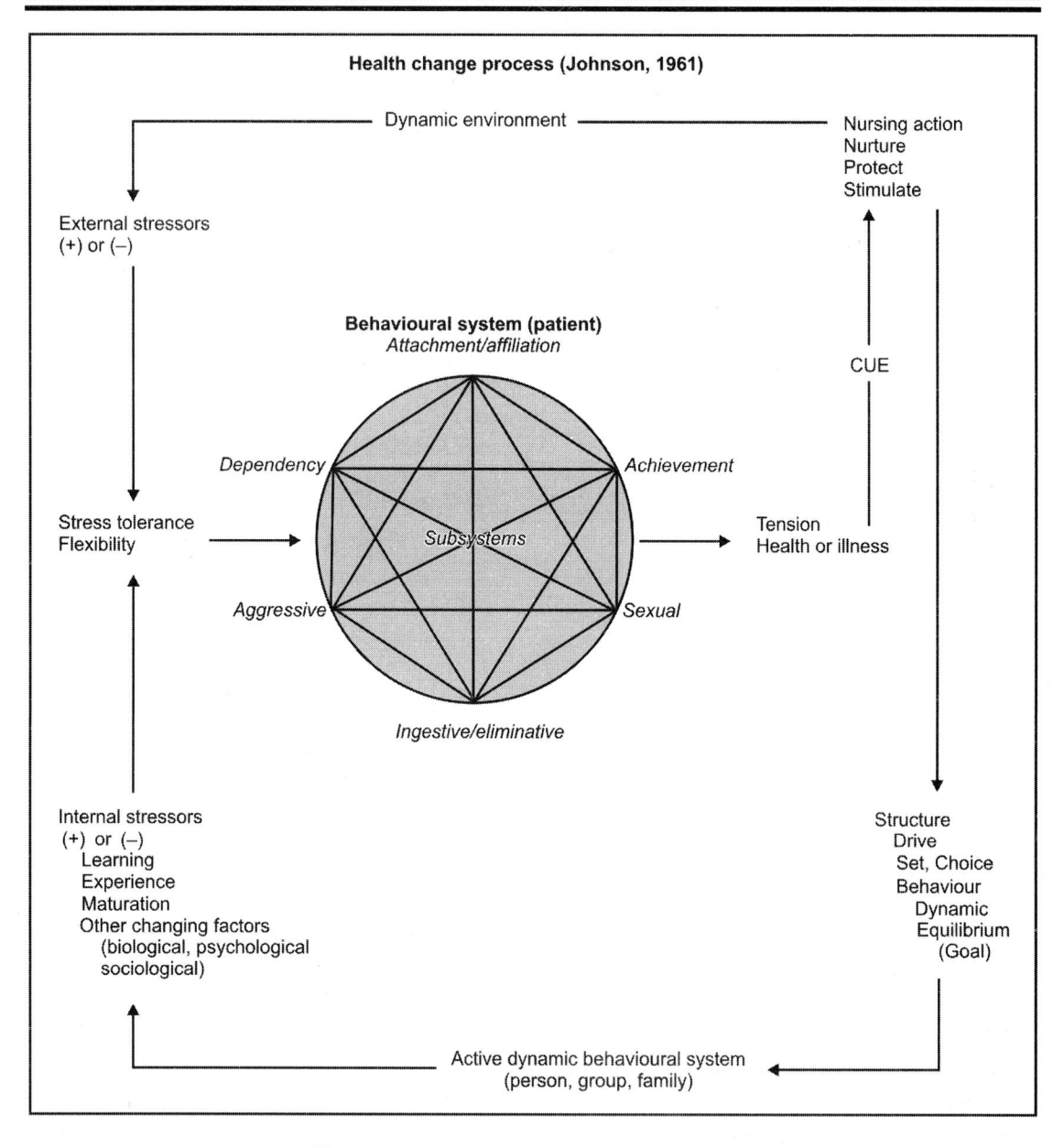

Figure 15.2: Johnson seven behavioural subsystem

threatened. This subsystem does not include those behaviours with a primary purpose of injuring other individuals, but rather those whose purpose is to protect and preserve self and society.

7. *The achievement subsystem* provokes behaviours that attempt to control the environment. Intellectual, physical, creative, mechanical and social skills are some of the areas (Johnson 1980). Other

areas of personal accomplishment or success may also be included in this system.

Paradigm and Behavioural System Model

Human Being

Johnson views man as a behavioural system with patterned repetitive and purposeful ways of behaving that link him to the environment. Man's specific response pattern forms an organised and integrated whole. Person is a system of interdependent parts that require some regularity and adjustment to maintain a balance. Further, assumed, that behavioural system is essential to man and when strong forces or lower resistance disturb behavioural system balance, man's integrity is threatened. Man's attempt to reestablish balance may require an extraordinary expenditure of energy which leaves a shortage of energy to biological and behavioural systems when some type of dysfunction occurs in one or other of the systems.

Environment

According to Johnson, the environment consists of all the factors that are not part of the individual's behavioural system but that influence the system and some of which can be manipulated by the nurse to achieve the health goal for the patient. Society relates to the environment in which an individual exists. An individual's behaviour is influenced by all the events in the environment. Cultural influences on the individual behaviour are viewed as profound. However, it is felt that there are many paths, varying from culture to culture, that influence specific behaviours in a group of people, although the outcome for all the groups or individual is the same. When the environment is stable, the individual is able to continue with successful behaviours.

Health

Johnson perceives health as an elusive dynamic state influenced by biological, psychological and social factors. Health is a desired value by health professionals and focusses on the person rather than illness.

Health is reflected by the organization, interaction, interdependence and integration of subsystems of the behavioural system. Man attempts to achieve a balance in this system, which will lead to functional behaviour. A lack of balance is the structural or functional requirements of the subsystems leads to poor health. When the system requires a minimal amount of energy maintenance, a larger supply of energy is available to affect biological process and recovery.

Johnson model supports the idea that the individuals attempting to maintain some balance or equilibrium.

Nursing

Nursing, as perceived by Johnson, is an external force acting to preserve the organizations of the patient's behaviour while the patient is under stress by means of imposing regulatory mechanisms or by providing resources. An art and science, Nursing, suggests external assistance both before and during system balance disturbance, and therefore requires knowledge of order, disorder, and control. Nursing activities do not depend on medical authority but are complementary to medicine.

Nursing's primary goal is to foster equilibrium within the individual, which allows for the practice of nursing with individuals at any point in the health-illness continuum. Nursing implementation may focus on alterations of a behaviour that is not supportive to maintaining equilibrium for the individual. Nursing is concerned with organized and integrated whole, but that the major focus is on maintaining a balance in the behavioural system when illness occurs in the individual.

Nursing Process and Johnson Work

This behavioural system model easily fits the nursing process model.

Assessment

Assessment focusses on the subsystem related to the presenting health problem. An assessment based on the behavioural system does not easily permit the nurse to gather detailed data about biological system. Use of subsystems provide actual data are:

- *Affiliative subsystem* might focus on the presence of significant others or on the social system of which the individual is a member.
- *Dependency subsystem* in which attention is placed on understanding how the individual makes needs known to significant others, so that the significant others in the environment can assist the individual in meeting those needs.
- *Ingestive subsystem* examines patterns of food and fluid intake, including social environment in which food and fluid are ingested.
- *Eliminative subsystem* generates the question related patterns of defecation and urination and the social context in which the patterns occurs.
- *Sexual subsystem* includes about sexual pattern and behaviour.
- *Aggressive system* generates questions about how individuals protect themselves from perceived threats to safety.
- *Achievement subsystem* allows for assessment of how the individual changes the environment to facilitate the accomplishment of goals.

Although there are many gaps in information about the whole individual if only behavioural system models are used to guide the assessment, some of them used this in the nursing process. Grubbs (1980) developed an assessment tool based on Johnson's seven subsystems plus subsystem she labelled 'restorative' which focussed on activities of daily living (ADL). Holiday, and others also proposed the model useful in nursing process.

Diagnosis

A diagnosis can be made related to insufficient or discrepancies with a subsystem or between subsystems. Diagnosis tends to be general to a subsystem rather than specific to a problem. Johnson never wrote about the use of nursing diagnosis with her model. They are extension of her work by Grubbs. Grubbs has proposed four categories of nursing diagnosis derived from Behavioural system modes as follows:

- *Insufficiency*—as a state which exists when particular subsystem is not functioning or developed to its fullest capacity due to inadequacy of functional requirements.
- *Discrepancy*—a behaviour that does not meet the intended goal. The incongruity usually lies between the action and the goal of the subsystem, although the set and choice may be strongly influencing the ineffective action.

- *Incompatibility*—the goals or behaviours of two subsystems in the same situation conflict with each other to the detriment of the individual.
- *Dominance*—the behaviour in one subsystem is used more than any other subsystem regardless of the situation or to the detriment of the other subsystems.

Planning

Planning for the implementation of nursing care should start at the subsystem level with the ultimate goal of effective behavioural functioning of the entire system. This is related to the diagnosis may be difficult because of the lack of client input into the plan. The plan focuses on the nurse's action to modify client behaviour. These plans that have a goal, to bring about homeostasis in a subsystem that is based on the nurse's assessment of the individual's drive, set, behavioural report to read observable behaviour. The plan may include protection nurturance, or stimulation of the identified subsystem.

Implementation

Implementation by the nurse present to the client on external force for the manipulation of the subsystem back to the state of equilibrium, i.e. Johnson's model focusses on maintaining or returning an individual's subsystem to a state of equilibrium. Implementation focusses on achieving the goals of nursing as identified by Johnson.

Evaluation

Evaluation is based on the attainment of a goal of balance, in the identified subsystem. If base-line data are available for the individual to return to the baseline behaviour. If the alterations in behaviour that are planned do occur, the nurse should be able to observe the return to previous behaviour pattern. Evaluation of the result of this implementation is readily possible if the state of balance that is the goal has been defined during the planning phase before the implementation.

Johnson's Work and Characteristics of a Theory

Using the characteristics of a theory discussed earlier as a guide, it is clear that Johnson has indeed developed a model. Johnson's Behavioural System Model is based on general system concepts. However, the definitions related to the terms used to label her concepts have not been made explicit by Johnson. Grubbs (1980) has presented her definitions of Johnson's terms, and to those are the definitions most often reflected in the literature of other investigators claiming to use Johnson's terms, and those are the definitions most often reflected in the literature of other investigators claiming to use Johnson's terms, and those are the definitions most often reflected in the literature of other investigators claiming to use Johnson's model.

1. Theories can interrelate concepts in such a way as to create a different way of looking at a particular phenomenon. Johnson does not clearly interrelate her concepts of subsystem that comprise the Behavioural System Model.
2. Theories must be logical in nature. The lack of clear interrelationships among the concepts creates difficulty in following the logic of Johnson's work. The definitions of the concepts are so abstract that they are difficult to use. For example, intimacy

is identified as an aspect of the affiliative subsystem, but the concept is not defined or described. An advantage of the abstract definition is that individuals using the model may identify an assessment tool that most specifically fits a problem and use it in their work. There are two major disadvantages. First, the abstract level and multiplicity of definitions make it difficult to compare the same subsystem across studies. Second, the lack of clear definitions for the interrelationships among and between the subsystems makes it difficult to view the entire behavioural system as an entity.

3. Theories should be relatively simple yet generalizable. Johnson's behavioural model can be generalized across the lifespan and across cultures. However, the focus on the behavioural system may make it difficult for nurses working with physically impaired individuals to use the model. Johnson's model is also very individual oriented, so that nurses working with groups of individuals with similar problems would have difficulty using the model. The subsystems in Johnson's Behavioural System Model are individual oriented to such an extent that the family can be considered only as the environment in which the individual presents behaviours and not as the focus of care.

4. Theories are the bases for hypotheses that can be tested or for theory to be expanded, and

5. Theories contribute to and assist in increasing the general body of knowledge within the discipline through the research implemented to validate them. It is difficult to test Johnson's model by the development of hypotheses. Subsystems of the model can be examined because relationships within the subsystems can be identified. The lack of definitions and connections between the subsystems creates a barrier for stating relationships in the form of hypotheses to be tested. Although such relationships may be predicted, the lack of definitions in the original work makes impossible to identify whether it is Johnson's work or someone's interpretation of her work that is being tested.

6. Theories can be used by practitioners to guide and improve practice. Johnson does not clearly define the expected outcomes when one of the subsystems is being affected by nursing implementation. An implicit expectation is made that all humans in all cultures will attain in the same outcome—homeostasis. Because of the lack of definitions the model does not allow for control of the areas of interest, so it is difficult to use the model to guide practice. The authors reportedly using the model to guide practice have not integrated the subsystems to the degree necessary to label this model a theory.

7. Theories must be consistent with other validated theories, laws, and principles but will leave open unanswered questions that need to be investigated. Johnson's Behavioural System Model provides a framework for organising human behaviour. However, it is a different framework from that provided by other nursing theorists, such as Roy (1989) or Rogers (1970). Johnson believes that she is the first person to view "man as a behavioural system." Others have viewed the behavioural subsystem as just one piece

of the biopsychosocial human being. Johnson's framework does contribute to the general body of nursing knowledge but needs further development. Johnson's Behavioural System Model is based on principles of general system theory. Her statements on the multiple modes of attaining the same subsystem goal, regardless of culture, are an example of the principle of "equifinality." As with Rogers (1970), this allows individuals to develop and change through time at unique rates but with the same outcomes at the end of the process mature, adult behaviours that is culturally acceptable.

Johnson's Behavioural System Model is congruent with many of the nursing models in the belief that the individuals is influenced by the environment. Since Nightingale (1859) first presented her beliefs about Nursing, nurses have been concerned with the individual's relationship with the environment. In practice, nurses often have the necessary control over the environment to promote a healthier state for the individual.

In general, the Johnson Behavioural System Model does not meet the criteria for theory. However, it must be stressed that Johnson does not suggest that she has developed a theory, although other nurses scholars have identified and used Johnson as a theorist. Although Johnson's Behavioural System Model has many limitations, she does provide a framework of reference for nurses concerned with specific client behaviours. She also views the behavioural system as active rather than merely reactive. Because the model allows for this belief, it can be studied. The theory has been associated primarily with individuals. Johnson believes groups of interactive behavioural systems. Use of her theory with families and other groups needs more visibility. As a result of the current emphasis on health promotion and maintenance and on illness and injury prevention, the theory could be developed further by recognizing behaviour disorders in these areas.

It should be noted that preventive nursing, i.e. to prevent behavioural system disorder, is not the same as preventive medicine, i.e. to prevent biological system disorders; and that disorders in both cases must be identified and explicated before approaches to prevention can be developed. At this point not even medicine has developed very many specific preventive measures (immunizations for some infectious diseases, and protection against some vitamin deficiency diseases are notable exceptions). There are a number of general approaches to better health, of course—adequate nutrition, safe water, exercise, etc. which are applicable contributing to prevention of some disorders. Small wonder then that preventive nursing remains to be developed, and this is true no matter what model or theory for nursing is used. Further development could identify nursing actions that would facilitate appropriate functioning of the system towards disease prevention and health maintenance. Instead of expending energy developing nursing interventions in response to the consequences of disequilibrium, nurses need to learn how to identify precursors of disequilibrium and respond with preventive interventions.

How can Johnson's theory be used in community health nursing? Assuming that a community is a geographical area, a subpopulation, or any aggregate of people, and assuming that a community can benefit from nursing interventions, the behavioural system framework can be applied to community health. A community can be described as a behavioural system with interacting subsystems that have structural elements and functional requirements. Communities have goals, norms, choices, and actions in addition to needing protection, nurturance, and stimulation. The community reacts to internal and external stimuli, which result in functional or dysfunctional behaviour. An example of an external stimulus is health policy, and an example of dysfunctional behaviour is a high infant mortality. Somewhere between is the behavioural system, consisting of yet undefined subsystems that are organized, interacting, interdependent, and integrated. Physical, biological, and psychosocial factors also affect community behaviour.

EVALUATION OF THEORY

- Johnson's theory is relatively simple in relation to the number of concepts. Man is described as a behavioural system composed of seven subsystems. Nursing is an external regulatory force. However, the theory is potentially complex because of the number of possible interrelationships between and among the behavioural system and its subsystems and the forces impinging on them. At this point, however, only a few of the potential relationships have been explored.
- Johnson's theory is relatively unlimited when applied to sick individuals, but it has not been used as much with well individuals or groups. Johnson perceives man as a behavioural system comprised of seven subsystems, aggregates of interactive behavioural systems. The role of nursing in nonillness situations is not clearly defined in the theory, but Johnson does address it.
- Empirical precision is difficult to achieve when a theory contains highly abstract concepts and has only potential generality. Empirical precision can improve when the subconcepts and the relationships between and among the subconcepts are well defined and reality indicators are introduced. The units and the relationships between the units in Johnson's theory are consistently defined and used. However, Johnson's theory has only a moderate degree of empirical precision because the highly abstract concepts need to be better defined. Throughout Johnson's writings terms such as balance, stability and equilibrium, adjustments and adaptations, disturbances, disequilibrium, and behavioural disorders are used interchangeably, which confounds their meanings. The introduction of subsystems improves the theory's empirical precision.
- Johnson's theory could guide nursing practice, education, and research; generate new ideas about nursing, and differentiate nursing from other health professions. By focusing on behaviour rather than biology, the theory clearly differentiates nursing from medicine although the concepts overlap with the psychosocial professions.

Johnson's behavioural systems theory provides a conceptual framework for nursing education, practice, and research. The theory has directed questions for nursing research. It has been analysed and judged to be appropriate as a basis for the development of a nursing curriculum. Practitioners and patients have judged the resulting nursing actions to be satisfactory. The theory has potential for continued utility in nursing to achieve valued nursing goals.

Chapter 16

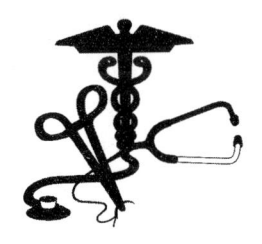

Roy's Adaptation Model

Sister Callista Roy, a member of the Sisters of Saint Joseph of Carondeler, was born October 14, 1939, in Los Angeles, California. She received a Bachelor of Arts in Nursing in 1963 from Mount Saint Mary's College in Los Angeles and a Master of Science in Nursing from the University of California at Los Angeles in 1966. After earning her nursing degrees, Roy began her education in sociology, receiving both an M.A. in sociology in 1973 and a Ph.D. in sociology in 1977 from the University of California.

While working toward her master's degree, Roy was challenged in a seminar with Dorothy E. Johnson to develop a conceptual model for nursing. Roy had worked as a pediatric staff nurse and had noticed the great resiliency of children and their ability to adapt in response to major physical and psychological changes. Roy was impressed by adaptation as an appropriate conceptual framework for nursing. The basic concepts of the model were developed while Roy was a graduate student at UCLA from 1964 to 1966.

Roy began operationalizing her model in 1968 when Mount Saint Mary's College adopted the adaptation framework as the philosophical foundation of the nursing curriculum. Roy was an associate professor and chairperson of the Department of Nursing at Mount Saint Mary's College until 1982. From 1983 to 1985, she was a Robert Wood Johnson Post Doctoral Fellow at the University of California in San Francisco as a clinical nurse scholar in neuroscience. During this time she conducted research on nursing interventions for cognitive recovery in head injuries and on the influence of nursing models on clinical decision making. In 1988 Roy began the newly created position of graduate faculty nurse theorist at Boston College School of Nursing.

Roy has published many books, chapters, and periodical articles and has presented numerous lectures and workshops focussing on her nursing adaptation theory. She is a member of Sigma Theta Tau, having received the National Founder's Award for Excellence in Fostering Professional Nursing Standards in 1981. Her achievements include a 1984 Honorary Doctorate of Humane Letters by Alverno College, a 1985 Honorary Doctorate from Eastern Michigan University, and a 1986 AJN Book of the Year Award for Essentials of the Roy Adaptation Model. Roy has been recognized in the *World Who's Who of Women, Personalities of America*, and as a Fellow of the American Academy of Nursing.

EVOLUTION OF THEORY

Roy's Adaptation Model for Nursing was derived in 1964 from Harry Helson's work in psychophysics. In Helson's Adaptation Theory, adaptive responses are a function of the incoming stimulus and the adaptive level. The adaptation level is made up of the pooled effect of three classes of stimuli: (i) focal stimuli, which immediately confront the individual; (ii) contextual stimuli, which are all other stimuli present; and (iii) residual stimuli, those factors that are relevant but that cannot be validated. Helson's work developed the concept of the adaptation level zone, which determines whether a stimuli will elicit a positive or negative response. According to Helson's theory, adaptation is a process of responding positively to environmental changes.

Roy combines Helson's work with Rapoport's definition of system and views the person as an adaptive system. With Helson's Adaptation theory as a foundation, Roy developed and further refined the model using concepts and theory from BP Dohrenwend, RS Lazarus, N Malaznik D. Mechanic, and H. Selye. Roy gave special credit to co-authors Driever, for outlining subdivisions of self-integrity, and Martinez and Sato, for identifying both common and primary stimuli affecting the modes. Other co-workers also elaborated the concepts: M. Pousch and J. Van Landingham for the interdependence mode and B. Randall for the role function mode.

After the development of her theory, Roy developed the model as a framework for nursing practice, research, and education. According to Roy, more than 1500 faculty and students have contributed to the theoretical development of the adaptation model.

In *Introduction to Nursing: An Adaptation Model*, Roy discussed self-concept. She and her collaborators used the work of Coombs and Snygg regarding self-consistency and major influencing factors of self-concept. Social interaction theories in Epstein's publication that self-perception is influenced by one's perceptions of other's responses. Mead expanded the idea by hypothesizing that self-appraisal uses the "generalized other." Sullivan suggests that self arises from social interaction. Gardner and Erickson provide developmental approaches. The other modes physiological, role functioning, and interdependence were drawn similarly from biological and behavioural sciences for an understanding of the person.

Roy is developing the humanism value base of her model. The model uses concepts from A.H. Maslow to explore beliefs and values of persons. According to Roy, humanism in nursing is the belief in the person's own creative power or the belief that the person's own coping abilities will enhance wellness. Roy's holistic approach to nursing is grounded in humanism.

The use of Roy's adaptation model in nursing practice led to further clarification and refinement. A 1971 pilot research study and a survey research study from 1976 to 1977 led to some result is attainment of an optimum level of wellness by the person.

As an open, living system, the person receives inputs or stimuli from both the environment and the self. The adaptation level is determined by the combined effect of the focal, contextual, and residual stimuli. Adaptation occurs when the person responds positively to environmental changes. This adaptive response promotes the integrity of the person, which leads to health. Ineffective responses to stimuli leads to disruption of the integrity of the person (Fig. 16.1).

There are two interrelated subsystems in Roy's model (Fig. 16.1). The primary, functional, or control processes subsystem consists of the regulator and the cognator. The secondary, effector subsystem consists of four adaptive modes: physiological needs, self-concept, role function, and interdependence.

Roy views the regulator and cognator as methods of coping. Perception of the person links the regulator with the cognator in that "input into the regulator is transformed into perceptions. Perception is a process of the cognator. The responses following perception are feedback into both the cognator and the regulator."

The four adaptive modes of the second subsystem in Roy's model provide form or manifestations of cognator and regulator activity. Responses to stimuli are carried out through these four modes. The mode's purpose is to achieve physiological, psychological, and social integrity. Interrelated propositions of the cognator and regulator subsystems link the systems of the adaptive modes.

Man as a whole is made up of six subsystems. These subsystems the regulator, cognator, and the form a complex system for the purpose of adaptation. Relationships between the four adaptive modes occur when internal and external stimuli affect more than one mode; when disruptive behaviour occurs in more than one mode; or when one mode becomes the focal, contextual, or residual stimulus for another mode.

The person is an adaptive system. System inputs include (i) three classes of stimuli (focal, contextual, residual) that arise from within the person and the external environment and (ii) the adaptation level. Adaptation level is fluid, is composed of all three classes of stimuli, and represents the person's standard or range of stimuli in which response will be adaptive.

Inputs are mediated by the control process subsystems of cognate and regulator coping mechanisms. The regulator mechanism is an automatic neuroendocrine response, whereas

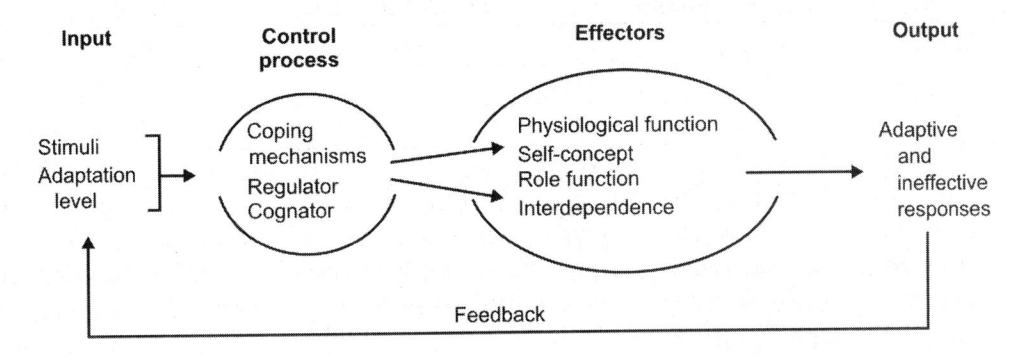

Figure 16.1: Person as an adaptive system

the cognator subsystems represent perception, information processing and judgements influenced by learning and emotions. Coping activity may or may not be adequate to maintain integrity. A system difficulty is present when coping activity is inadequate as a result of need excess or deficits.

The system effectors are the adaptive modes. These modes (physiologic, self-concept, role function, and interdependence) are the form in which regulator and cognator subsystems manifest their activity.

The adaptive system (person's) output is a response that may be adaptive or ineffective, Adaptive responses are those that contribute to adaptation goals (i.e. responses that promote growth, survival, reproduction, and self-mystery). Adaptation is an ongoing purposive response. Adaptive responses contribute to health and the process of being and becoming integrated; ineffective responses do not.

Using nursing process, the nurse promotes adaptive resposes in the adaptive modes during health and illness. Thus energy is freed from inadequate coping to promote health and wellness. System responses in each mode are assessed (i.e. described according to objective and subjective data; first-level assessment). Behaviours can be assessed by observation, measurement, and interview. A tentative judgement about whether the behaviour is adaptive or ineffective is then made, and stimuli influencing the adaptive systm are then identified (second-level assessment). A nursing diagnosis follows, goals are set, and interventions are selected. Goals are mutually agreed on, and a goal-setting hierarchy is proposed. Survival is a priority goal, followed by goals that promote growth, ensure continuation of the species or society, and promote attainment of full potential. Factors precipitating ineffective behaviour are changed, and coping behaviour (i.e. adaptation level) is broadened. The person's level of coping is continuously revised. Evaluation of interventions requires returning to the first steps in the nursing process (i.e. noting behaviours manifested by the adaptive system or person).

Roy's Adaptation Model for nursing is derived in 1964 from Bertalanffy's (1968) General system theory and Harry Helson's (1964) Adaptation theory. Other experts who influenced Roy in the development of her model included Dohernwend, Lazarus, Mechanic and Selye. Rapports ideas in the area of systems and Maslow's thoughts on human needs also contributed to the model. The Roy Adaptation model has evoked much interest and respect since its inception in 1964 by Roy on part of her graduate work at the University of California, Los Angeles under the guidance of Dorothy E. Johnson. In 1970 the faculty of Mount Saint Mary's College in Los Angeles adopted Roy's Adaptation Model as the conceptual framework of the undergraduate nursing curriculum. A text was written by Roy and fellow faculties describing the Roy's Adaptation Model (RAM) and presenting nursing assessment and intervention reflective of the distinctive focus of the Model.

In 1981, Roy and Sharon Roberts wrote "Theory construction in Nursing: Adaptation Model, to discuss the use of the Roy model to construct nursing theory. Roy works extremely well with other nurse scholars on national and international basis, mentioning them in the use of her model in education service, practice and research. Roy's contribution to nursing science are commendable and significant. The reader who is excited by the model will find that a rich response has been made and continue to be made by nurse practitioners, educators and researchers in the analysis, testing and application of the model for nursing.

In 1991 Roy and Andrews wrote a clinical text "The Roy Adaptation Model: The definitive statement. It presents the collective experiences of several contributing authors who have taught and practised using the Roy's Model for the last 20 years.

Concepts Used by Roy

System

A system is "a set of units so related or connected as to form a unity or whole and characterised by inputs, outputs, and control and feedback processes."

Adaptation Level

A person's adaptation level is "a constantly changing point, made up of focal, contextual, and residual stimuli, which represent the person's own standard of the range of stimuli to which one can respond with ordinary adaptive responses."

Adaptation Problems

Adaptation problems are "the occurrences of situations of inadequate responses to need deficits or excesses." In the second edition of *Introduction to Nursing*, Roy states:

It can be noted at the point that the distinction being made between adaptations and nursing diagnosis is based on the developing work in both of these fields. At this point, adaptation problems are seen not as nursing diagnosis, but as areas of concern for the nurse related to adapting person or group (within each adaptive mode).

Focal Stimulus

A focal stimulus is "the degree of change or stimulus most immediately confronting the person and the one to which the person must make an adaptive response, that is the factor that precipitates the behaviour."

Contextual Stimuli

Contextual stimuli are "all other stimuli present that contribute to the behaviour caused or precipitated by the focal stimuli."

Residual Stimuli

Residual stimuli are "factors that may be affecting behaviour but whose effects are not validated."

Regulator

A regulator is a "subsystem coping mechanism which responds automatically through neural-chemical-endocrine processes."

Cognator

A cognator is a "subsystem coping mechanism which responds through complex processes of perception and information processing learning judgement and emotion."

Adaptive (Effector) Modes

Adaptive or effector's modes are a "classification of ways of coping that manifest regulator and cognator activity, that is, physiological, self-concept, role function, and interdependence."

Adaptive Responses

Adaptive responses are "responses are "responses that promote integrity of the person in terms of the goals, that is, survival, growth, reproduction and mastery."

Physiological Mode

"Physiological needs involve the body's basic needs and ways of dealing with adaptation in regard to fluid and electrolytes; exercise and rest, elimination, circulation and oxygen; and regulation which includes the senses, temperature, and endocrine regulation."

Self-concept Mode

"Self-concept is the composite of beliefs and feelings that one holds about oneself at a given time. It is formed from perceptions, particularly of other's reactions, and directs one's behaviour. Its components include; (i) the physical self, which involves sensation and body image; and (ii) the personal self, which is made up of self-consistency, self-ideal or expectancy, and the moral, ethical self.

Role Performance Mode

Role function is the performance of duties based on given positions in society. The way one performs a role is dependent on one's interaction with the other in the given situation. The major roles that one plays can be analysed by imagining a tree formation. The trunk of the tree is one's primary role, that is, one's development level—for example, generative adult female. Secondary roles branch off from this—for example, wife, mother, teacher, finally, tertiary roles branch off from secondary roles—for example, the mother role must involve other associates for a given period of time. Each of these roles is seen as occurring in dyadic relationship, that is, with a reciprocal role.

Interdependence

"The interdependence; mode involves one's relations with significant others and support system. In this mode one maintains psychic integrity by meeting needs for nurturance and affection."

Roy Adaptation Model

As stated earlier, Roy credits the works of Von Berthalanffys, and Helson's theories on formatting basis of scientific assumptions underlying the Roy model. The assumption underlying the Roy model are as given below.

Assumptions from Systems Theory

- *Holism:* A system is a set of units so related or connected as to form a unity or whole.
- *Interdependence:* A system is a whole that functions on a whole by virtue of the interdependence of its parts.
- *Control processes:* A system have inputs, output, and control and feedback processes.
- *Information feedback:* Input, in the form of a standard or feedback often is referred to as information.
- *Complexity of living system:* Living systems are more complex than mechanical systems and have standards and feedback to direct their functioning as a whole.

Assumption from Adaptation Level Theory

- *Behaviour as adaptive:* Human behaviour represents adaptation to environmental and organism forces.

- *Adaptation as a function of stimuli and adaptation level:* Adaptive behaviour is a function of the stimulus and adaptation level, that is, the pooled effect of the focal contextual and residual stimuli.
- *Individual, dynamic adaptation level:* Adaptation is a process of responding positively to environmental changes. This positive response decreases the response necessary to cope with the stimuli and increases sensitivity to respond to other stimuli.
- *Positive and active process of responding:* Response reflects the state of the organism as well as the properties of stimuli, and hence, are regarded as active processes.

Scientific Assumptions

Roy has drawn eight assumptions which are based on systems and adaptation level theories, and are as follows:
1. The person is a biopsychosocial being.
2. The person is in constant interaction with changing environment.
3. To cope with a changing, world the person uses both innate and acquired mechanisms, which are of biologic, psychological, and social origin.
4. Health and illness are one inevitable dimensions of life.
5. To respond positively to environmental changes, the person must adapt.
6. The person's adaptation is function of the stimulus exposed to and one's adaptation level.
7. The person's adaptation level is such that it comprises a zone indicating the range of stimulations that will lead to a positive response.
8. The person is conceptualised as having four modes of adaptation-physiologic; self-concept, role function; and interdependence.

Philosophical Assumptions

Roy (1988) addressed the thoughtful explication of eight philosophical assumptions. Four based on the philosophical principle of **Humanism** and four based on the philosophical principle of veritivity (a word coined by Roy).

Assumption from Humanism

Creativity—Persons have their own creative power and shares in creative power.

Purposefulness—A person's behaviour is **purposeful** and not merely a cause and effect. (Behaves purposefully, not in sequence of cause and effect).

Holism—Person in holistic, i.e. individual possesses intrinsic holism.

Interpersonal process—A person strives to maintain integrity and to realise the need for relationship, viz. individual's options and view points are of value in the interpersonal relationship is significant.

Assumptions Based on Veritivity

The veritivity derived from the Latin **Veritas**, meaning truth was coined by Roy. The premise underlying Roy's term is that there is an absolute truth. Roy defines veritivity as "a principle of human nature that affirms a common purposefulness of human existence..." A person is viewed in the context of:
- Purposefulness of human existence.
- Unity of purpose of humankind.
- Activity and creatively for the common good.
- Values and meaning of life.

Elements of the Roy's Adaptation Model (RAM)

The four essential elements of the RAM are the following:
- The person who is recipient of nursing care.
- The concept of environment.
- The concept of health.
- Nursing.

Person Theory (Person as an Adaptive System)

Roy (1984) states that the recipient of nursing care may be the person, a family, a group, a community, or a society. Each considered by the nurse as holistic adaptive system. According to Roy, "a person, a family, a group, a community, or a society, each considered by the holistic adaptive system." According to Roy "a person is bio-psychosocial being in constant interaction with a changing environment." She defines the person, the recipient of nursing care, as a living, complex, adaptive system, with internal processes (the cognator and regulator) acting to maintain adaptation in the four adaptive modes (Physiological needs, self concept, role function and interdependence). The person as living system is "whole made up of parts or subsystems that function as unity for some purpose."

The idea of an **adaptive system** combines the concepts of system and adaptation as follows:

System

In her model, Roy conceptualises the person in a holistic perspectives. Individual aspects of parts act together to form a unified being. Additionally, on living systems, persons are in constant interaction with their environments. Between the system and the environment occurs an exchange of information, matter and energy. Characteristics of a system include inputs, controls and feedback (Fig. 16.1).

For example, cell is a living open system, has its inner and outer world. From its outer world, it must draw forth the substance it needs to survive. Within itself, the call must maintain order over its vast number of molecules.

Adaption

Roy (1991) used diagram shown in Figure 16.1 above to represent the adaptive system of a person. The adaptive system has inputs of stimuli and adaptation level, output as behavioural responses that serve as feed back and control and process known as coping mechanisms. The adaptive system has input coming from the external environment as well as from the person. She identifies in its as stimuli and adaptation level. Stimuli are conceptualised as falling into three classifications focal, contextual and residual.
- *Focal stimulus*—The internal or external stimulus most immediately confronting the person, the object or event that attracts one's attention; "a degree of change that precipitates adaptive behaviour; stimulus most immediately confronting the person, the one to which he must make an adaptive response, stressor.
- *Contextual stimuli*—are all other stimuli of the persons internal and external world that can be identified as having a positive or negative influence on the situation.
- *Residual stimuli*—are those internal or external factors having an indeterminate effect on the person's behaviour, that effect

has not or cannot be validated: Environmental factors within or outside the person whose effects in the current situation are unclear, possible yet uncertain, influencing stimuli, includes beliefs, attitudes, experience or traits.

Input

Along with the stimuli, the adaptation level of the person, act as input to that person as an adaptive system. The focal, contextual and residual stimuli combine and interface to set the adaptation level of the person at a particular point in time. This range of response is unique to the individual; each person's adaptation level constantly changing. Significant stimuli that comprise the focal, contextual and residual stimuli include the factors such as the degree of change, past experiences, knowledge level, strengths and/or limitations.

Output and Feedback

Output of the person as a system are the responses of the person. Output responses can be both external and internal. Thus these responses are the persons' behaviours. They can be observed, intuitively perceived by the nurse, measured and subjectively reported by the person. Output responses become feedback to the person and to the environment. Roy has categorized outputs of the system as either adaptive response or ineffective responses.
- Adaptive responses are those that promote the integrity of the person. The person's integrity or wholeness, is behaviourally demonstrated when the person is able to met the goals in terms of survival, growth, reproduction and mastery.
- Ineffective responses do not support these goals.

Coping Mechanism

Roy has used the term coping mechanism to describe control processes of the person as an adaptive system. Some coping mechanisms are inherited or genetic. Such as WBC defense system against bacteria that seek to invade the body (or mental mechanisms—which she has not used). Other mechanisms are learned, such as use of antiseptics to cleanse a wound. She presents a unique nursing science concept of control mechanisms, that are called the "regulator" and "cognator." Her model considers the regulator and cognator coping mechanism to be subsystems of the person as an adaptive system.

Regulator Subsystem

Has the components of input, internal process and output. Input stimuli may originate externally or internally to the person. The transmitters of regulatory system are chemical, neural, or endocrine in nature. Autonomic reflexes which are neural responses originating in the brainstem and spinal cord, are generated as output responses of the regulator subsystem. Target organs and tissues under endocrine control also produce regulator output responses. Finally, Roy presents psychomotor responses originating from the central nervous system as regulator subsystem responses. Many physiological processes can be viewed as regulator subsystem responses. For example, several regulatory feedback mechanisms of respirations have been identified. One if these is increased carbon dioxide, the end product of metabolism, which stimulates chemoreceptors in the medulla to increase respiratory rate. Strong stimulation of these centres can increase ventilation six-to-seven fold.

An example of regulator process when a noxious external stimulus is visualised and transmitted via the optic nerve to higher brain centres and taken to lower brain autonomic centres. The synapathetic neurons from these origins have multiple visceral effects including increased blood pressure and increased heart rate. Roy's schematic representation of the regulatory process seen in Figure 16.1.

Cognator Subsystem

Stimuli to the cognator subsystem is also both external and internal in origin. Output responses of the regulator subsystem can be feedback stimuli to the cognator subsystem. Cognator control process are related to the higher brain function is of perception or information processing, in relation to the internal processes of selective attention coding and memory. Learning is correlated to the processes of imitation, reinforcement, and insight. Problem-solving and decision-making are the internal processes relating to judgement and finally, emotions have the processes of defence to seek relief, affective appraisal, and attachment.

In maintaining the integrity of the person the regulator and cognator are postulated as frequently acting together. The adaptation level of the person as an adaptive system is influenced by the individual's development and use of these coping mechanisms. Maximal use of coping mechanisms broadens the adaptation level of the person and increases the range of stimuli to which the person can positively respond.

Adaptive Modes

Although cognator and regulator processes are essential to the adaptive responses of the person, these processes are not directly observable. Only the responses of the person can be observed, measured or subjectively reported. Roy (1991) identified four adaptive modes or categories for assessment of behaviour that results from the regulator and cognator mechanism of response. The adaptive modes are the *physiological, self-concept, role function* and *interdependence modes*. Behaviour related to the modes is the manifestation of the stimuli; the person's adaptation level and coping processes. By observing the person's behaviour in relation to the adaptive modes, the nurse can identify adaptive or ineffective responses in situations of health and illness.

The four adaptive modes for assessment are as follows:

Physiological Mode

The physiological mode represents physical response to environmental stimuli and primarily involves the regulator subsystem. The basic need of this mode is physiologic integrity and is composed of the needs associated with oxygenation, nutrition, elimination, activity and rest and protection. The complex processes of this mode are associated with the senses, fluids and electrolytes, neurological function and endocrine functions. These needs and process may be defined as follows.

- *Oxygenation:* The pattern of oxygen use related to respiratory and cardiovascular physiology and pathophysiology.

- *Nutrition:* Patterns of nutrient use for maintaining human functioning, promoting growth, and repairing injured tissue.
- *Elimination:* Patterns of elimination of waste products.
- *Acting and rest:* Patterns of activity and rest.
- *Protection:* Patterns related to skin integrity and immunity.
- *Senses:* The input channel of the person through which sensory-perceptual information is processed.
- *Fluid and electrolytes:* The complex process of maintaining body fluids and electrolytes in balance for the persons.
- *Neurological function:* Key neural process and complex relationship of neural function to regulator and cognator coping mechanism.
- *Endocrine function:* Patterns of endocrine control and regulation that act in conjunction with nervous system to maintain control of the body processes.

Self-concept Mode

The self-concept mode relates to the basic need for psychic integrity. Its focus is on the psychological and spiritual aspects of the person. Attention given to the subcategories of physical self and personal self. The *physical self* has the component of body sensation and body image. The *personal self* has the components of self consistency, self ideal, and moral-ethical-spiritual self. Body-sensation is how the person experiences the physical self, and body image how the person views the physical self. Self-consistency represents the person's efforts to maintain self-organization and to avoid disequilibrium. Self-ideal represents what the person expects to be and do, and moral-ethical-spiritual self represents the persons' belief system and self-evaluation.

Role Function Mode

The role function mode identifies the patterns of social interaction of the person in relation to others reflected by primary, secondary, and tertiary roles. The basic need met is social integrity. The *primary* role determines the majority of person's behaviours and is defined by the persons' sex, age, and developmental stage, *Secondary* roles are assumed to carry out the tasks required by the stage of development and primary role. *Tertiary* roles are temporary, feely chosen, and may include activities related to hobbies. Behaviours in this mode are described as instrumental or expressive. Instrumental behaviours are usually physical, have a long-term orientation, and focus on role mastery. Expressive behaviour represents feelings or attitudes are usually emotional, and seek immediate response.

Interdependent Mode

The interdependent mode is where affectional needs are met. Strongly reflective of the humanistic values held by Roy the interdependence mode identifies pattern of human value, affection, love and affirmation. These processes occur through interpersonal relationship on both individual and group levels.

Metaparadigm and RAM

Human Being

Person is a biopsychosocial being in constant interaction with a changing environment and recipient of nursing care as living system.

Environment

Roy has broadly defined environment as "all conditioning circumstances and influences that surround and effect the development and behaviour of the person's or group." Thus all stimuli, whether internal or external are part of the person's environment. Within her model, Roy specifically categorizes stimuli as focal, contextual, and residual. Changes in the environment act as catalysts, stimulating person to make adaptive responses. Thus stimuli from within the person and stimuli from around the person represent the element of environment. To quote an example, elderly person admitted to hospital, all the conditions of influence on him.

Health

Health is been defined as "a state and process of being and becoming an integrated and whole person." Holism and integrated functioning are not only basic premises of systems theory, but are also congruent with the philosophical assumptions of Roy's Adaptation Model (RAM).

Health is a state reflects the adaptation process and is demonstrated by adaptation in each of your integrated adaptive modes: physiologic, self-concept, role function and interdependence. The integration of these four adaptive modes reflects wholeness.

Health is a process, whereby individuals are striving to achieve their maximum potential. This process can be readily seen in healthy people, who exercise regularly, do not smoke, and pay attention to dietary habits. The process of health can also be seen in persons in the terminal stages of cancer as they seek to control over symptoms, such as pain, and strives for integration within themselves and in relation to significant others.

The integrity of the person is expressed as the ability to meet the goals of survival, growth, reproduction and mastery. The aim of the nurse practising under the Roy model is to promote the health of the person by promoting adaptive responses.

Nursing

Roy defines the 'goal of nursing' as the promotion of adaptive responses in relation to the four adaptive modes. *Adaptive responses* are those that positively affect the health. Stimuli and the person's adaptation level are inputs to the person as any adaptive system. The person's adaptive level determines whether a positive response to internal or external stimuli will be elicited. Nursing seeks to reduce ineffective responses and promote adaptive responses as output behaviour of the person. The nurse, therefore, promotes health in all life processes, including dying with dignity. A person's ability to cope varies with the state of the person at different times.

Nursing activities or interventions are delineated by the model on those that promote adaptive responses in situations of health and illness. As a rule, these approaches are identified as action taken by the nurse to manage the focal, contextual, or residual stimuli on the person. By making these adjustments, the total stimuli fall within the adaptive level of the person. Whenever possible, the focal stimulus—that which represents the greatest degree of changes—is the focus of nursing activity. For a person with chest pain, the focal stimulus is the imbalance between the demand for oxygen by the body and the supply of oxygen that the heart can provide. To alter the focal stimuli, the nurse manages the stimuli of demand so that an adaptive response can be made. In turn, when focal stimuli cannot be altered, the nurse promotes an adaptive response by altering contextual stimuli.

In addition, the nurse may anticipate that the person has a potential for ineffective response secondary to stimuli, likely to be present in a particular situation. The nurse acts to prepare the person for anticipated changes through strengthening regulator and cognator coping mechanism. Plans that broaden the person's adaptation levels correlate with the ideas of health promotion currently found in the literature. Finally nursing actions suggested by the model include approaches aimed at maintaining adaptive responses that support the person's effort to creativity use his or her coping mechanisms.

Nursing Process and Roy's Adaptation Model

The last key concept in the Roy's Adaptation Model is nursing activities, which have been described as the nursing process. This RAM offers guidelines to the nurse in application of the nursing process. The elements of the Roy's Nursing Process include assessment of behaviour, assessment of stimuli, nursing diagnosis, goal setting intervention and evaluation.

Behaviour Assessment

Behaviour assessment is considered to be the gathering of responses or out put behaviours of the person as an adaptive system in relation to each of the four adaptive modes: physiological, self-concept, role function, and interdependence. The specific data are gathered by the nurse through the processes of observation, careful measurement, and skilled interview techniques.

Assessment of the client in each of the four adaptive modes enhances a systematic and holistic approach. Such assessment clarifies the focus that the nurse or nursing teach will take in caring for the client. Ideally, thoroughly conducted and recorded nursing assessment in the four adaptive modes sets the tone of understanding for an entire health care team of the particular situation of a client. Proficiency in the practice of nursing requires skilled assessment of behaviours and the knowledge to compare the person to specific criteria to evaluate behavioural response as adaptive or ineffective.

For example, an indications of adaptive difficulty includes the following:

Signs of pronounced regulator activity

1. Increase in heart rate of blood pressure.
2. Tension.
3. Excitement.
4. Loss of appetite.
5. Increase in serum cortisol.

Signs of cognator ineffectiveness include

1. Faulty perception/information processing.
2. Ineffective learning.
3. Poor judgement.
4. Inappropriate effect.

Guide questions related to each adaptive mode can be developed to reflect the age or acuity of the client population being assessed. Information collected includes subjective, objective, and measurement data. Behaviour that varies from expectations, norms, and guidelines frequently represents ineffective responses. Roy has identified frequently occurring signs of pronounced regulator activity and cognator ineffectiveness. The presence of these behaviours also suggests ineffective responses.

Assessment of Stimuli

After behavioural assessment, the nurse analyses the emerging themes and patterns of client behaviour to identify ineffective responses or adaptive responses requiring nurse support. When ineffective behaviours or adaptive behaviours requiring support are present, the nurse makes an assessment of internal and external stimuli that may be affecting behaviour. In this phase of assessment, the nurse collects data about the focal, contextual, and residual stimuli impacting on the client. This process clarifies the etiology of the problem and identifies significant contextual and residual factors, common influencing stimuli have been identified by Roy and her colleagues and are listed in Table 16.1.

Table 16.1: Common stimuli affecting adaptation

Culture	Socio-economic status, ethnicity, belief system.
Family	Structure, take.
Developmental stage	Age, sex tasks, heredity, and genetic factors.
Integrity of adaptive modes	Physiological (including diseases pathology), self-concept, role function, interdependence.
Cognator effectiveness	Perception, knowledge and skill.
Environment considerations	Change in internal or external environment, medical management, use of drugs alcohol, tobacco.

Nursing Diagnosis

Roy describes three methods of making a nursing diagnosis. One method is to use a typology of diagnoses developed by Roy and related to the four adaptive modes.

The second method is to make a diagnosis by stating the observed response within one mode along with the most influential stimuli. Using this method, a diagnosis for Mr. Ananth could be stated as "chest pain caused by a deficit of oxygen to the heart muscle associated with an over exposure to hot weather."

The third method summarizes responses in one or more adaptive modes related to the same stimuli. For example, if the person experiencing chest pain is a farmer, working outside in hot weather is necessary for success in his or her work. In this case, an appropriate diagnosis might be: "Role failure associated with limited physical (myocardial) ability to work in hot weather."

On the other hand, a nursing diagnosis using any of the foregoing methods can also be a statement of adaptive responses that the nurse wishes to support. For example, if Mr. Ananth is seeking help through vocational counselling to adapt to his physical limitation, the nurse may diagnose a need to support this behaviour. In this case, an appropriate diagnosis would be: "Adaptation to role failure by seeking an alternative career." Roy and others also have developed a typology of indicators of positive adaptation.

Planning (Goal Setting)

Goals are the end point behaviours that the person is to achieve. They are recorded as client behaviours indicative of resolution of the adaptation problem. The goal statement includes the behaviour, the change expected, and a time frame. Long-term goals reflect resolution of adaptive problems and the availability of energy to meet other goals (survival, growth, reproduction, and mastery). Short-term goals identify expected client behaviours that indicate cognator or regulator coping. Whenever possible, goals are set mutually with the person. Mutual goal setting respects the privileges and rights of person.

Implementation

Nursing interventions are planned with the purpose of altering or managing the focal or contextual stimuli. Implementation may also focus on broadening the person's coping ability, or adaptation level, so that the total stimuli fall within that person's ability to adapt. The nurse plans specific activities to alter the selected stimuli appropriately.

Evaluation

The nursing process is completed by evaluation. Goal behaviours are compared to the person's output responses, and movement toward or away from goal achievement is determined. Readjustments to goals and interventions are made on the basis of evaluation data.

The Roy Nursing Process Applied to Nursing in a Recovery Room

The Roy model can be applied to nursing assessment and interventions in various clinical situations. In the following case study, the Roy model is applied to a person during the period of immediate recovery from surgery and anaesthesia.

Behavioural assessment focuses on the physiological mode responses during the first hour of recovery time after person experiences surgery and general anaesthesia. By applying the Roy model, significant behaviours can be conceptualized as regulator system activity. Regulator output responses that vary from baseline values determined for the person may be the first warning of an ineffective response to postoperative stimuli. Key baseline values are the person's presurgery measures of heart rate, blood pressure, and respiratory rate. Immediately, upon observation of changes from the baseline, assessment of stimuli is done. Goals are set with the basic survival of the person as a priority. Interventions are taken so that focal and contextual stimuli are altered and adaptation is promoted. The evaluation of goal achievement is made, and further actions are taken as necessary.

Situation

Mrs. Anitha is received from surgery after a major abdominal operation. Before surgery, her baseline vital signs were: heart rate, 80 beats per minute; blood pressure, 120/80 mmHg; and respiratory rate, 16 per min. After 45 minutes in recovery, her vital signs are: heart rate, 150/min. blood pressure 90/60 mmHg; respiratory rate, 32 per minute. Increased regulator output response is signalled by sympathetic nervous system stimulation of the heart in response to decreased blood pressure. The nurse decides that Mrs. Anitha is showing an ineffective response. Therefore, assessment of stimuli is done.

The focal stimulus is a decrease of arterial blood pressure secondary to an unknown underlying cause. The contextual stimuli are: age 45 years, cool extremities, poor nail blanching, no food or drink for 12 hours, intravenous infusion (IV) of dextrose 5% in water with lactated Ringer's solution at 100 cc per hour. Also contextual stimuli include 200 cc of IV fluids infused during surgery, 10 cc of urine excreted during the first

45 minutes in recovery, 1½ hours of general anaesthesia, estimated blood loss of 500 cc during surgery, no operative site bleeding, and level of consciousness slow to respond to tactile stimuli after 45 minutes in recovery. The residual stimuli include history of renal infections.

The nursing diagnosis of a decreased arterial blood pressure secondary to fluid volume deficit is made. A fluid volume loss is suggestion both by the contextual data and by the changes in the baseline heart rate, blood pressure, and urine output. The nurse then intervenes by altering contextual stimuli so that an adaptive response is promoted. The goal of a circulatory volume adequate to maintain a blood pressure of plus 90-20 mm Hg of baseline levels within 15 minutes is set. The nurse plans and then takes the following intervention steps. The IV rate is increased to 300 cc per hour. The foot of the bed is elevated to increase venous return. Forty percent oxygen is given by mask. Mrs. Anitha is verbally and tactilely stimulated and told to take slow deep breaths. The nurse prepares vasopressor medications for immediate use and applies an external continuous blood pressure cuff for constant blood pressure monitoring. The nurse also consults with other team members as to Mrs. Anitha's clinical presentation.

A constant evaluation of the effectiveness of the nursing actions is made. The nurse holds Mrs. Anitha in recovery until the goal of adequate circulation volume is met. Evaluation criteria include urine output greater than 30 cc per hour, mental alertness, rapid nail bed blanching, blood pressure plus or minus 20 mm Hg of presurgery levels, pulse plus or minus 20 beats per minute of baseline, and respirations plus or minus 5 per minute of baseline, and respirations plus or minus 5 per minute of presurgery levels.

Roy's Work and the Characteristics of a Theory

1. Theories can interrelate concepts in such a way as to create a different way of looking at a particular phenomenon. The Roy model does interrelate concepts in such a way as to present a new view of the phenomenon being studies. It identifies the key concepts relevant to nursing: the person, environment, health and nursing. The person is viewed as constantly interacting with internal and external stimuli. The person is active and reactive to these stimuli. Stimuli are defined as focal, that which invokes invokes the greatest degree of change; contextual; and residual. The theory suggests the influence of multiple causes in a situation, which is a strength when dealing with multifaceted human beings. Adaptation is a positive response made by the person to the experience being encountered. Adaptation is facilitated by the use of the regulator and cognator coping mechanisms. The adaptation level represents the range of stimuli that the person can tolerate and continue to maintain adaptive responses. The areas of response where the effects of coping are evidenced include the four adaptive modes; physiological, self-concept, role function, and interdependence. Thus, by a quick review of the concept of the person who is the recipient of nursing care, one sees that a very specific perspective or image has been defined by the Roy model. Beginning work in the development of theory related to these concepts has been

done by Roy, Roberts, and others. The view suggests a holistic framework as opposed to a view of the ill person as a biological entity with a disease process. It reflects a view of nursing that is concerned with many aspects of the person—physiological, self-concept, role function and interdependence.

2. Theories must be logical in nature. The sequence of concepts the Roy model follows logically. In the presentation of each of the key concepts there is the recurring idea of adaptation to maintain integrity. The definition of health is based on the idea of integrity, which in turn is operationalized to mean responses that meet the person's goals of survival, growth, reproduction, and mastery. Promoting adaptive responses in situation of health and illness is the goal of nursing. The person is conceptualized as a holistic, adaptive system.

3. Theories should be relatively simple yet generalizable. The concepts of the Roy model are stated in relatively simple terms. However, the concept of the person as an adaptive system does present a challenging use of specific terms, including cognator and regulator mechanisms and adaptation level. The four adaptive modes may be the first aspect of the model that the student or nurse is able to assimilate. Based upon nursing tradition, assessment of fluid and electrolytes, elimination, oxygenation, roles, and such evoke familiar images. As one nurse studying the theory stated, "It's what we've always done. I don't know that the big deal is perhaps, she failed to realize that such a statement was compliment any of the model's fit to clinical practice.

Let us also consider the generalised ability of the model in various settings. Use of the Roy model to organize curriculum has been demonstrated by the faculty at Mount Saint Mary's College in Los Angeles. Similarly, extensive use of the model as well as pictorial representations of it have been made by the faculty and students of the Royal Alexandra Hospitals School of Nursing. Use of the model for the care of various client populations is exemplified by the works of Farkas (1981). Giger, Bower, & Miller (1987), and Janelli (1980). Research studies examining the use of the model in nursing practice include the work of Fredrickson et. al. (1991), Hoch (1987), Limandri (1986), and Pollock (1993).

4. Theories can be the bases for hypotheses that can be tested or for theory to be expanded, and

5. Theories contribute to and assist in increasing the general body of knowledge of a discipline through the research implemented to validate them. The testing of a theory in practice is the basis for scientific development of a profession. Because Roy presents her work as a model, subtheorizing is present when application of the model is made for predictive understanding in a clinical situation. The model must be able to clearly identify the connecting relationships between underlying theories. Testable hypotheses are thus generated. Hill and Roberts (1981) discuss "relevant theory derivations" in their study of nursing interventions to promote the health of children with birth defects who are in need of habitation. Developmental and social learning concepts related to the Roy

premises and hypotheses for testing are proposed. Multiple examples of hypotheses for testing are generated by Roy and Roberts (1981). Because the model is an umbrella that can link theories, its contributions in the future to the body of nursing knowledge may be considerable.

6. Theories can used by practitioners to guide and improve their practice. Perhaps the most important aspect of a theory is its usefulness in practice. How does application of the Roy model guide and improve the work of the practitioner? A major strength of the model is that it guides nurses to use observation and interviewing skills in doing and individualized assessment of each person. Behaviour related to the four adaptive modes is collected during behavioural assessment. In considering all the adaptive modes—physiological, self-concept, role function, and interdependence—the nurse is likely to have comprehensive view of the person.

The concepts of the Roy model are applicable within many practice settings of nursing. Literature cited throughout this chapter reflects application of the model by nurse educators, practitioners, and researchers in a variety of educational and clinical settings.

The use of the model may demand a change in the allocation of time, and resources. Painstaking application of the model requires significant input of time and effort. The benefit to the client of complete assessment and implementations in areas of concern, however, justifies the effort and allocation of resources. Even in practice settings that require quick action, the elements of the model are still compatible with quality care. Especially useful is the guide for the assessment of stimuli which helps identify focal, contextual, and residual stimuli. The development by Roy of a typology of nursing diagnosis of common adaptation problems is an exciting outflow of the model. Further integration of Roy's work with that of Nanda is to be seen.

Goal setting and achievement in nursing are likely to be facilitated by application of commonly defined concepts and direction of focus. Because the model encourages identification of the local, contextual, and residual stimuli within a situation, it immediately indicates, the course of nursing action. Nursing actions are geared to altering these stimuli. This aspect of the model helps the practitioner in making specific decisions about what actions to take. In another way, practitioners can see the importance of their actions in influencing the adaptation of the person. For example, the nurse can view nursing actions such as maintaining bed rest or relieving pain or fears as significant in maintaining an adaptive response for the person.

7. Theories must be consistent with other validated theories, laws and principles but will leave open unanswered questions that need to be investigated. By its structure, the Roy model requires the integration of further theorizing for explanatory and predictive information in clinical situations. The concept of adaptation as developed by the model appears to have good linkage qualities. Theory development has been undertaken by Roy, her co-author, and others as cited throughout this chapter. Future nursing research and field

application will continue to validate and adjust the Roy model.

EVALUATION OF THE THEORY

According to Chinn and Jacobs "clarity requires the semantic and structural organization of goals, assumptions, concepts, definitions, relationships, and structure into a logically coherent whole." Duldt and Giffin state that Roy's arrangement of concepts is logical, but that the development of definitions is in adequate related to her original format. Terms and concepts borrowed from other disciplines are not redefined for nursing. Roy's theory examples tend to use a biopsychosocial set as the principle for organizing, instead processors. One limitation these authors cite is that Roy claims to follow a holistic view, but leaves out "spiritual, humanistic, and existential aspects of being a person." Instead," man is defined as a survival-oriented, behaviourist (condition-response), amoral, living system."

Mestal and Hammond discussed difficulties with Roy's model in classifying certain behaviours due to overlapping of concept definitions. The problem identified dealt with theory conceptualisation and the need for mutually exclusive categories to classify human behaviour. Their problem with the person's position on the health-illness continuum has been clarified by Roy in the redefining of health as personal integration. However, other researchers have also referred to difficulty in classifying behaviour exclusively in one adaptive mode.

A part of the structural inconsistency of the model occurs because a series of assumptions borrowed from behaviouristic thought and systems theory are difficult to reconcile with the assumptions of humanism. This combination of such divergent theoretical roots may be a basis for a part of the internal tension of the Roy model, but these assumptions of humanism are what makes the model applicable to nursing.

- The Roy model includes the concepts of nursing, person, health-illness, environment, adaptation, and nursing activities. It also includes the subconcepts of regulator, cognator, and the four effector modes of physiological, self-concept, role function, and interdependence. Because this theory has several major concepts and subconcepts and numerous relational statements, it is complex.
- Roy defines her model as drawn from multiple middle range theories and advocates multiple middle range theories for use in nursing Middle range theories are testable, but have sufficient generality to be scientifically interesting. Roy's model has been classified as a grand theory. The broad scope is an advantage because the model may be used for other theory building and testing in studying smaller ranges of phenomena. Roy's model is generalizable to all settings in nursing practice, but is limited in scope because it primarily addresses the concept of person-environment adaptation and focuses primarily on the client; information on the nurse is implied.
- Increasing complexity within theories often helps increase empirical precision. When subcomponents are designated within the theory, the empirical precision increases, assuming the broad concepts are based in reality. Because Roy's broad concepts stem from theory in physiological psychology, psychology, sociology, and nursing, empirical data indicate that this

general theory base has substance. Roy studied and analysed 500 samples of patient behaviour collected by nursing students. From this analysis, Roy proposed her four adaptive models in man. This is the least supported of Roy's concepts.

Roy's assumptions can also be analysed to determine what type of statements they are. The eight assumptions of the Adaptation Model of Nursing are as follows:

1. The person is a biopsychosocial being.
2. The person is in constant interaction with a changing environment.
3. To cope with a changing world, the person uses both innate and acquired mechanisms, which are biological, psychological, and sociological in origin.
4. Health and illness are one inevitable dimension of the person's life.
5. To respond positively to environmental changes, the person must adapt.
6. The person's adaptation is a function of the stimulus he is exposed to and his adaptation level.
7. The person's adaptation level is such that it comprises a zone indicating the range of stimulation that will lead to a positive response.
8. The person is conceptualised as having four modes of adaptation: physiological needs, self-concept, role function, and interdependence relations.

Of the eight basic assumptions presented in the model, assumptions 1 through 5 are existence statements. Assumptions 6 and 7 are associational statements can be either associational or causal. The relational statements are the relations that may be tested.

Roy identifies many propositions in relation to the regulator and cognator mechanisms and the self-concept, role function, and interdependence modes. These propositions have varying degrees of support from general theory and empirical data. The majority of the propositions are relational statements and can also be tested. 48 Testable hypotheses have been derived from the model.

Derivable consequences refer to how practically useful, important, and generally sufficient the theory is in relation to achieving valued nursing outcomes. The theory needs to guide research and practice, generate ideas, and differentiate the focus of nursing from other service professions.

The Roy adaptation model has a clearly defined nursing process and can be useful in guiding clinical practice. The model is also capable of generating new information through the testing of the hypotheses that have been derived from it.

Meleis asserts that there are three types of nursing theorists: those who focus on needs, those who focus on interaction, and those who focus on outcome. Roy's Adaptation Model is classified as an outcome theory, defined by this author as "a well-articulated conception of man as a nursing client and of nursing as an external."

Chapter 17

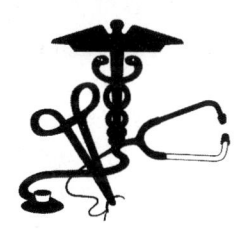

Neuman's Systems Model

Betty Neuman was born in 1924 on a farm near Lowell, Ohio. Her father was a farmer and her mother a homemaker. She developed a love for the land while growing up in rural Ohio, and this rural background developed her compassion for people in need. Dr. Neuman's initial nursing education was completed with double honors at Peoples Hospital School of Nursing (now General Hospital), Akron, Ohio, in 1947. She then moved to Los Angeles to live with relatives. In California she held various positions including hospital staff and head nursing, school nursing, and industrial nursing. She was also involved in clinical teaching in what is now the USC Medical Center, Los Angeles, in the areas of medical-surgical, communicable disease, and critical care. Because she had always been interested in human behaviour, she attended the University of California at Los Angeles with a double major in public health and psychology. She completed her baccalaureate degree with honors in nursing in 1957 and then helped establish and manage her husband's obstetrical and gynaecological practice. In 1966 she received her master's degree in Mental Health, Public Health Consultation from UCLA. She received a doctoral degree in Clinical Psychology from Pacific Western University in 1985.

Neuman was a pioneer of nursing involvement in mental health. She developed, taught, and refined a community mental health programme for postmaster level nurses at UCLA. Dr. Neuman and Donna Aquilina were the first two nurses to pioneer development of the nurse counsellor role within Los Angeles based community crisis centers. She developed her first explicit teaching and practice model for mental health consultation in the late 1960s, before the creation of her systems model. This teaching and practice model is cited in her first book publication in 1971. Neuman then designed a conceptual model for nursing in 1970 in response to requests from UCLA graduate students who requested a course emphasizing breadth rather than depth in understanding the variables in nursing. The model initially was developed to integrate student learning of client variables extending nursing beyond the medical model. It included such behavioural science concepts as problem identification and prevention. Dr. Neuman first published her model in 1972. She spent the following decade further defining and refining various aspects of the model in preparation for her book entitled The *Neuman Systems Model: Application to Nursing Education and Practice*. A second edition (1989) illustrates further development and revision of the model.

Since developing the Neuman Systems Model, she has been involved in a wide variety of professional international activities, including numerous publications, paper presentations, consultations, lectures, and conferences. Dr. Neuman has a wide range of teaching areas, having taught nurse continuing agencies for 14 years. She has remained an active private practice therapist as a licensed clinical member of the American Association of Marriage and Family Therapist as a licensed clinical member of the American Association of Marriage and Family Therapists since 1970. Dr. Neuman maintains her role as consultant internationally for nursing schools and practice agencies adopting the model.

EVOLUTION OF THEORY

The model has some similarity to Gestalt theory. Gestalt theory maintains that the homoeostatic process is the process by which an organism maintains its equilibrium, and consequently its health, under varying conditions. Neuman describes adjustment as the process by which the organism satisfies its needs. Because many needs exist and each may disturb client balance or stability, the adjustment process is dynamic and continuous. All life is characterized by this ongoing interplay of balance and imbalance within the organism. When the stabilizing process fails to some degree, or when the organism remains in a state of disharmony for too long and is consequently unable to satisfy its needs, illness may develop. When this compensatory process fails completely, the organism may die. The Gestalt approach, then, considers the individual as a function of the organism-environmental field and considers behaviour a reflection of relatedness within that field.

The model is also derived from philosophical views of deChardin and Bernard Marx. Marxist philosophy suggests that the properties of parts are determined partly by the larger wholes within dynamically organized systems. Along with this, Neuman confirmed that the patterns of the whole influence awareness of the part, which is drawn from deChardin's philosophy of the wholeness of life. She used H. Selye's definition of stress, which is the non-specific response of the body to any demand made on it. Stress increases the demand for readjustment. This demand is non-specific; it requires adaptation to a problem, irrespective of what the problem it. The essence of stress is therefore the non-specific demand for activity. Stressors are tension producing stimuli with the potential for causing disequilibrium, such as situational or maturational crises.

Neuman's model also reflects general systems theory, that is, the nature of living open systems. This theory states that all the elements are in interaction in a complex organization. From Caplan's conceptual model for levels of prevention, Newman relates these prevention levels to nursing.

The person is a unique, wholistic system yet possesses a common range of normal characteristics and responses. Persons are a dynamic composite of physiologic, psychologic, socio-cultural, developmental, and spiritual variables. These variables interact with internal and external environmental stressors. The wholistic system of the person is open. As an open system it interacts with, adjusts to, and is adjusted by the environment. The external environment is defined as all that interfaces with the person's system. The internal and external environments are a source of stressors that have different potentials to disturb the normal line of defense and disrupt the system. The normal line of defense is essentially the usual steady state of the individual and is composed of the normal range of responses to stressors within people that evolve over time. The flexible line of defense cushions and protects individuals from stressor. Lines of resistance are conceptualized as internal factors that help people defend against stressors, and they protect the core structure and stabilize and return individuals to a normal line of defense when stressors break through.

The system's model is based on an individual's relationship to stress, reaction to it, and reconstitution factors that are dynamic in nature. The nurse assesses, manages, and evaluates patient systems. Nursing's focus is the variables that affect a person's response to stressors. Assessment of individuals considers knowledge of factors influencing a patient's perceptual field, the meaning stressors have to a patient as validated by patient and caregiver, and factors the caregiver believes influence the patient situation. Basically, nursing focusses on the occurrence of stressors, the organism's response to them, and the state of the organism. Primary prevention identifies and allays risk factors associated with stressors; it focuses on protecting the normal line of defense and strengthening the flexible line of defense. Secondary prevention is related to symptomatology, intervention priorities, and treatment; it helps to strengthen internal lines of defense. Death occurs if the basic core structure of the system fails to support the intervention. Tertiary prevention protects reconstitution or return to wellness following treatment.

Nursing acts to impede or arrest an entropic state or a state of disorder and disorganization. Health is a state of movement toward negentropy or evolution; it is a state of inertness free from disrupting needs. Health implies a homeostatic balance. This balance depends on free energy flow between the organism and the environment. In health the system's normal line of defense is maintained, and the lines of resistance are intact; the basic structural elements of the system are preserved.

The Neuman Systems Model (NSM) was originally developed in 1970 on request of the Graduate students of UCLA in order to provide an overview of the physiological, psychological, socio-cultural and developmental aspects of human being as an introductory course. **Neuman** says that her personal philosophy of "helping each other live" was supportive in developing the wholistic systems perspective of NSM. She drew upon her clinical experiences from variety of health care and community settings and the theoretic perspectives of stress and systems. The model has some similarities to **Gestalt** theory which maintains that the homeostatic process is the process by which an organism maintains its equilibrium, and consequently, its health, under varying conditions. Neuman describes adjustment as the process by which the organism satisfies its needs. Because many needs exist and each may disturb client balance or stability, the adjustment process is dynamic and continuous.

The Neuman system model derived philosophical views from Dacharden and Bernard Mark (1955), stress from Selye (1950), Systems from Von Bertalanffy (1968), levels of prevention from Caplan (1964) and etc. Neuman conceptualized the model from sound theories rather than from nursing research.

B. Neuman (1955) considered "nursing" as a system because nursing practice contains elements in interaction with one another. Advantages of an open systems perspectives in nursing include the use of systems as unifying force across various scientific fields as well as the increasing complexity of nursing, which calls for on organizational system that can respond to change. A system perspective supports recognition of the complex while valuing the importance of the parts. The relationships between the parts and the interaction of the parts or the whole with the environment provide a mechanism. For viewing the system environment exchanges, which support the dynamic and constantly changing nature of the systems. And she views wholism as both philosophical and a biological concept. Wholism includes relationship that arise from wholeness, dynamic freedom, and creativity as the system responds to stressors from the internal and external environments.

The Neuman System Model (NSM)

In the Neuman System Model, the two major components are *stress* and the *reaction to stress*. In this, client is viewed as an open system, in which repeated cycles of impact, process, output and feedback constitute a dynamic organizational pattern. Using the systems prospective, the client may be an individual, a group, a family, a community or any aggregate. In their development toward growth and survival, open systems continuously become more differentiated and elaborate or complex. As they become more complex, the internal conditions of regulation become more complex. Exchanges with the environment are reciprocal; both the client and the environment may be affected either positively or negatively, by each other. The system may adjust to the environment or adjust the environment to itself. The environment influences are identified as intra-, inter- and extrapersonal. The ideal is to achieve *optimal system* stability. When a system achieves stability a revitalization occur. As an open system, the client system has a propensity to seek or maintain balance among the various factors, both within and outside the system, that seeks to disrupt it. These forces called as *stressors* and views them as capable of having either positive or negative effects. *Reactions* to the stressors may be possible or not yet occurring, or actual, with identifiable responses and symptoms.

The major concepts identified in the Neuman System Model are:
- Wholesale client approach
- Open system
- Basic structure
- Environment
- Created environment
- Stressors
- Lines of defense and resistance
- Degree of reaction
- Preventions as intervention and

- Reconstructions and later she added
- Content
- Input and output
- Feedback
- Negentropy
- Entropy
- Stability
- Wellness and illness.

Wholistic Client Approach

The NSM is a dynamic, open, system approach to client care originally developed to provide an unifying focus or nursing problems definition and for best understanding the client interaction with the environment. The client as a system may be defined as a person, family, group, community issue. Here the clients are viewed as whole whose parts are in dynamic interaction. The model considers all *variables* simultaneously affecting the client system. *Physiological, socio-cultural*, developmental and spiritual variable. In other words she views the individual client wholistically and considers the variable simultaneously and comprehensively. In the ideal situation, these variable functions are in harmony with stability in relation to internal and external environmental stressors. Each of the variables should be considered when assessing system reaction to the stressors for each of the concentric circles in the model diagram (Fig. 17.1). It is vital to avoid fragmentation of optimum stability of the client system is to be promoted through nursing care. Meanings of these variables are as follows:

- The physiological variable refers to the structure and functions of the body.
- The psychological variables refers to mental processes and relationships.
- The socio-cultural variable refers to system functions that relate to social and cultural expectations and activities.
- The development variables refer to those processes related to development over the life span.
- The spiritual variables refer to the influence of spiritual beliefs.

Neuman indicates that the first four variables are commonly understood by nursing. The spiritual variable added recently because it is viewed as an innate component of the basic structure that may or may not be acknowledged or developed by the client and it permeating all the other variables of the client system and existing on a developmental continuum from complete awareness of the presence and potential of the variable to a highly developed spiritual understanding that supports optimal wellness.

Open System

A system is open when its clients are exchanging information energy within its complex organization. Stress and reaction to stress are basic components of open system. (Explained in the beginning portion of NSM)

Environment

Neuman defines environment as "all the internal and external forces affecting and being affected by the client at any time comprise the environment."

- The *internal* environment exists with in the client system. All forces and interactive influences that are solely within the boundaries of the client system make up this environment.
- The *external* environment exists outside the client system. Those forces and interactive

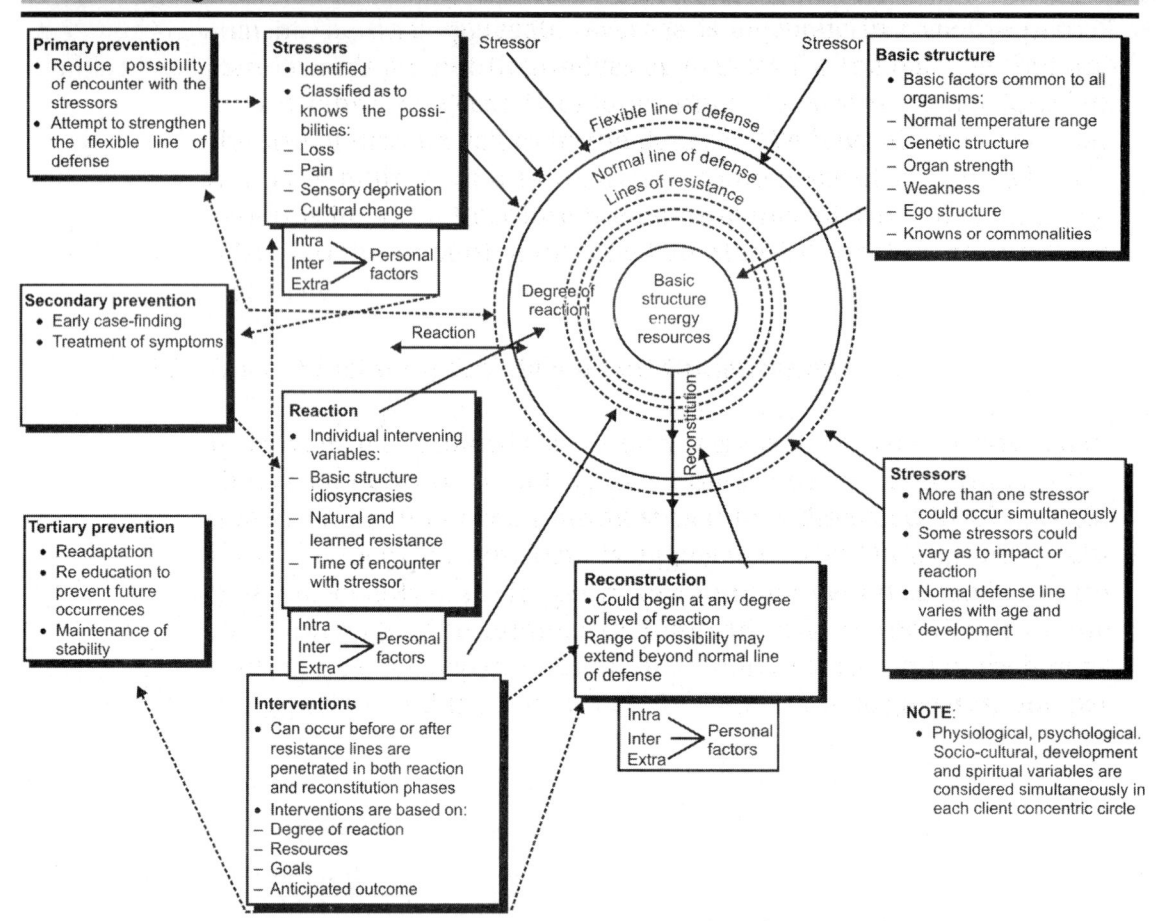

Figure 17.1: The Neuman systems model

influences that are outside the system boundaries are identified as external.

The influence of the client on the environment and the environment on the client may be positive or negative at any time. Variation in both the client systems and environment can affect the direction of the reaction. For example, individual who experiences sleep deprivation are more susceptive to viruses of the common cold from the environment than those who are well rested.

Created environment, identified by Neuman (1989) meant that it is the client's unconscious mobilization of all system variables toward system integration, stability and integrity. It is symbolic system of wholeness, as it represents the open system exchange of energy with both internal and external environment. It is dynamic and depicts the unconscious mobilization of all system variable, particularly the psychological and socio-cultural variables. The purpose of this mobilization is the integration, integrity and stability of the system.

A major objective of the created environment is to provide a positive stimulus toward health for the client. It is developed to be protective but may have a negative effect on the system if it uses energy needed to react to environmental stressors. While providing nursing, nurse has to identify created environ by why, what, what extent, what is ideal in the created environment.

Contents

The five variables (physiological, psychological, socio-cultural developmental and spiritual) of man is interaction with the environment comprise the whole system of the client.

Basic Structure

The basic structure consists of all variables as survival factors common to man, as well as unique individual characteristics. The inner circle of the diagram (Fig. 17.1) represents the basic survival factors or energy sources of the client.

The basic structure or central care is made up of those survival factors common to the species. These factors include the system variables genetic features and strength and weakness of the system parts. If the client system is human being, the basic structures contain such features as the ability to maintain body temperatures within a normal range, genetic features, such as hair colour and response to stimuli, and the functioning of the various body systems and their interrelationships. There are also the baseline characteristics associated with each of the five variables, such as physical strength, cognitive ability and value systems.

Neuman identifies system stability or homeostasis as occurring when the amount of energy that is available exceeds their being used by the system. This stability preserves the character of the system. Since the system is an open system, the stability is dynamic. As output, becomes feedback and input, the system seeks to regulate itself. A change in one direction is countered by a compensating movement in the opposite direction. When the system is disturbed from its normal or stable, state there is a rapid surge in the amount of energy needed to deal with the disorganization that results from the disturbance.

Process or Function

The exchange of matter, energy, and information with the environment and the interaction of the parts and supports of the system of man. A living system tends to move toward wholeness.

Input and Output

"The matter, energy and information exchanged between man and environment, which is entering or leaving the system at any point in time.

Feedback

The process within which the matter, energy and information as a system output provides feedback for corrective action to change, enhance, or stabilize the system.

Negentropy

A process of energy utilization that assists system progression toward stability or wellness.

Entropy

A Process of energy depletion that moves the system to illness or death.

Stability

The client or system successfully copes with stressors, it is able to maintain an adequate level of health. Functional harmony or balance preserves the integrity of the system.

Stressors

Stressors are environmental forces that may alter system stability. Neuman views stressors as:
- Interpersonal forces occurring within the individual (e.g. conditioned response auto-immune response).
- Interpersonal forces occurring between one or more individuals (e.g. role expectations).
- Extrapersonal forces occurring outside the individual (e.g. financial circumstances a social policy).

Stressors are "stimuli which might penetrate both the client's flexible and normal lines of defense: the potential outcome of an interaction with a stressor may be beneficial positive or noxious (negative).

Wellness

Wellness exists when the parts of the client system interacts in harmony. System needs are met.

Illness

Disharmony among the parts of the system is considered illness in varying degrees reflecting unmet needs.

Normal Line of Defenses

The normal line of defense is the model's outer solid circle. It represents a stability state for the individual, system or the condition following adjustment made to stressors and maintained over time that is considered uniquely normal (Fig. 17.1).

This is a result or composite of several variables and behaviours such as the individuals usual coping pattern, lifestyle, and developmental stage, it is basically the way in which an individual copes with stressors while functioning within the cultural pattern of birth and which he/she attempts to conform.

This is considered to be the usual level of stability for the system or the normal wellness state and is used as the baseline for determining deviation from wellness for the client system. The normal line of defense has changed overtime as a result of coping with a variety of stressors. The stability represented by the normal line of defense is actually a range of responses to the environment. For example, any stressor may invade the normal line of defense when the flexible line of defense offers inadequate protection, when the normal line of defense offers inadequate protection. When the normal line of defense is invaded, or penetrated, the clients system reacts. The reaction will be apparently in symptoms of instability or illness and may reduce the systems ability to withstand additional stresses.

Flexible Lines of Defense

The model's outer broken ring is called the flexible line of defense. It is the outer boundary and initial response, or protection, of the system to stressors. It serves as a cushion and is described as accordion like as it expands away from or contracts closer to the normal line of defense. It is dynamic and can be rapidly altered over a short period of time. It is perceived as a protective buffer for preventing stressors from breaking through the solid line of defense. The relationship of the variables can affect the degree to which an individual is able to use their flexible line of defense against possible reaction to a stressor such as loss of sleep. It is important to strengthen this flexible line of defense to prevent a possible reaction.

Line of Resistance

The series of broken rings surrounding the basic core structure are called the flexible line of resistance. These rings represent resource factors that help the client defend against a stressor. An example is the body's immune response system. The lines of resistance protect the basic structure and become activated when the normal line of defense is invaded by environmental stressors. If the lines of resistance are effective in their response, the system can reconstitute, if the line of resistance are not effective, the resulting energy depletion may lead to death.

Degree of Reaction

The degree of reaction is the amount system instability resulting from stressor invasion of the normal line of defense. Neuman does not discuss this reactions separately, but she points out that reactions and outcomes may be positive or negative and she discusses system movement toward negentropy or entropy.

Prevention of Intervention

Interventions are purposeful actions to help the client retain, attain, and/or maintain system stability. They can occur before and/or after resistance lines are penetrated in both reaction and reconstitution phases. Neuman supports beginning intervention when a stressor is either suspected or identified. Interventions are based on possible or actual degree of reaction, resources, goals and the anticipated outcome. Neuman identifies three levels of intervention—primary, secondary and tertiary—which are used to retain, attain and maintain system balance. More than one prevention mode may be used simultaneously.

Primary Prevention

Primary prevention is carried out when a stressor is suspected or identified. A reaction has not yet occurs but the degree of risk is known. Neuman states, "The actor or intervener would perhaps attempt to reduce the possibility of the individuals encounter with the stressor or attempt to strengthen the individual's flexible line of defense to decrease the possibility of a reaction.

Primary prevention occurs prior to system reacting to a stressor; it includes health promotion and maintenance of wellness. It focuses on strengthening flexible line of defense through preventing stress and reducing risk factors. This intervention occurs which the risk or hazard is identified, but before the reaction occurs. Strategies that might be used include immunization, health education, exercise and lifestyle changes.

Secondary Prevention

Secondary prevention occurs after the system reacts to a stressor and is provide in terms of existing symptoms, i.e. it in involves interventions or treatment initiated after symptoms from stress have occurred. It focusses on strengthening the internal lines of resistance and thus protects the basic structure through appropriate treatment of symptoms. The intent is to regain optimal system stability and to conserve energy in doing so. Here, both the clients' internal and external resources would be used toward system stabilization to strengthen internal lines of resistance, reduce the reaction, and increase the resistance factors.

Tertiary Prevention

Tertiary prevention occurs after the active treatment or secondary prevention strategies. It focusses on readjustment towards optimal client system stability. A primary goal is to strengthen resistance to stressors by reduction to help prevent recurrence of reaction and regression. Its purpose is to maintain wellness or protect the client system reconstitution through supporting existing strengths and continuing to conserve energy. Tertiary prevention may begin at any point after system stability has begun at any point after system stability has begun to be reestablished (Reconstitution has begun). This process leads back in a circular fashion toward primary prevention. An example would be avoidance of stressors known to be hazardous to the client.

Reconstitution

Reconstitution is the state of adaptation to stressors in the internal and external environment. Reconstitution begins at any degree or level of reaction and may progress beyond or stabilize somewhat below the client's previous normal line of defense. Included in reconstitution are, interpersonal, interpersonal, extrapersonal and environmental factors interrelated with physiological, psychological, socio-cultural, developmental and spiritual variables.

Reconstitution is the increase in energy that occurs in relation to the degree of reaction to the stressors. It may expand the normal line of defense beyond its previous level, stabilize the system at lower levels, or return it to the level that existed before the illness. It depends on successful mobilization of client resources to prevent further reaction to the stressor, and it represents a dynamic state of adjustment.

Neuman (1995) also discusses nursing as a part of the model. The major concern for nursing is to help the client system attain, maintain or retain system stability. This may be accomplished through accurate assessment of both the actual or potential effects of stressor invasion and assisting the client system to make those adjustments necessary for optimal wellness. In supplementing system stability, the nurse provides the linkages between the client system the environment, health and nursing.

Paradigm of Neuman's Model

The four major concepts in Nursing's metaparadigm are identified by Neuman as part of her model and have been discussed. The brief summary of each is as follows:

Human Being

The Neuman model presents the client as a Whole person, that is, a dynamic composite of interrelationship among physiological, psychological, socio-cultural, developmental and spiritual factors. The client (human being) is defined as an open system, that interacts with both internal and external environmental forces of stressors. The human is in constant charge, moving towards a dynamic state of system stability or toward illness of varying degrees, i.e. viewed as an open system in reciprocal interaction with environment.

Environment

Environment is a vital arena that is germane to the system and its functions; it includes internal, external and created environment. The environment may be viewed as all factors that affect and are affected by the system.

Health

Neuman equates health to wellness and defines health or wellness as " the condition in which all parts and supports (variables) are in harmony with the whole of the client. It is condition as degree of system stability and is viewed as a continuum from wellness to illness. Stability occurs when all the systems parts and subparts are in balance or harmony so that the whole system is in balance. When system needs are met, optimal wellness exists. When needs are not satisfied, illness exists. When the energy needed to support life is not available, death occurs.

Man is an interacting open system with the environment and is either in a dynamic state of wellness or in experiencing same degree of illness. Reconstitutions wellness may occur after adaptation to stressors with a return to maintenance and stability of the client system.

Nursing

Neuman believes nursing is concerned with the whole person. She views nursing as a "Unique profession in that it is concerned with all of the variables affecting an individual's response to stress." Because the nurse's perceptions influence the care given. Neuman states that the care given as well as the client's perceptual field must be assessed. She has developed an assessment and Intervention tool to help with this task.

Propositions of the Neuman Systems Model

Neuman (1974) presented the assumptions that she identified as underlying the Neuman Systems Model. She has now labelled these as propositions (Neuman 1995). These proposit-ions follow:

1. Although each individual client or group as a client system is unique, each system is a composite of common known factors or innate characteristics within a normal, given range of response contained within a basic structure.

2. Many known, unknown, and universal environmental stressors exist. Each differs in its potential for disturbing a client's usual stability level or normal line of defense. The particular interrelation-ships of client variables,—physiological, psychological, socio-cultural, developmental and spiritual —at any point in time can affect the degree to which a client is protected by the flexible line of defense against possible reaction to a single stressor or a combination of stressors.

3. Each individual client/client system has evolved a normal range of response to the environment that is referred to as a normal line of defense, or usual wellness/stability state. It represents change over time through coping with diverse stress encounters. The normal line of defense can be used as a standard from which to measure health deviation.

4. When the cushioning, accordion-like effect of the flexible line of defense is no longer capable of protecting the client/client system against an environmental stressor, the stressor breaks through the normal line of defense. The interrelationships of variables—physiological, psychological, socio-cultural, developmental, and spiritual—determine the nature and degree of the system reaction or possible reaction to the stressor.
5. The client, whether in a state of wellness or illness, is a dynamic composite of the interrelationships of variables—physiological, psychological, socio-cultural, developmental, and spiritual. Wellness is on a continuum of available energy to support the system in an optimal state of system stability.
6. Implicit within each client system is a set of internal resistance factors known as lines of resistance, which function to stabilize and return the client to the usual state of wellness (normal-line of defense) or possibly to a higher level of stability following an environmental stressor reaction.
7. Primary prevention relates to general knowledge that is applied to client assessment and intervention in identification and reduction or mitigation of possible or actual risk factors associated with environmental stressors to prevent possible reaction. The goal of health promotion is included in primary prevention.
8. Secondary prevention relates to symptomatology following a reaction to stressors, appropriate ranking of intervention priorities, and treatment to reduce their noxious effects.
9. Tertiary prevention relates to the adjustive processes taking place as reconstitution begins and maintenance factors move the client back in a circular manner toward primary prevention.
10. The client as a system is in dynamic, constant energy exchange with the environment.

The Neuman Systems Model and the Nursing Process

Neuman (1982-1995) presents a three step nursing process format. The first step is entitled *"Nursing diagnosis"* and includes the use of a data base to identify variances from wellness and development or hypothetical interventions. The second step, *"Nursing Goals,"* includes caregiver-client negotiation of intervention strategies to retain, attain or maintain system stability. The third step, *"Nursing Outcomes,"* includes nursing intervention using the prevention models, confirming that the desired change has occurred or reformulating the nursing goals, using the outcomes of short-term goals to determine longer-term goals and validating the nursing process through client outcomes. Neuman's first step parallels the assessment and diagnosis phases of the five phase nursing process. Her second step equates to the planning phase, and her third step equates to the implementation and evaluation phases.

Using the Neuman Systems Model, in the *Assessment* phase of the nursing process the nurse focusses on obtaining a comprehensive client data base to determine the existing state of wellness and the actual or potential reaction to environmental stressors.

The collected data are priorized and compared to or synthesized with, relevant theories to explain the client's condition. Variances from the usual state of wellness are identified and a summary of impressions developed. The summary includes intra-, inter-and extrapersonal factors.

The synthesis of data with theory also provides the basis for the *Nursing Diagnosis*. In the Neuman model, the diagnostic statement should reflect the entire client condition.

Planning involves negotiation between the caregiver and the client, or recipient of care. The overall goal of the caregiver is to guide the client to conserve energy and to use energy as a force to move beyond the present, ideally in a way that preserves or enhances the client's wellness level. More specific goals will be derived from the nursing diagnoses. The perceptions of both the client and the caregiver must be considered in setting goals.

According to Neuman (1995), nursing actions *(Implementation)* are based on the synthesis of a comprehensive data base about the client and the theory (ies) that are appropriate in light of the client's perceptions and possibilities for functional competence within the environment. The modes for identifying these actions are the levels of prevention as intervention.

It is more explicitly identified in the "Nursing Outcomes" step of Neuman's three step nursing process. According to this third step, evaluation confirms that the anticipated or prescribed change has occurred. If this is not true, then goals are reformulated. Immediate and long range goals are then structured in relation to the short-range outcomes.

The Neuman Systems Model and the Characteristics of a Theory

1. Theories can interrelate concepts in such a way as to create a different way of looking at a particular phenomenon. Neuman has presented a view of the client that is equally applicable to an individual, a family, a group, a community or any other aggregate. The systems view she presents in conjunction with the prevention modalities as intervention, are a unique way of viewing health care phenomena. The interaction of the client system and its environment as they relate to health provide a useful view of the world. The emphasis on primary prevention, including health promotion, is specific to the model and increasingly important in today's health care environment.

2. Theories must be logical in nature. The Neuman Systems Model, particularly as presented in the model diagram (see Fig. 17.1), is logically consistent. The three step nursing process is also logical, with its emphasis on a comprehensive data base, mutual decision making between caregiver and client system, and use of outcomes. However there are some inconsistencies between the diagram and the verbal presentation of the model. The diagram includes reaction that is not specifically discussed in the text. Conversely, the verbal presentation incorporates health, environment, and nursing, which do not appear in the diagram. It is inferred that the diagram is considered to be the most important representation of the model because it is changes in the diagram that require unanimous agreement of the Neuman

trustees. Logically based upon this reference, the concepts in the verbal presentation should be derived from the diagram.

Other inconsistencies relate to Neuman's emphasis on a wholistic approach and a comprehensive view of the client system and her discussion of health and illness. The wholistic and comprehensive view is associated with an open system. Health and illness are presented on a continuum with movement toward health described as negentropic and toward illness as entropic. Entropy is a characteristic of a closed rather than an open, system. She does speak of levels of wellness, rather than levels of illness, but does not make it clear if health and illness are dichotomous.

3. Theories should be relatively simple yet generalizable. Once understood, the Neuman Systems Model is relatively simple, and has readily acceptable definitions of its components. Its generalizability is supported by the more than three dozen chapters in the third edition of the *Neuman Systems Model* that discuss the use of the model in curriculum, nursing practice, and nursing administration in the United States and Internationally. Neuman (1995) also indicates that although the model was designed for nursing, it can be use by other health care providers.

An initial drawback to simplicity is the diagram of the model (Fig. 17.1). In its efforts to represent multiple relationships and components, the diagram has become awesome. With a guide to the diagram, the components can be clearly understood, and the initial sense of over whelping complexity overcome.

4. Theories can be the bases for hypotheses that can be tested or for theory to be expanded, and

5. Theories contribute to and assist in increasing the general body of knowledge within the discipline through the research implemented to validate them. Hypotheses can be and have been derived from the Neuman Systems Model and the relationships within the model. The third edition of *The Neuman Systems Model* cites multiple published research articles, doctoral dissertations, and masters theses that have reported research based on the model. The areas of research have included client systems of individuals, families, and groups of practicing nurses and nursing students in educational settings, hospitals, and the community.

6. Theories can based by practitioners to guide and improve their practice. Neuman has provided tools that are specifically designed to assist practitioners in using the model in practice. The model is congruent with the increasing emphases on home health care and health promotion. It has been widely used by practitioners in nursing education, practice and administration nationally and internationally.

7. Theories must be consistent with other validated theories, laws and principles but will leave open unanswered questions that need to be investigated. Neuman identifies the theories upon which she drew to develop the systems model. Her work appears to be consistent with these theories, and there is no apparent conflict with other theories. There are many questions yet to be answered including; Does the use of the Neuman Systems

Model increase the effectiveness of communication with other health care providers? What is the most effective way to identify client system's optimal level of wellness?

The Neuman Systems Model does not fully meet all the characteristics of a theory. Since it is presented as a model, this is not surprising. Neuman (1995) reports that she and A. Koertvelyessy have found that the major theory of the model is that of optional client system stability. This theory is that the health of the client system is represented by stability. Neuman cites an unpublished papers as the only reference for the theory.

Two significant areas have been identified for further exploration and development: created environment and the spiritual variable within person. Created environment has been addressed earlier in this chapter under both major concepts and definitions and major assumptions. The spiritual variable as a dimension of person was added before 1989 to the four variables of physiological, psychological, sociocultural, and developmental and is currently being researched. Dr. Neuman believes the spiritual variable is necessary for a truly wholistic perspective.

Buchanan has used the concepts of the Neuman Systems Model in community health nursing to develop a "macro systems" nursing view (i) to facilitate a community approach to relationships between the client and the environment and (ii) to intervene with preventive, corrective, and rehabilitative measures.

Neuman and Koertvelyessy have identified the theory of optimal client system stability as a major theory for the model. Neuman views the prevention as intervention concept as having potential for theoretical formulation and states that several other theories are inherent within the model. Nursing research is needed to validate the Neuman Systems Model and the newly defined theory of optimal client system stability.

The validity of the model in the future depends on the testing of mid-range theory developed from the model. Lowry and Anderson demonstrated how the model could be used to guide mid-range theory research studies and their prototype was used to investigate the variables that affect weaning of mechanically ventilated patients. Breckenridge is continuing her work with renal clients and developing midrange theory.

The model is being used and studied by other disciplines. Peter Twomey, Health Director at the Division School of Health and Community Studies in Sheffield, England, uses the model in physiotherapy and occupational therapy curricula. The University of Michigan is using the model as a potential base for their physical therapy programme.

A Neuman Systems Model Trustee Group has been established to preserve, protect, and perpetuate the integrity of the model for the future of nursing. Its international members, personally selected by Neuman, are dedicated professionals. The home of the Neuman Archives has been established at Neuman College Library at Aston, Pennsylvania.

EVALUATION OF THEORY

- Neuman developed a comprehensive nursing conceptual model that operationalizes systems concepts for nursing relevant to the breadth of nursing phenomena. It should remain relevant as well to future nursing needs as identified by the American Nurses Association and World Health Organization. Its lack of specificity allows for a wide range of nurse creativity in its use. Neuman's own critique notes that prior criticisms, such as "its concepts are too broad," have been discounted. It is most congruent with the general trend toward wholistic systemic thinking in nursing. The model's comprehensive and flexible nature will allow for future structuring of all nursing activities "as it has proven to do in the past."

- Neuman presents abstract concepts that are familiar to nursing. Although additional definitions could be helpful, the model's concepts of client, environment, health, and nursing are all inherent and congruent with traditional values. Concepts defined by Neuman and those borrowed from other disciplines are used consistently throughout the model.
- Multiple interactions and interrelationships comprise this broad systemic model; they are organized in complex yet logical manner, and variables tend to overlap to some degree. The concepts coalesce, but a loss of theoretical meaning would occur if they were completely separated. Neuman states that the concepts can be separated for analysis, specific goal setting, and interventions. The model can be used to delineate further the systems concept for nursing and also describe various other health care systems. It can be used to explain the client's dynamic state of equilibrium and the reaction or possible reaction of stressors as a result of environmental conflict. Using the prevention concept within the framework, one can predict the origin of stressors. The model can be used to describe, explain, or predict nursing phenomena. Because of the complex nature of the model, it cannot be described as a simple framework, yet nurses using the model describe it as easy to understand and adapt within a variety of cross-cultural groups.
- The Neuman Systems Model's has been used in a wide variety of nursing situations; it is readily adaptable and comprehensive enough to be useful in all health care settings, including administration and research. Other related health fields can use this framework because of its systemic nature and emphasis on the client system as a whole. The social goals and utility of the model, for example, wholistic care, prevention, and systems concepts, are congruent with present social values.

  Some concepts are broad and represent the phenomena of one person as client, or a larger system, and others are more definitive and identify specific modes of action, such as primary prevention. The subgoals can be identified as broad nursing actions. Because of the broad scope of this model, it can be considered general enough in nature and includes all nursing phenomena under consideration.
- Although the model has not been completely tested to date, nursing scientists are demonstrating major interest in and use of the model to guide nursing research. Hoffman described a list of variables and selected operational definitions that were derived from the Neuman model. Ziegler's nursing diagnosis taxonomy is a useful contribution to further research and theory

development. Findings by Hoch suggest that planned nursing interventions based on the Neuman model are more effective than the absence of planned intervention in decreasing dysphasia and increasing life satisfaction among elderly retirees. Louis and Koertvelyessy's 1987 survey on the utilization of the model in nursing research provides further documentation of increasing empiricism with the model. Continued testing and refinement will increase the model's empirical precision as the research process, analysis, and synthesis of findings from multiple studies are completed.

- Neuman's conceptual model provides the professional nurse with important guidelines for assessment of the whole person, utilization of the nursing process, and implementation of preventive intervention. The focus on primary prevention and interdisciplinary care facilities improved quality of care and is futuristic. Active client participation and negotiation of nursing goals illustrated in the Neuman nursing process fulfil current health mandates.

Another derivable consequence of the model is its potential to generate nursing theory. With continued theory development through research with the model, nursing can expand its scientific knowledge. According to Fawcett the model meets social considerations of congruence, significance, and utility. The model is broad and systemically based. It lends itself well to a comprehensive view within which nursing can be responsive to the world's rapidly changing health care needs. The greatly expanded nursing roles and information base now requires a broad organizing principle (framework) for adequate direction. The increasing number of doctorally prepared nurses are just beginning to validate nursing models and develop a scientific theory base from them for the nursing field.

The Neuman Systems Model provides an appropriate nursing framework and comprehensive approach to contemporary and future goal phenomena and concerns facing nursing and health care delivery in the twenty-first century. The role of the nurse in the future can become dominant if the nursing profession accepts the challenge to assume leadership in the unification of health care delivery using the broad systems perspectives of the Neuman Systems Model. A letter written to Dr. Neuman in 1991 by a recently deceased Manitoba Trustee member, Linda Drew, appropriately draws closure to this chapter yet shares a flavor of the excitement felt as the discipline and science of nursing advances towards the next century.

The Neuman model is not only alive and well, but will have a very long shelf-life because it is so adaptable and continues to provide a very pragmatic framework for dealing with a whole host of issues in nursing practice, education, administration and research. This along with the commitment of nurses and other health care providers to continue using this framework will guarantee a very healthy, exciting future for the model.

Chapter 18

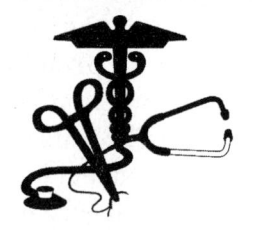

Levine's Four Conservation Principles

Myra Estrin Levine obtained a diploma from Cook County School of Nursing in 1944, an S.B. from the University of Chicago in 1949, and an M.S.N. from Wayne State University in 1962, and has taken postgraduate courses at the University of Chicago. Hutchins' curriculum was being taught to undergraduate students at that time. All students took a year-long survey in the biological, physical, and social sciences and the humanities. The students read and analyzed primary work under the guidance of distinguished professors. Irene Beland became Levine's mentor while she was a graduate student at Wayne State and directed her attention to many of the authors who greatly influenced her thinking.

Levine has enjoyed a varied career. She has been a private duty nurse (1944), a civilian nurse in the U.S. Army (1945), a preclinical instructor in the physical sciences at Cook County (1947-1980), the director of Nursing at Drexel Home in Chicago (1950-1951), and a surgical supervisor at the University of Chicago Clinics (1951-1952) and at Henry Ford Hospital in Detroit (1956-1962). She worked her way up the academic ranks at Bryan Memorial Hospital in Lincoln, Nebraska (1951), Cook County School of Nursing (1963-1967), Loyola University (1967-1973), Rush University (1974-1977), and the University of Illinois (1962-1963, 1977-1987). She chaired the Department of Clinical Nursing at Cook County School of Nursing (1963-1967) and coordinated the graduate nursing programme in oncology at Rush University (1974-1977). Levine was the director of the Department of Continuing Education at Evanston Hospital (March-June 1974), and a consultant to the department (July 1974-1976). She was an adjunct associate professor of Humanistic Studies at the University of Illinois 1981-1987. She is now a Professor Emerita, Medical Surgical Nursing, University of Illinois at Chicago, In 1974 Levine went to Tel-Aviv University, Israel, as visiting associate professor and returned as a visiting professor in 1982. She was also a visiting professor at Recanati School of Nursing, Ben Gurion University of the Negev, Beer Sheva, Israel (March-April, 1982).

Levine has received numerous honors, including being a charter fellow of the American Academy of Nursing (1973), honorary membership in the American Mental Health Aid to Israel (1976), and honorary recognition from the Illinois Nurses' Association (1977). She was the first recipient of the Elizabeth Russell Belford Award for excellence in teaching from Sigma Theta Tau (1977). Both the first and second editions of her book *Introduction to Clinical Nursing* received AJN Book of the Year awards and her 1971 book, *Renewal for Nursing* was translated into Hebrew. Levine was listed in *Who's Who in American Women* (1977-1988) and in *Who's Who in American Nursing* (1987). She was elected fellow of the Institute of Medicine of Chicago (1987-1991). Levine was recognized for her outstanding contributions to nursing by the Alpha Lambda chapter Sigma Theta Tau (1990). In January 1992, she was awarded an honorary doctorate of humane letters from Loyola University Chicago. Levine was an active leader in the American Nurses' Association and the Illinois Nurses' Association. After her retirement in 1987, she remained active in theory development and encouraged questions and research about her theory.

A dynamic speaker, she was a frequent presenter on programmes, workshops, seminars, and panels, and a prolific writer regarding nursing and education. Levine has also served as a consultant to hospitals and schools of nursing. Although she never intended to develop theory, she provided an organizational structure for teaching medical-surgical nursing and a stimulus for theory development. "The Four Conservation Principles of Nursing" was the first statement of the conservation principles. Other preliminary work included "Adaptation and Assessment: A Rationale for Nursing Intervention, For Lack of Love Alone, and "The Pursuit of Wholeness. The first edition of her book using the conservation principles, *Introduction to Clinical Nursing,* was published in 1969. She addressed the consequences of the four conservation principles in "Holistic Nursing. The second edition of the book was published in 1973. Since then, Levine has presented the conservation principles at nurse theory conferences, some of which have been audiotaped, and at the Allentown College of St. Francis de Sales Conferences in April 1984.

In 1989 substantial change and clarification about her theory were published in her chapter "Four Conservation Principles: Twenty Years Later" in Riehl's book *Conceptual Models for Nursing Practice.* She elaborates on how redundancy characterizes availability of adaptive responses when stability is threatened. Adaptation processes establish a body economy to safeguard the individual's stability. Adaptation is the essence of conservation.

EVOLUTION OF THEORY

A person is a wholistic being whose open and fluid boundaries coexist with the environment, which may be perceptual, operational, and conceptual, and is a unity who is to remain conserved and integral. He or she sends messages that reflect his or her current adaptive state. Adaptation is a method of change, and change is life process. When adaptation fails, conservation is threatened, and adaptation needs occur. Adaptive needs are reflected in messages sent.

Nursing occurs at the interface between the open and fluid boundaries of whole persons and environments. The nurse receives and interprets messages and intervenes supportively or therapeutically.

Intervention is guided by the four principles of conservation: conservation of energy, structural integrity, personal integrity, and social integrity. Conservation, based on an assessment of a person's adaptive needs, aids adaptation. When a patient's energy and structural, personal, and social integrity are conserved—that is, when the nurse acts therapeutically—adaptation can better occur, and the person achieves a state of unity and integrity. When conservation cannot be effected in the face of overwhelming adaptation needs, death ensues. Supportive interventions, such as assisting a client toward peaceful death, are appropriate when adaptation is failing without hope of reversal. The goal for nursing is the wholeness of the patient, brought about by conservation in the four areas when adaptive needs are manifested.

Myra Levine, herself told that she never intended to develop theory, but she provided an organizational structure for teaching Medical-Surgical Nursing and stimulus for theory development. In the beginning, she used to putting her ideas about nursing into writing. "The Four Conservation Principles" was the first statement of the conservation principles." The first edition of her work using the conservation principles, *Introduction to Clinical Nursing* was published in 1969. She addressed the consequences of four conservation principles in "Holistic Nursing." In fact more than two decades after the initial publication of her book (1969). She has referred to her work as a theory but prefers to identify it as a conceptual model. She states that she was looking for a way to teach all the major concepts in medical surgical nursing in three quarters and for a way to generalize the content, to move away from a procedurally oriented educational process. She was interested in helping nurses realize that every nurse-patient contact leads to a puzzle in relation to nursing care that needs to be solved in an individualized manner. Her work evolved over the year, with the most recent comprehension update the theory published in 1989.

Myra Levine believed that entry into the health care system is associated with giving up some measure of personal independence. To designate the person who has entered the health care system, a client reinforces the state of dependency, for a client is a follower. She supports the term patient, because patient means sufferer, and dependency is associated with suffering. It is the condition of suffering that makes it possible to set independence aside and accept the services of another person. It is the challenge of the nurse to provide the individual with appropriate care without losing sight of the individuals integrity, to honour the trust that the patient has placed in the nurse, and to encourage the participation of the individual in his or her own welfare. The patient comes in trust and dependence only for as long as the services of the nurse are needed. The nurse's goal is always to impart knowledge and strength so that the individual can ... walk away ... as an independent individual.

Concepts Used by Myra Levine

Holistic

"Whole, health, hale are all derivations of the Anglo-Saxon word HAL." Levine quotes Erikson, who says, "Wholeness emphasizes a sound, organic, progressive, mutuality between diversified functions and parts within an entirety, the boundaries of which are open and fluent."

Holism

Holism means that "human beings are more than different from the sum of their parts. "Perceiving the "wholes' depends upon recognizing the organization and interdependence of observable phenomena.

Integrity

Integrity is from the Latin *Integer*, meaning one. Integrity means being in control of one's life.

Conservation

Conservation is from Latin word *Conservation*, meaning to keep together. "Conservation describes the way complex systems are able to continue to function even when severely challenged. Through conservation, individuals are able to confront obstacles and adapt accordingly while maintaining their uniqueness. "The goal of conservation is health, "while" the rules of conservation and integrity hold" in all situations where nursing is required. The primary focus of conservation is on the integrity of "oneness" of the individual. Although nursing interventions may deal with one particular aspect, it must also recognize the influence of the other conservation principles.

Conservation Principles

Levine's model stresses nursing interactions and interventions that are intended "to keep together the unique and individual resources that each individual beings to his predicament." Those interactions are based on the scientific background of the conservation principles. Nursing care is based on scientific knowledge and nursing skills. There are four conservation principles:

1. *Conservation of energy*: The individual requires a balance of energy and a constant renewal of energy to maintain life activities. That energy is challenged by processes such as healing and aging. This second law of thermodynamic applies to everything in the universe including people.

   Conservation of energy has long been used in nursing practice even with the most basic procedures. Nursing interventions "scaled to the individual's ability are dependent upon providing care that makes the least additional demand possible."

2. *Conservation of structural integrity:* Healing is a process of restoring structural integrity. Nurses should limit the amount of tissue involved in disease by early recognition of functional changes and by nursing interventions.

3. *Conservation of personal integrity*: Self-worth and a sense of identity are important. Nurses can show patients respect by calling them by names respecting their wishes, valuing personal possessions, providing privacy during procedures, supporting their defenses, and teaching them. "The nurse's goal is always to impart knowledge and strength so that the individual can resume a private life—no longer a patient, no longer a dependent."

4. *Conservation of social integrity:* Life gains meaning through social communities, and health is socially determined. Nurses fulfill professional roles, provide for family members, assist with religious needs, and use interpersonal relationships to conserve social integrity.

Adaptation: Adaptation is a process of change, whereby the individual retains his integrity within the realities of his environment. Some adaptations are successful, some or not. Adaptation is a matter of degree not an all-or-nothing process.

Levine speaks of three characteristics of adaptation: history, specificity, and redundancy. Levine states ... "every species has fixed patterns of responses uniquely designed to ensure success in essential life activities, demonstrating that adaptation is both historical and specific." In addition, adaptive patterns may be hidden in the individual's genetic code. Individuals use deliberate redundant options in maintaining or achieving health. Loss of redundant choices either through trauma, age, disease, or environmental conditions make it difficult for the individual to maintain life. Levine suggests that "the possibility exists that aging itself is a consequence of failed redundancy of physiological and psychological processes."

Environment

Environment is "where we are constantly and actively involved. The person and his relationship to the environment is what counts.

Levine also views each individual as having his own environment, both internally and externally. The internal environment can be related by nurses as the physiological and patho-physiological aspects of the patient. Levine uses a definition of the external environment from Bates, who suggests three levels. The perceptual level includes the aspects of the world about us that we are able to intercept and interpret with our sense organs. The operational level contains things that affect us physically even though we cannot directly perceive them, such as micro organisms. At the conceptual level, the environment is constructed from cultural patterns, characterized by a spiritual existence, and mediated by the symbols of language, thought, and history. There are four levels of integration that safeguard the end and help a person maintain his integrity or wholeness.

Organismic Response

The capacity of the individual to adapt to his environmental condition has been called the organismic response. It can be divided into four levels of integration: fight or flight, inflammatory response, response to stress, and perceptual response.

Fight or Flight

The most primitive response is the fight or flight, syndrome. The individual perceives that he is threatened, whether or not a threat does actually exist. Hospitalisation, illness, and new experiences elicit a response. The individual responds by being on the alert to find more information and to assure his safety and well-being.

Inflammatory Response

This defense mechanism protects the self from insult in a hostile environment. It is a way of healing. The response uses available energy to remove or keep out unwanted irritants or pathogens. But it is limited in time because it drains the individual's energy reserves. Environmental control is important.

Response to Stress

Selye described the stress response syndrome to predictable, nonspecifically induced organismic changes. The wear and tear of life is recorded on the tissues and reflects long-term hormonal responses to life experiences that cause structural changes. It is characterized by irreversibility and influences the way patients respond to nursing care.

Perceptual Response

This response is based on the individual's perpetual awareness. It occurs only as the individual experiences the world around him. This response is used by the individual to seek and maintain safety for himself. It is information seeking.

Trophicognosis

Levine recommended trophicognosis as an alternative to nursing diagnosis. It is a scientific method to reach a nursing care Judgment.

THEORY OF LEVINE

Myra Levine discusses adaptation, conservation and integrity. Adaptation is the process by which conservation is achieved, and the purposes for conservation is integrity. The case of her theory are her four principles of conservation.

Adaptation

Adaptation is the life process by which, over time, people maintain their wholeness or integrity as they respond to environmental challenges. It is the consequence of interaction between the person and the environments. Successful engagement with the environment depends on an adequate store of adaptations. Both physiological and behavioural responses are different under different conditions. For example, responses to very quick or very noisy environments will differ. It is possible to anticipate certain kinds of reactions, but the individuality of responses prevents accurate prediction.

Adaptation includes the concepts historicity, specificity and redundancy.

Historicity

Adaptation is a historical process, responses are based on past experiences, both personal and genetic.

Specificity

Adaptation is specific. Each system has very specific responses. For example, the physiological responses that defend oxygen supply or the brain are distinct from those that maintain the appropriate blood glucose level. Particular responses are called into action by a particular challenge, responses are task specific. They are also synchronized.

Redundancy

One of the most remarkable things about living species in the number of levels of response which permit them to confront the reality of their environment in ways that somehow maintain their well being. These redundant systems are both protective and adaptive. If one system does not adapt, another can take over. Redundant system may function in a timeframe; some are corrective whereas others permit a previously failed response to be re-established.

Levine describes adaptation as the best "fit if the person with his or her predicament of time and space.

Conservation

Conservation is the product of adaptation. It is a universal concept, a natural law, that deals with defense of wholeness and system integrity. Conservation defends the wholeness of giving systems by ensuring their ability to confront change appropriately and retain their unique identity.

Conservation describes how complex systems continue to function in the face of several challenges, it provides not only for current survival but also for future vitality through facing challenges in the most economical way possible. For example, thermostat is a set at a selected temperature. As long as the temperature in the room is the same as the set temperature, nothing occurs. When room temperature falls below that selected temperature, the thermostat activities the heating system but only until the room temperature again reaches the thermostat setting. When the setting is reached, the thermostat turns the heating system. Levine (1990) describes this a conserving energy using it in the most frugal, economic and energy-sparing fashion.

The essence of conservation is the successful use of responses that cost the least. "Conservation is clearly the consequence of the multiple, interacting, and synchronized negative feedback systems that provide for the stability of the living organism (Levine 1989 p. 329) As long as systems are physiologically stable, or in balance, negative feedback systems can function at minimal cost. Energy resources are conserved for use when needed to restore balance. Homeostasis is a state of conservation, a state of synchronized sparing of energy.

Levine states that physiological and behavioural responses are essential components of the same activity. They are not parallel or simultaneous, but part of the same whole. She also recognizes that it is difficult to breakdown a body of knowledge and that often information must be gathered piece by piece. Thus, physiological and behavioural responses are often identified and described as separate things. Since they represent the same whole it is important to put the pieces together to represent the whole.

Levels of Behaviours

Levine (1989) describes four levels of behaviour, which are as follows:

1. *Fight or flight response:* The adrenocortical-sympathetic reactions that provide both physiological and behavioural readiness in the face of sudden and unexplained challenges in the environment.
2. *Inflammatory response:* which we relay upon for restoration of physical wholeness and healing.
3. *Stress response:* It described as an integrated defense that occurs over tire, and is influenced by accumulated experience of the individual.
4. *Perceptual response:* Perceptual system in which the senses not only provide access to environmental energy sources but also convert these sources into meaningful experiences. People not only see, they look; they not only hear, they listen.

These levels of behaviour suggest the individual as an active participant with the environment, not mere by as a reactive being. The levels of responses are not sequential but rather redundant and integrated within the individual.

Integrity Principles of Conservation

Nurses' role in conservation is to help the person with the process of "Keeping together" the total person through the lease expense of

effort. Levine (1989) proposed the following fair principles of conservation:
- The conservation of energy of the individual.
- The conservation of the structural integrity of the individual.
- The conservation of the personal integrity of the individual.
- The conservation of the social integrity of the individual.

Conservation of Energy

The conservation of energy is basic to the natural, universal law of conservation. Levine states that energy is not hidden; it is eminently identifiable, measurable, and manageable. Within nursing practice, the measurement of vital signs is a daily measurement of energy parameters. For example, body temperature is an indication of the heat (energy) generated by living cells as they accomplish their work. Energy conservation is encouraged through the limitation of activities for coronary patients of the planned gradual resumption of activities postoperatively. It is important, that even at rest, energy costs are incurred through the activities necessary to support living. Levine identifies these as those activities involved in growth, transport and biochemical and bioelectrical charge. She states "the conservation of energy is clearly evident in the very sick, whose lethargies, withdrawal and self concern are manifested while in its wisdom the body is spending its energy resources on the process of healing. She describes the conservation of energy continue the theme of conservation by including structural integrity, personal integrity and social integrity and also describes the conservation of energy as protecting functional integrity. It is concerned with the integrity of the whole person, the essence of wholeness is integrity.

Conservation of Structural Integrity

The conservation of structural integrity focusses on the healing process. Through multiple experiences with scraped knees and such that heal with no scarring, human develops a mind-set that expects perfect restoration of structural integrity throughout life. 'Healing is the defense of wholeness.' Nurses suggest structural integrity throughout efforts to limit injury and thus, limit scarring, through proper positioning and range of motion to prevent skeletal deformity, pressure areas or loss of muscle tone. To Levine the phantom limb phenomenon suggest the idea that sense of structural integrity is more than a psychological need.

Conservation of Personal Integrity

The conservation of personal integrity focuses on a sense of self. Levine describes identification of self-actualization as observed in efforts of severely brain injured person to retain their personal identity. She points out tat both Maslow and Rogers discussed self-actualization as reaching beyond, but supported Goldstein's concept, i.e. reaching in to the person rather than a reaching beyond. She believes that human have both a public and a very private self. At least some portion of the private self is not known even to those who are closest to the person. The self is "defined, defended, and described only by the soul that own it; that private self is unique and whole. A person can share mere fragments of it with others." In this way, a separation between self and others is maintained. She states that efforts at collecting a complete psychosocial data base may well violate personal integrity. She state: "the most generous psycho-social approach would be to limit the recording of confidences to only those generalizations that actually make a difference in the choice of treatment plans." She likens the awareness of self to independence.

Conservation of Social Integrity

The conservation of social integrity involves a definition of self that goes beyond the individual. Individuals use their relationships to define themselves. One's identity is connected to family, community, culture, ethnicity, religion, vocation, education and socio economic status. To function successfully in this wide variety of social environment, requires a broad behavioural repertoire. The ultimate direction for social integrity is derived from the ethical values of the social system. The health care system is a vast social order with its own rules, but it is an instrument of society and must guarantee privacy, personhood and respect as moral imperatives. She points out that disease prevention is an issue of social integrity and discusses the need both to discuss and to fund studies and programs to deal with overwhelming health problem such as smoking, alcohol, drug abuse, AIDS and cancer.

The conservation principles do not, of course, operate simply in isolation from each other. They are joined with in individual as a cascade of life events, churning and changing on the environmental challenge is comforted and resolved in each individual's unique way. The nurse as a caregiver becomes part of that environment, bringing the every nursing opportunity his or her own cascading repertoire of skill, knowledge, and compassion. It is a shared enterprise and each participant is rewarded.

Paradigm of Levine Theory

Levine skillfully weaves her beliefs about human body, environment, health and nursing, throughout her discussion of conservation and adaptation as follows.

Human Being

She assumed person is who we know out self to be or a sense of identity. When a person is being studied, the focus should be on wholeness. She also maintains that a person cannot be understood outside the context of the place and time in which he or she is functioning or separated from the influence of everything, that is happening around him or her. Not only human beings influenced by their current surroundings/circumstances, they also are "hardened by a lifetime experience' which has been recorded on the tissues of the body as well as on the mind and spirit." Human beings are continually adapting them. Interactions with their environment. The process of adaptation results in conservation. Human beings have need for nursing when they are suffering and can set aside independence and accepts the services of others.

Health

Levine assumes health is socially determined. It is predetermined by social groups and is not just an absence of pathological conditions, change in characteristics of life, and adaptation is the method of change. The organism retains its integrity in both the internal and external environment through its adaptive capability.

She indicates that health and diseases are patterns of adaptive change. Some adaptations are more successful than others; all adaptations are the ones that achieve the best fit in the most conserving manner.

Health is the goal of conservation. She discussed the words health, whole and integrity as all being derived from the same root word and that, even with a multiplicity of definitions of health, each individual still defines health for him or herself.

Environment

Environment is the "context in which we live ourselves." It is not a passive backdrop. We are active participants in it." Levine draws the classification of Bates (1967), i.e., three aspects of environment.
  i. The operational environment—It consists of those undetected natural forces that impinge on the individual.
  ii. The perceptual environment—It consists of information that is recorded by the sensory organs.
  iii. The conceptual environment—It is influenced by language, culture, ideas and cognition.

According to her, it is difficult to measure the environment, because adaptations and conservation are based upon the human beings' interaction with the environment, efforts to understand the environment and role it plays in an individual's predicament are vital. It is important to consider the wholeness of the individual, which includes the individual's ethnic and cultural heritage, economic niche, the opportunities ignored or seized" in social context. She states, it is the social systems that, in every place and in every generation, establishes the values that direct it and sets the rules by which its members are judged. The social integrity of the individual mirrors the community to which he or she belongs.

Nursing

Nursing is human intervention. Professional nursing should be reserved for those few who can complete a graduate program as demanding as that expected of professional in any other discipline. There will be a very few professional nurses. The purpose of nursing is to take care of others when they need to be taken care of. The dependency created by this need is a very temporary state. Nursing takes place wherever there is an individual who needs care to some degree.

Levine discusses the fact that the person who provides nursing care has special burden of the concern since the "permission to enter into the life goals of another human being bears onerous debts of responsibility of choice. The nurse-patient relationship is based on the willful participation of both parties, and in such a relationship there cannot be a "substitute for honesty, fairness, and mutual respect." It is the nurses' tasks to bring a body of scientific principles on which decisions depend into the precise situation which she shares with the patient. Sensitive observation and the selection of relevant data form the basis for her assessment of his nursing requirements. The nurse participates activity in every patient's environment, and much what she does, supports his adjustments as he struggles in the predicament of illness.

The essence of Levine's theory is that "when nursing intervention influences adaptation favourably, or toward renewed social well being, then the nurse is acting in a therapeutic sense. When the response is unfavourable, the nurse adds supportive care." The goal of nursing is to promote wholeness.

Nursing theory is tested finally in the pragmatic, humble daily exchanges between nurse and patient. (its) success (is demonstrated in its ability to) equip individuals with renewed strength to pursue their levels in independence, fulfillment, hope and promise.

Nursing Process and Levine's Theory

Myra Estrin Levine's concepts of adaptation, conservation and integrity can be used to guide patient care with in the nursing process.

Assessment

Assessment is an understanding of the wholeness of the patient needs to be his end result, Levine's principles of conservation can be used as a guide to structure the assessment. The assessment would not be initiated unless the person is suffering and willing to become to some degree dependent upon the nurse. The overarching question could be what adaptation is needed or has not been successful? The history, specificity, and potential for redundancy in this area of adaptation need to be investigated. For example, for assessment of cardiac patient when brought to hospital, nurse uses the principle of conservation as below.

　i. Assessment data in relation to principles of conservation of energy will include energy resources and expenditure. For example, vital signs, laboratory values, use of oxygen and nutrients, activities of daily living, nutrition, exercise, elimination, menstrual cycle, etc are any aspects of living that require energy. Information about the balance between energy input and output, are recorded.

　ii. Assume data in relation to principles of conservation of structural integrity would relate to information about injury and disease process, which include laboratory values that reflect the immune/inflammatory response, direct observation of wounds and any visible indication of disease, e.g. rashes in case of measles and information from the patient about symptoms which are not observable, i.e. nausea pain.

　iii. Data in relation to conservation of personal integrity need to be collected very carefully. Levine warns about the threat to self of the patient that can be created if the nurse seeks a too through investigation of the self of the patient. Her guidelines to use "only those generalizations that actually make a difference in the choice of treatment plans."

　iv. Assessment data related to the conservation of social integrity includes information about others who have influenced the person's identification of self. Again, the kind and amount of data collected in this area needs to be constructed carefully with due sensitivity to the needs of the person to maintain privacy. Information may be obtained about family, community in which the person lives and works religious preferences, cultural and ethnic influences and any other social information that the person deems important to share and that could influence the plan of care.

Nursing Diagnosis

Levine proposed the use of the term 'trophicognosis' as an alternative to nursing diagnosis. Trophicognosis is a nursing care judgment that is arrived at through the use of scientific method. She stated that "No diagnosis should be made that does not include the other persons whose lives are entwined with that of individual. The nursing diagnosis focusses on the course of the patient's suffering—what has put him or her in the predicament of need—and on the area in which adaptation needs to be supported in order to achieve conservation and integrity.

Planning

Planning focuses on what the nurse to do to aid the patient in again becoming independent. The goals that are set will reflect the patient's behaviour and planned activities will include both willing participants—the nurse and the patient. Levine has make no effort to be prescriptive about the kinds of actions that would be planned, but she is very clear, however, that the intent is to return the patient to a state of independence as quickly and fully as possible.

Implementation

Implementation is designed according to the four conservation principles.
- For conservation of energy, action will seek to balance energy input with energy output. The actions may focus on increasing energy input through improved nutrition or in deceased output in full bed rest. At rest also, body using energy that will less compared to other activities.
- For structural integrity, nursing action will be based on limiting the amount of tissue involvement in infections and disease. Such actions will include appropriate positioning to prevent formation of bedsores, change of dressings, and administration of antibodies.
- For personal integrity, efforts will be based on helping the person to preserve his or her identity and selfhood. These actions may begin in deciding to project the private self by not collecting complete psychosocial data and continue through the design of treatment plans that take individual characteristics to account. Here it is better to observe strict moral approach.
- For social integrity, nursing actions are based on helping the patient to preserve his or her place in a family, community and society. Such nursing actions may include teaching the family about the patient care needs (e.g. teaching persons with new colostomies how to handle food and fluid intake).

Evaluation

Levine has not discussed evaluation, but her emphasis on the importance of assisting the person to return to independence as soon as possible supports the need for evaluation. The evaluation data focus on the effectiveness of adaptation in achieving conservation and integrity in the four areas of energy, structural integrity, personal integrity and social integrity.

Levine's Work and Characteristics of a Theory

1. Theories can interrelate concepts in such a way as to create a different way of looking at a particular phenomenon.
   Levine interrelated concepts of adaptation, conservation and integrity in a way that provides a nursing view different from that

of the adjunctive disciplines with which nursing shares these concepts. Adaptation is identified as a process the product of which is conservation. The purpose of conservation is integrity or wholeness. Levine's writings clearly discuss the interrelationships of these concepts and specify how they influence the practice of nursing.

2. Theories must be logical in nature. Levine's work is logical. One thought or idea flows from the previous one and into the next. She is attuned to the original use of words and takes care in her use of words and how they relate to one another.

3. Theories should be relatively simple yet generalizable. There are only three major concepts in Levine's theory. This is the essence of simplicity. Because these three concepts apply to all living human beings and according to Levine, nursing is not setting specific, the theory is generalizable. It can be used in any setting with any human being who is suffering and willing to seek assistance from a nurse.

4. Theories can be the bases for hypotheses that can be tested or for theory to be generated, and

5. Theories contribute to and assist in increasing the general body of knowledge within the discipline through the research implemented to validate them. Hypotheses have been developed from Levine's theory, and research has been conducted to test these hypotheses. The results of these research studies have contributed to the general body of knowledge in nursing. Levine (1989) discusses the studies conducted by Wong (1968) and Winslow, Lane, and Gaffney (1985) that support the importance of energy conservation for patients with myocardial infarctions. Research has also been conducted in using Levine's theory with confused patients over age 60 and caring for neonates and for women in labour (Foreman 1989 1991, Newport, 1984; Yeates and Roberts, 1984). Other studies have also been conducted. A number of these are included in Schaefer and Pond (1991) others are unpublished master's theses or doctoral dissertations, and thus are less accessible than published materials.

6. Theories can be used by practitioners to guide and improve their practice. Levine developed her work to teach nursing students the practice of medical-surgical nursing. She had a practice-oriented focus in doing so. The work certainly provides a guide to practice and if used consistently can improve practice. Areas of nursing practice that have been reported in the literature as using Levine's work include the homeless; patients with burns, congestive heart failure, chronic pain, and epilepsy; and clinical settings which include critical care, emergency room, long term care, pediatrics, and perioperative nursing (Bayley 1991).

7. Theories must be consistent with other validated theories, laws, and principles but will leave open unanswered questions that need to be investigated. Levine has clearly identified those ideas from adjunctive disciplines that she has used in her work. These include Cannon's (1966) perceptual systems, Erikson's (1969, 1975) discussions of the influence of environment on development, Bates's (1967) three types of environment, and the works, of Dubos (1966), Cohen (1968), and Goldstein (1963)

in relation to adaptation. Her work is consistent with these works but builds on them in a way that creates questions to be answered. Such questions could include; Does change in one type of environment have as greater effect on adaptation than changes in the other two types? Why are some people more (or less) effective than others in adapting, conserving and thus maintaining integrity? What are the most effective ways of conserving social integrity through disease prevention activities?

Levine wrote a textbook for beginning students that introduced new material into curricula. She presented an early discussion of death and dying and believed that women should be awakened after a breast biopsy and consulted about the next step.

Introduction to Clinical Nursing provides an organizational structure for teaching medical-surgical nursing. In both the 1969 and 1973 editions, Levine presents a model at the end of each of the first nine chapters. Each model contains objectives, essential science concepts, and nursing process to give nurses foundation for nursing activities. The nine models are as follows:

1. "Vital signs," including temperature, pulse, and respirations.
2. "Body movement and positioning," including body posture, body mechanics, bed rest, and ambulation.
3. "Ministration of personal hygiene needs," including personal and environmental hygiene.
4. "Pressure gradient systems in nursing intervention," specifically fluids.
5. "Nursing determinants in provision for nutritional needs," including psychological, cultural, religious, socioeconomic, and therapeutic needs for fluids and nourishment.
6. "Pressure gradient systems in nursing," specifically gases and pulmonary ventilation.
7. "Local application of heat and cold," stressing patient's safety and comfort.
8. "The administration of medications.
9. "Establishing an aseptic environment," including teaching patients principles of asepsis.

Critics argue that although the text is labeled introductory, a beginning student would need a fairly extensive background in physical and social science to use it. Another critic suggests a definite strength is the emphasis of scientific principles, but a weakness of the text is that it does not present adequate examples of pathological profiles when disturbances are discussed. For this reason, one reviewer recommends the text as supplementary or complementary, rather than as a primary text. Levine wrote a teacher's manual to assist in the use of her book.

Hall indicates Levine's model is one used as a curriculum model. Several graduate students are using Levine's model for theses and dissertations.

Fitzpatrick and Whall state, "All in all, Levine's model served as an excellent beginning. Its contribution has added a great deal to the overall development of nursing knowledge." However, Fawcett states that to establish credibility "more systematic evaluations of the use of the model in various clinical situations are needed, as are empirical studies that test theories directly derived from or linked with the conservation principles." Many research questions can be generated from Levine's model. Several graduate students are using the conservation principles as a framework for their research.

Levine and others have worked on using the conservation principles as the basis of a taxonomy of nursing diagnosis. However, further development of this concept has been deferred since the American Nurses Association took over nursing diagnosis.

EVALUATION OF THEORY

- Levine's model possesses clarity. Fitzpatrick and Whall believe Levine's work to be both internally and externally consistent. Fawcett states that "this conceptual model is consistent in its approach to the person as a holistic being and provides nursing with a logically congruent, holistic view of the person."
- The model has numerous terms. However, Levine adequately defines them for clarity.
- Although the four conservation principles initially appear simple, they contain subconcepts and multiple variables. Nevertheless, this model is still one of the simpler ones that has emerged.
- The four conservation principles can be used in all nursing contexts.
- Levine used deductive logic to develop her model, which can be used to generate research questions.
- Various authors disagree as to the level of contributions provided by Levine's model. The four conservation principles constituted one of the earliest models and seems to be receiving increasing recognition.

Chapter 19

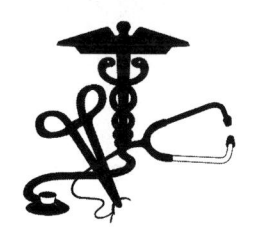

Leininger's Cultural Care Theory

Madeleine M. Leininger is the founder of transcultural nursing and a leader in transcultural nursing and human care theory. She is the first professional nurse with graduate preparation in nursing to hold a Ph.D. in cultural and social anthropology. Born in Sutton, Nebraska, she began her nursing career after graduating from a diploma program at St. Anthony's School of Nursing in Denver. She was a Cadet Corps nurse while pursuing the basic nursing program. In 1950 she obtained a B.S. degree in biological science from Benedictine College, Atchison, Kansas, with a minor in philosophy and the humanistic studies. After graduation she served as an instructor, staff nurse, and head nurse on a medical-surgical unit and opened a new psychiatric unit as director of the nursing service at St. Joseph's Hospital in Omaha. During this time she did advanced study in nursing, nursing administration, teaching and curriculum in nursing, and test and measurement at Creighton University in Omaha.

In 1954 Leininger obtained an M.S.N. in psychiatric nursing from Catholic University of America in Washington, D.C. She then moved to the University of Cincinnati, where she began the first graduate clinical specialist programme in child psychiatric nursing in the country. She also initiated and directed the first graduate nursing programme in psychiatric-mental health nursing at the University of Cincinnati. During this time she wrote one of the first basic psychiatric nursing texts with Hofling, entitled *Basic Psychiatric Nursing Concepts* (1960), which was published in 11 languages and used worldwide.

While working in a child guidance home in the mid-1950s, Leininger identified in the staff a lack of understanding of cultural factors in-*Nursing* (1985), *Care: Clinical and Community Uses of Care* (1988), *Ethical and Moral Dimensions of Care* (1990), *The Caring Imperative in Education* (1990), and *Culture Care Diversity & University: A Theory of Nursing* (1991), which is a full account of her theory with the method. She has published more than 265 articles and 40 chapters plus numerous films and research projects focussed on transcultural nursing, human care and health phenomena, and other topics relevant to nursing and anthropology. She also served on editorial boards of 10 major publications. She is known as one of the most creative and productive authors in nursing, providing new and substantive nursing content with futuristic ideas and trends to advance nursing as a discipline and profession.

Leininger has received many awards and recognition of her accomplishments. She is listed in *Who's Who of American Women, Who's Who in Health Care, Who's Who in Community Leaders, The World's Who's Who of Women in Education, The International Who's Who in Community Services, The Who's Who in International Women,* and other such listings. Her name appears on *The National Register of Prominent Americans and International Notables, international Women,* and *The National Register of Prominent Community Leaders.* She received an Honorary Doctorate of Human Letters from Benedictine College, Atchison, Kansas, in 1975, and in 1976 was presented an Award of Recognition for unique and significant contributions to the American Association of Colleges of Nursing. Leininger is a Fellow in the American Academy of Nursing and is a Fellow of the American Anthropological Society and the Society for Applied Anthropology. Her other affiliations include Sigma Theta Tau, the National Honor Society of Nursing; Delta Kappa Gamma, the National Honorary Society in Education; and the Scandinavian College of Caring Science in Stockholm. She has served as distinguished visiting scholar or lecturer in 48 universities in this country and abroad and was recently visiting professor at six universities in Sweden, in two universities in Japan, and five in Australia and New Zealand. While at Wayne State University, she has received the Board of Regents' Distinguished Faculty Award, Distinguished Researcher Award, and the President's Excellence in Teaching Award.

EVOLUTION OF THEORY

Leininger's theory is derived from the discipline of anthropology, but she conceptualized the theory to be relevant to nursing. She has defined *transcultural nursing* as a major area of nursing that focusses on a comparative study and analysis of different cultures and subcultures in the world with respect to their caring behaviour; nursing care; and health-illness values, beliefs, and patterns of behaviour with the goal of developing a scientific and humanistic body of knowledge to provide culture-specific and culture-universal nursing care practices.

The goal of transcultural nursing extends beyond an awareness state or appreciation of different cultures. It means making professional nursing knowledge and practices culturally based, conceptualized, planned, and practiced. Leininger has stated that in time there will be "a new taxonomy of nursing practice that will reflect different kinds of nursing care, which are culturally defined, classified, and tested as a guide to provide nursing care." She makes this prediction because culture is the broadest and the most holistic means to conceptualize, understand, and be effective with people. In addition, she states that "transcultural nursing is becoming one of the most important, relevant, and highly promising areas of formal study research and practice because of the multicultural world in which we live." She predicts that for nursing to be relevant to clients and the world, transcultural nursing knowledge will be imperative to guide all nursing decisions and actions.

Caring is postulated as the central and unifying domain for nursing knowledge and practices. Diverse factors influence patterns of care and health or well-being in different cultures. Caring includes assistive, supportive, and facilitative acts for another individual or a group with evident or anticipated needs. Caring serves to ameliorate or to improve human conditions through behaviours, techniques, processes, and patterns. Professional nursing care embodies scientific and humanistic modes of helping or enabling receipt of personalized service to maintain a healthy condition for life or death.

Caring emphasizes healthful, enabling activities of individuals and groups that are based on culturally defined ascribed or sanctioned helping modes. Caring behaviours include comfort, compassion, concern, coping behaviour, empathy, enabling, facilitating, interest, involvement, health-consultative acts, health-instruction acts, health-maintenance acts, helping behaviours, love, nurturance, presence, protective behaviours, restorative behaviours, sharing, stimulating behaviours, stress alleviation, succorance, support, surveillance, tenderness, touching, and trust. Culture determines personal life or worldviews that are mediated through language. Contextual factors such as technology, religion, philosophic beliefs, social and kinship lines and patterns, values and life ways, political and legal factors, economic factors, and educational factors all influence care patterns. Likewise, these factors affect are patterns and the health of individuals and families, as well as groups. Diverse health systems mediate the expression of health. Nursing is one health system that overlaps with folk systems and professional health care systems.

Human caring is a universal phenomenon, and every nursing situation has transcultural nursing care elements. Caring is essential to human development, growth, and survival, and caring behaviours vary transculturally in priorities, expression, and needs satisfaction. Caring plays a more important role in recovery than cure but receives less reward. If effective, caring reflects professional concern, compassion, stress alleviation, nurturance, comfort, and protection. Nursing should provide care consistent with its emergent science and knowledge, with caring as a central focus. Caring and culture are inextricably linked, and nursing care should be culturally congruent and aimed at preserving, maintaining, accommodating, negotiating, repatterning, and restructuring care patterns.

Leininger's theory is derived from the discipline of anthropology, but she conceptualized the theory to be relevant to nursing. She has defined 'transcultural nursing as a major area of nursing that focuses on a comparative study and analyses of different cultures and subculture in the world with respect to their caring behaviours, nursing care, and health-illness values, beliefs, patterns of behaviour with the goal of developing a scientific and humanistic body of knowledge to provide culture-specific and culture-universal nursing care practices.

Leininger's goal of transcultural nursing extends beyond an awareness state or appreciation of different cultures. It means making professional nursing knowledge and practices culturally based, conceptualized, planned and practices. She has stated that in time, there will be "a taxonomy of nursing practice that will reflect different kinds of nursing care, which are culturally defined, classified, and tested and guide to provide nursing care. She makes this prediction because culture is the broadest and the most holistic means to conceptualize, understand and be effective with people. In addition, she states that "transcultural nursing is becoming one of the most important relevant, and highly promising areas of formal study research, and practice because of the multicultural world in which we live.' She predicts that for nursing to be relevant to clients in the world, transcultural nursing knowledge will be imperative to guide all nursing decisions and actions.

During 1940s, Leininger recognized the importance of caring to nursing. Statements of appreciation for nursing care made by patients alerted her to caring values and led to her long-standing focus on care as the dominant ethos of nursing, In mid 1950 s, the experienced what she describes as cultural shock while she was working in a child guidance clinic, as a clinical nurse specialist with disturbed children and parents.

The child guidance clinic she observed recurrent behavioural difference among the children and concluded that these differences had cultural base. She identified a lack of knowledge of children's cultures on the missing link in nursing to understand the variations in care of clients. This experience led her to become the first professional nurse in the world to earn a doctorate in anthropology, and led to the development of transcultural nursing as subfield of nursing.

Transcultural Nursing

Leininger (1960) first used the terms "transcultural nursing," 'ethnonursing' and 'cross-cultural nursing.' She offered the first transcultrual nursing course with field experience at the University of Colorado in 1966, has been in the development of similar courses at a number of other institutions. She defined "transcultural nursing" as a learned subject or branch of nursing, which focuses upon the comparative study and analysis of cultures with respect to nursing and health-illness caring practices, beliefs, and values with the goal to provide meaning for and efficacious nursing care services to people cultural values and health illness context." And she also defined "ethnonursing as the study of nursing care beliefs, values and practices as cognitively perceived and known by a designated culture through their direct experiences, beliefs and value systems."

Now the term "transcultural nursing" (rather than Cross-cultured) is used to refer to the evolving knowledge and practices related to this new field of study and practice. Leininger developed her theory of transcultural nursing on the premise that the peoples of each culture not only can know and define the ways in which they experience and perceive their nursing care world but also can relate these experiences and perceptions to their general health beliefs and practices. Based on this premises, nursing care is derived and developed from the cultural context in which it is to be provided.

Cultural Care Theory

Leininger (1991) asserts that human care is central to nursing as a discipline and as profession. She and others have studied the phenomena of care for over four decades. They recognize and are proponents of the preservation of care as the essence of nursing. With this increasing recognition of care as essential to nursing knowledge and practice, Leininger labelled her theory culture care. She drew upon anthropology for the culture component and upon nursing for the care component. Her belief that cultures have both health practices that are specific to one culture and prevailing patterns that are common across cultures led to the addition of the terms "diversity" and "universality" to the title of her theory. Thus most current title of Leininger's theory is 'culture care' or culture care diversity and universality."

In 1985, Leininger published her work on a theory and in 1988 and 1991, she presented further explication of her ideas. In 1991 presentation, she provided orientational definitions for the concepts of culture, culture care, cultural care diversity, environmental context, ethno-history, generic (folk or lay) care system, professional care system, cultural congruent nursing care, health care/caring, cultural care preservation, cultural care accommodation and cultural care repatterning.

The major orientational definitions for the theory are as follows:

1. Care (noun) refers to abstract and concrete phenomena related to assisting, supporting, or enabling experiences or behaviours toward or for others with evident or anticipated needs to ameliorate or improve a human condition or lifeway.
2. Caring (gerund) refers to actions and activities directed toward assisting, supporting, or enabling another individual or group with evident or anticipated needs to ameliorate or improve a human condition or lifeway or to face death.
3. Culture refers to the learned, shared, and transmitted values, beliefs, norms, and lifeways of a particular group that guides their thinking, decisions, and actions in patterned ways.
4. Culture care refers to the cognitively learned and transmitted values, beliefs, and patterned lifeways that assist, support, facilitate, or enable another individual or group to maintain their well-being or health, to improve their human condition and lifeway, or to deal with illness, handicaps or death.
5. Health refers to a state of well-being that is culturally defined, valued, and practiced, and that reflects the ability of individuals (or groups) to perform their daily role activities in culturally expressed, beneficial, and patterned lifeways.
6. Environmental context refers to the totality of an event, situation, or particular experiences that give meaning to human expressions, interpretations and social interactions in particular physical, ecological, sociopolitical, and /or cultural settings.
7. Cultural care diversity refers to the variabilties and/or differences in meanings, patterns, values, lifeways, or symbols of care within or between collectivities that are related to assistive, supportive or enabling human care expressions.
8. Cultural care universality refers to the common, similar, or dominant uniform care meanings, patterns, values, lifeways, or symbols that are manifest among many cultures and reflect assistive, supportive, facilitative or enabling ways to help people (The term *Universality* is not used in an absolute way nor as a fixed statistical finding).

9. Generic folk or lay system refers to culturally learned and transmitted, indigenous (or traditional), folk (home-based) knowledge and skills used to provide assistive, supportive, enabling, or facilitative acts towards or for another individual, group, or institution with evident or anticipated needs to ameliorate or improve a human lifeway, health condition (or well-being), or to deal with handicaps and death situations.
10. Professional systems refers to formal and cognitively learned professional knowledge and practice skills that are taught in professional institutions to a number of multidisciplinary personnel in order to serve consumers seeking health services.
11. Cultural care preservation or maintenance refers to those assistive supportive, facilitative, or enabling professional actions and decisions that help people of a particular culture to retain and/or preserve relevant care values so that they can maintain their well-being, recover from illness, or face handicaps and/or death.
12. Culture care accommodation or Negotiation refers to those assistive, supportive, facilitative, or enabling creative professional actions and decisions that help people of a designated culture to adapt to, or to negotiate with, others for a beneficial or satisfying health outcome with professional care providers.
13. Cultural care repatterning or restructuring refers to those assistive, supportive, facilitative, or enabling professional actions and decisions that help clients reorder, change, or modify their lifeways for new, different, or more beneficial health care patterns while respecting the client's cultural values and beliefs and providing a better (or healthier) lifeway than before.
14. Cultural congruent (Nursing) care refers to those cognitively based assistive, supportive, facilitative, or enabling acts or decisions that are tailor-made to fit with an individual's group's or institutions' cultural values, beliefs and lifeways in order to provide meaningful beneficial and satisfying health care, or well-being services.

OTHER ORIENTATIONAL DEFINITIONS

1. Nursing refers to a learned humanistic and scientific profession and discipline that is focused on human care phenomena and activities in order to assist, support, facilitate, or enable individuals or groups to maintain or regain their well-being (or health) in culturally meaningful and beneficial ways, or to help people face handicaps or death.
2. World view refers to the way people tend to look out on the world or their universe to form a picture or a value stance about their life or world around them.
3. Cultural and social structure dimensions refers to the dynamic patterns and features of interrelated structural and organizational factors of a particular culture (subculture or society), which includes religious kinship (social), political (and legal), economic, educational, technologic, and cultural values, and how these factors may be interrelated and function to influence human behaviour in different environmental contexts.

4. Ethnohistory refers to those past facts, events, instances, and experiences of individuals, groups, cultures, and institutions that are primarily people-centred (ethno) and that describe, explain, and interpret human lifeways within particular cultural contexts and space-time referents.

In addition to the definitions, Leininger presented assumptions which support her prediction that different cultures perceive, know and practice care in different ways, yet there are some commonalities about care among cultures of the world. These assumptions to support her transcultural care theory, can be stated as follows:

1. Human caring is a universal phenomenon, but the expressions, processes structural forms, and patterns of caring very among cultures.
2. Caring acts, and processes are essential for human birth, development, growth, survival and peaceful death.
3. Caring is the essence of nursing and the distinct, dominant, and unifying nature of nursing.
4. Care has a biophysical, cultural, psychological, social, and environmental dimension, and the concept of culture provides the broadest means to know and understand care.
5. Nursing is a transcultural phenomenon as nurses interact with clients, staff and other groups and requires that nurses identify and use intercultural nurse-client and system data.
6. Care behaviours, goals and functions vary transculturally because of the social structure, world view, and cultural values of people from different cultures.
7. Self and other care practices vary in different cultures and in different folk and professional care systems.
8. The identification of universal and non-universal folk and professional caring behaviours, beliefs, and practices is essential to discover, the epistemological and ontological base of nursing care knowledge.
9. Care is largely culturally derived and requires culturally based knowledge and skills for satisfying and efficacious nursing practices.
10. There can be no curing without caring, but there can be caring without curing.

And she refers to the commonalities as universality and to the differences as diversity as given below:

1. Care is the essence of nursing and a distinct, dominant, central and unifying focus.
2. Care (caring) is essential for well-being, health, healing, growth, survival, and facing handicaps or death.
3. Culture care is the broadest holistic means to know, explain, interpret, and predict nursing care phenomena to guide nursing care practices.
4. Nursing is a transcultural humanistic and scientific care discipline and profession with the central purpose to serve human beings world wide.
5. Care (caring) is essential to curing and healing, for there can be no curing without caring.
6. Culture care concepts, meanings, expressions, patterns, processes, and structural forms of care have different (diversity) and similar (towards commonalities or universalities) characteristics among all cultures of the world.
7. Every human culture has generic (lay, folk, or indigenous) care knowledge and practices and usually professional care

knowledge and practices, which vary transculturally.

8. Cultural care values, beliefs, and practices are influenced by and tend to be embedded in world view, language, religion (or spiritual), kinship (social), politics (or legal), education, economic, technology, ethnohistory, and environmental context of a particular culture.
9. Beneficial, healthy, and satisfying culturally-based nursing care contributes to the well-being of individuals, families, groups and communities within their environmental context.
10. Culturally congruent nursing care can only occur when culture care values, expressions, or patterns are known and used appropriately and meaningfully by the nurse with individuals or groups.
11. Culture care differences and similarities between professional caregivers and clients (with their generic needs) exist in human cultures worldwide.
12. Clients who show signs of culture conflicts, noncompliance, stresses, and ethical or moral concerns need nursing care that is culturally-based.
13. The qualitative paradigm with naturalistic inquiry modes provides the essential means to discover human care transculturally.

Leininger (1991) points out that the model is not the theory but a depiction of the components of the theory of culture care diversity and universality. The purpose of this model is to aid the study of how the components of the theory influence the health status of, and care provided to, individuals, families, groups, communities and institutions within a culture. She presents cogent arguments for the use of the model to guide discovery research that uses qualitative and ethnographic method of study. She speaks strongly against the use of operational definitions and preconceived notions and the use of causal or linear prospective in studying cultural cars, diversity and universality. She supports the importance of finding out what is of exploring and discovering the essence and meanings of care (Fig. 19.1).

Paradigm and Leininger's Theory

Leininger presents an argument of care as the central concept in nursing's metaparadigm as follows:

Human Being

Human are believed to be caring and to be capable of being concerned about the needs, wellbeing, and survival of others. Human care is universal, that is seen in all cultures. Humans have survived within cultures and through place and time because they have been able to care for infants, children, and the elderly in a variety of ways and in many different environments. Thus humans are universally caring beings who survive in the diversity of cultures through their ability to provide the universality of care in a variety of ways according to differing cultures, needs and settings.

Health

Leininger speaks of health systems, health care practices, changing health patterns, health promotion and health maintenance. Health is an important concept in transcultural nursing. Because, of the emphasis on the need for nurses to have knowledge that is specific to the culture in which nursing is being practiced, it is

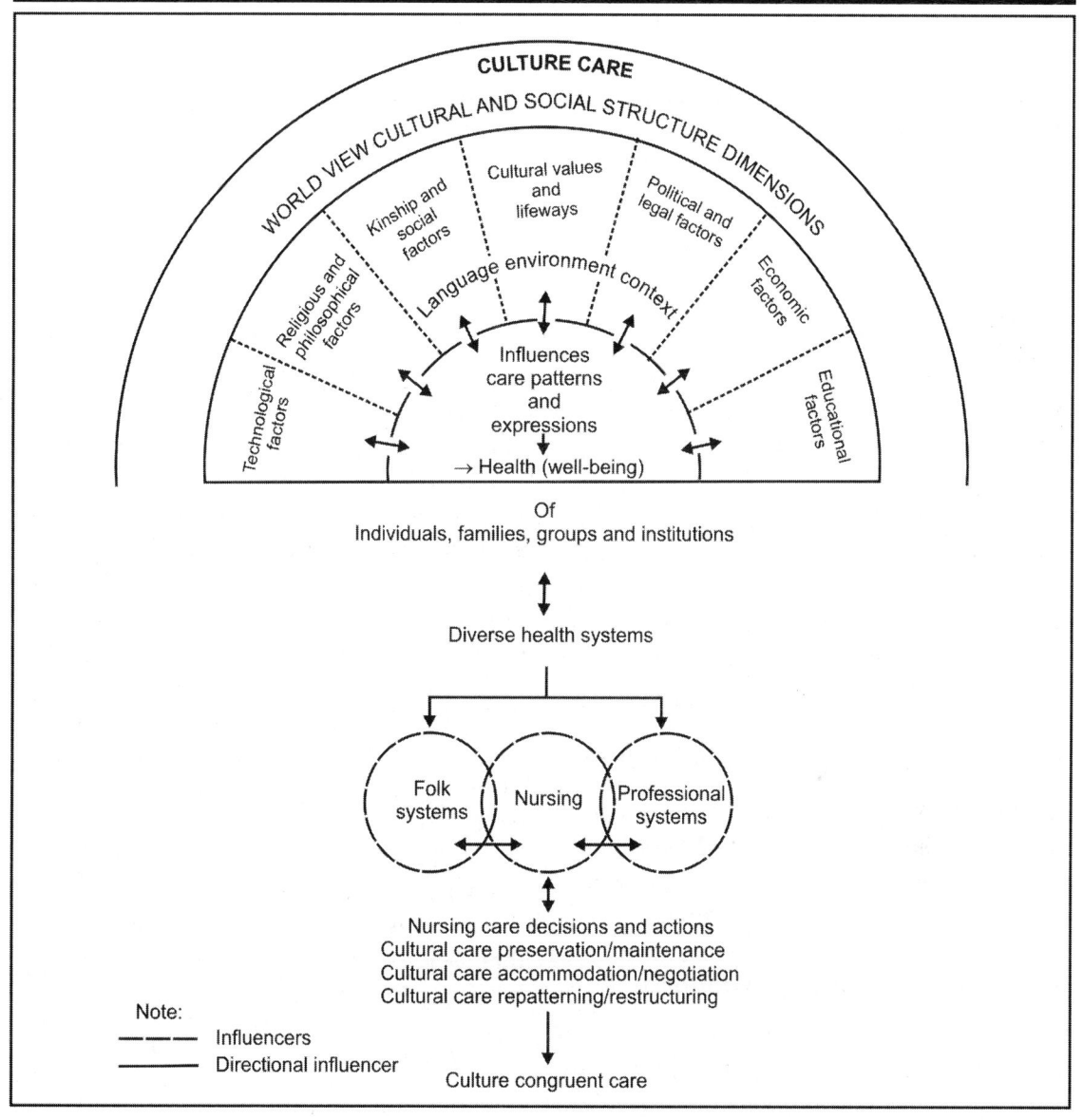

Figure 19.1: Leininger's sunrise model to depict theory of cultural care diversity and universality

presumed that health is viewed as "being universal across cultures burdefined within each culture in a manner that reflects the beliefs, values, practices of their particular cultures." Thus health is both universal and diverse.

Environment

Leininger speaks worldview, social structure, and environmental context instead of environment. Environment context is defined as being the totality of an event, situation and experience. Her definition of culture focuses on a particular group (society) and the patterning of actions, thoughts, and decisions that occur as a result of "learned, shared and transmitted values beliefs, norms and lifeways." Thus, Leininger does not use specific definition to environment, but the concept of cultural closely related to environment.

Nursing

Leininger defines nursing as "a learned humanistic art and science that focuses upon personalized (individual and groups) care behaviours, functions and processes directed towards promoting and maintaining health behaviours or recovery form illness which have physical psychocultural, and social significance or meaning for those being assisted generally by a professional nurse or one with similar role competences."

Nursing Process and Leininger's Theory

There are parallels between the Sunrise Model (Leininger) and Nursing Process. Both represents one problem-solving process and client who is recipient of nursing care.

Assessment of Nursing Diagnosis

When the Sunrise model is appropriately used, one is assessing or gathering knowledge and information about the social structure and world view of the client's culture. Other information as well as factors of technology, religion, philosophy, kinship, social structure, cultural values, beliefs, politics, legal systems, economics, and education. Much of this knowledge could be gathered before the identification of a particular client and would be useful in preventing both culture shock and cultural imposition. After analyzing these informations nurses identify the problem and state it in the form of nursing diagnosis.

Planning and Implementation

Occurs with nursing care decisions and actions. Again, nursing care decisions and actions need to be culturally based to best meet the needs of the client and provide culture congruent care. The three modes of actions are cultural care preservation/maintenance, cultural care accommodation/negotiations and cultural care repatterning/restructuring. In preservation and maintenance, the nurse's action focus on supporting, assisting, facilitating, and enabling of client or preserve or retain favourable health, to recover from illness, or to face handicap or death. Culture care accommodation/negotiation creates, professional efforts to facilitate, enable, assist or support action will help to client's adjustment to environment for facilitating satisfying health outcome, cultural repatterning, refers to professional actions that seek to help client change in meaningful health of life pattern.'

Evaluation

Leininger places a great deal of importance upon the need for nursing care to provide ways in which care will benefit the client and on the need to systematically study nursing care behaviour to determine which behaviours are appropriate to the lifeways and behavioural patterns of the culture is the equivalent to evaluation.

LEININGER'S WORK AND THE CHARACTERISTIC OF A THEORY

Beginning with the identification of a need to understand the culture of clients, through the introduction of the terms transcultural nursing and ethnonursing care, to the presentation of the sunrise model. Madelline Leininger has developed the theory. She calls it Culture Care Diversity and University.

1. Theories can interrelate concepts in such a way as to create a different way of looking at a particular phenomenon. Leininger has developed the sunrise model to demonstrate the interrelation-ships of the concepts in her theory of Culture Care Diversity and Universality. The worldview and social structure portion of the model does not differ significantly from any other view of culture and its interaction with human beings, with the possible exception of the inclusion of care and health patterns. The model focusses on individuals, families, groups, communities and socio-cultural institutions which is similar to other theories of nursing. The inclusion of the term "Cultural" does provide a distinguishing feature since no other nursing theory has this emphasis on culture. Health systems include generic, professional, and nursing care systems. The inclusion of the generic system is unique to the cultural care theory Nursing care decisions and actions are identified as supporting, accommodating or repatterning is specific to this theory. The sunrise model of Culture Care Diversity and Universality in itself supports the concepts of diversity and universality. The worldview, social structure, and description of individuals, families, groups, communities, and institutions are essentially universal as they have much in common with many other theories. The identified care systems and types of nursing care actions are diverse, or more specific and unique to this particular theory. Overall, the theory of Culture Care was the first to focus specifically on human care from a transcultural perspective (Leininger, 1991). It provides a holistic rather than a fragmented view of people. This view includes "worldview; biophysical state; religious (or spiritual) orientation; kinship patterns; material (and nonmaterial) cultural phenomena; the political, economic, legal, educational, technological, and physical environment; language; and folk and professional care practices." Thus, Leininger has interrelated concepts in a way which provides a different way of looking at the phenomenon of nursing care.

2. Theories must be logical in nature. There is an inherent logic in the thought that as more is known about a client, the opportunity to provide care that meets that client's needs increases. Leininger has focused on a particular area of knowledge as being important—that area is the culture of the client with culture having a broad definition. The sunrise model has a logical order to it. This order is reflected in the movement from a world view through language and environmental context, care patterns and expressions of individuals, families, groups, communities and institutions into diverse health systems to nursing care decisions and actions to culture congruent nursing care.

3. Theories should be relatively simple yet generalizable. Leininger's theory is essentially parsimonious in that the necessary concepts are incorporated in such a manner that the theory and its model can be applied in many different settings. The theory and model are not simple in terms of being easily understood upon first contact. However, Leininger's presentations of the theory and model support the need for each of the concepts and demonstrate how the concepts are interrelated. Once the interrelationships are grasped, simplicity is more apparent. The theory and model are excellent examples of being generalizable. The concepts and relationships that are presented are at a level of abstraction which allows them to be applied in many different situations. They provide a guide for knowledge that moves from initial generation of knowledge through affirmation of substantive knowledge to application of that knowledge in a caring process. While the knowledge is to be specific to the situation in which the nursing care is to occur, the process of generating and applying the knowledge is universal.
4. Theories can be the bases for hypotheses that can be tested or for theory to be expanded. During the development of the Culture Care Diversity and Universality theory many studies have been conducted that demonstrate the theory can be the basis for research. A number of these studies were presented during for national transcultural nursing conferences held from 1975 to 1978 at the College of Nursing, University of Utah. The proceedings of these conferences are presented in *Transcultural Nursing*. These proceedings reflect the importance of ethnographic research in the development of this theory. Leininger (1985) presented a number of relational statements that provide a foundation for further study. In addition, Leininger (1991) developed a method of study which she labelled ethnonursing research method. She includes examples of ethnonursing research studies of Filipino and Anglo American nurses, old order Amish, urban Mexican-Americans, Ukrainian pregnancy and childbearing, the Gadsup Akuna, dying patients, and Greek-Canadian Widows.

It is important to note that the theory of Culture Care Diversity and Universality is based upon, and calls for, qualitative rather than quantitative research. The development of hypotheses is characteristic of positivistic, quantitative research. The development of research questions and of relational statements is characteristic of qualitative research. Leininger (1991) states that nursing science should be defined "as the creative study of nursing phenomena which reflects the systematization of knowledge using rigorous and explicit research methods within either the qualitative or quantitative paradigm in order to establish a new or to advance nursing's discipline, knowledge." Therefore, from the viewpoint of qualitative research, this criterion is met.

The hypotheses derived from Leininger's theory are as follows:
- There is an identifiable, positive relationship between the way people of different cultures define, interpret and know care with their recurrent patterns of thinking and living.

- The EMIC (inside views) of cultural care values, beliefs and practices of cultures will show a close relationship to their daily life care patterns.
- The meaning and use of cultural care concepts varies cross-culturally and influences nursing care -giver and care-receiver practices.
- There is a meaningful relationship between social structure factors and worldview with generic (folk) and professional care practices.
- Nursing care sub systems are closely related to professional health care systems but differ markedly from generic health care systems.
- Nursing care decisions or actions that are based upon the use of clients cultural care values, beliefs, and practices will be positively related to client's satisfactions with nursing care.
- Nursing care actions or decisions that are based upon the use of cultural care preservation, accommodation, and/or repatterning in client care will be positively related to beneficial nursing care.
- Signs of intercultural care conflicts and stresses will be evident if caregivers and care recipients lead to dissatisfactions for both.
- Marked differences between the meanings and expressions of care givers and care recipients lead to dissatisfactions for both.
- High dependency of the clients upon technological nursing car activities will be closely related to cultural care that reflects decreased personalized care action.
- Religion and kinship care factors will be more resilient to change then technological factors.
- Western views of cultural care values will be markedly different from non-Western care values.
- Self-care practices will be evident in cultures that value individualism and independence, other care practices will be evident in cultures that support human interdependence.
- Anglo-American nurse-client teaching methods will be dysfunctional with clients of non-Western cultural value orientations.

5. Theories contribute to and assist in increasing the general body of knowledge within the discipline through the research implemented to validate them. The research that has been conducted on transcultural nursing has contributed to the general body of knowledge within the discipline of nursing. One of the outcomes of this research is the identification of major cultural care constructs. Leininger indicates that, as of 1991, ethnonursing research identified 172 care constructs from 54 cultures. These constructs have more diversity than universality of meaning. Included in these constructs are anticipation of, attentiveness to, comfort, compassion, coping, empathy, engrossment, helping, nurturance, protection, restoration, support, stimulation, stress, alleviation, succorance, surveillance, touch and trust.

6. Theories can be utilized by the practitioners to guide and improve their practice. In her presentation of the theory, Leininger presents examples of research findings which can guide and improve the

practice of nursing. One example presents the differences in the interpretations of care by American nurses in several general hospitals, Canadian nurses, and Polynesian nurses in Hawaii. The American nurses interpreted care as first dealing with stress alleviation and then comfort. Canadian nurses reported care as being primarily support. Polynesian nurses in Hawaai first identified care as sharing with others in personalized cultural ways and then added being generous to others to achieve signs of harmony among people and their environment. Knowing the diversity in nurses' interpretation of care supports the diversity which will be present in clients and reinforces the need to be knowledgeable about this diversity. Care is universal, the meaning of care is diverse. Leininger (1991) also presents the use of the theory in nursing administration. She states that "the goal of the theory is to improve and to provide culturally congruent care to people that is beneficial, will fit with, and be useful to the client, family or culture group healthy lifeways."

7. Theories must be consistent with other validated theories, laws, principles, but will leave open unanswered questions that need to be investigated. Leininger's theory is certainly consistent with all theories that include the concept of the importance of knowing the client as a person rather than as a problem. Leininger's discussion of the seriousness of unintentional cultural imposition practices by nurses, and of the nurse's need to be-aware of his or her own culture and its implications for the nurse-client situation, is very similar to King's (1981) emphasis on the importance of perceptions and the need for the nurse to be alert to both client and personal perceptions. This is but one example of areas of agreement with other theories. It is important to note that while Leininger Watson (1988) and Boykin and Schoenhofer (1993) all speak of the importance of caring they approach caring differently.

The unanswered questions that remain to be investigated are greater in number than those that have been answered. Since cultures are diverse not only among cultures but within them, and individuals, even within the same culture, respond differently to the same stimuli, each nurse-client situations provides new questions to be explored.

"It is reasonable to predict that all professional nurses in this country and abroad will come to recognize the need to know and use transcultural concepts in their practice, teaching, research, and consultation." Currently, the demand for prepared transcultural nurses far exceeds the number of faculty and clinical specialists in the field. More transcultural nurse theorists, researchers, and scholars are needed to develop and synthesize the new nursing knowledge and to change unicultural norms of nursing practice to multicultural ones. "By the year 2000, it is hoped that most nurses will have a basic knowledge of a number of cultural groups in the world and an in-depth knowledge of two or three cultures." Leininger believes transcultural nursing research will lead to some entirely new theories and different ways to conceptualize nursing education and to practice nursing. "Health disciplines will gradually become involved in transcultural studies and practices in the near future as health science courses and programs of study become established." Because of the increased need for nurses to know and understand cultures and related nursing care needs, there is an increasing demand for transcultural nurses prepared as educators, researchers, and consultants. "It is reasonable to predict that transcultural nurse specialists. . . will (and should be) tomorrow's leaders in national and international teaching, research, and service programmes."

Present and future research in the field of transcultural nursing will enhance theoretical development and will continue to identify culture-specific and universal care constructs. According to Leininger, universal and diverse care constructs are essential to establish a substantive scientific and humanistic body of transcultural and general nursing knowledge to make nursing a worldwide profession and discipline. Leininger's theory is rapidly gaining international interest because it is holistic, relevant, and futuristic and deals with multicultural nursing care conditions and needs.

EVALUATION OF THEORY

- Because the concepts of transcultural nursing theory are complex and multiple, the theory is not simple. Many questions are proposed in pursuit of a scientific body of nursing knowledge based on systematic investigation. The theoretical development and the research goals are to seek both universal and specific culturally defined care phenomena from diverse cultures and from the culture of nursing. The theory is truly transcultural, global in scope, and highly complex, requiring knowledge and appreciation of transcultural and anthropology insights. Leininger's theory is an evolving one with different but related models to guide the researcher in conceptualizing the theory and research approaches. Because of its holistic and comprehensive nature, several concepts and constructs related to social structure, environment, and language are important to understand to see how care and health are influenced by these dimensions. The theory shows multiple interrelationships of concepts and diversity of key concepts. It requires anthropological and transcultural nursing knowledge to be used fully and accurately by nursing researchers. Once the users of the theory have conceptualized the theory, Leininger finds that undergraduate and graduate nursing students find it highly practical, relevant, and more simple than complex.
- The transcultural nursing theory does purport to demonstrate the criterion of generality, as it is a qualitatively oriented theory that is broad, comprehensive, and worldwide in scope. In fact, transcultural nursing theory addresses nursing care from a multicultural and world view perspective. It is useful and applicable to both groups and individuals with the goal of rendering culture-specific nursing care. The broad or generic concepts are organized and operationalized for study in specific cultures. The research has led to a taxonomy of care with many subsets. Many aspects of culture, care, and health, as these factors impact on nursing, are being studied. From this culture-specific data, a few universal care constructs are being identified. More research is needed, and a greater number of the world's cultural groups need to be studied to

- validate the caring constructs. The theoretical model is a guide for the study of any culture and for comparative study of several cultures. Findings from the theory are being used in client care in a variety of health and community settings worldwide.
- The transcultural nursing theory is researchable, and qualitative research has been the primary paradigm to discover largely unknown phenomena of care and health in diverse cultures. This qualitative approach differs from the traditional quantitative research method, which renders measurement the goal of research. However, the ethnoscience research method is extremely rigorous and linguistically exacting in nature and outcomes. Eighty-five care constructs have been identified thus far, and more are being discovered. The important attribute is that accuracy of data derived with the use of ethnomethods or from an emic or people's viewpoint is leading to high validity and reliability of data. Ongoing and future research is hoped to lead to additional care and health findings as well as implications for ethnonursing practices and education to fit specific cultures as well as universal features. The qualitative criteria of credibility and confirmability from in-depth studies of informants and their contexts are becoming clearly evident.
- Transcultural nursing theory has important outcomes for nursing. Rendering culture-specific care is a necessary and essential new goal in nursing. It places the transcultural nursing theory well within the domain of nursing knowledge acquisition and use. The theory is useful and applicable to nursing practice, education, and research. The concept of care as the primary focus of nursing and the base of nursing knowledge and practice is long overdue and essential to advance nursing knowledge and practices. Leininger notes that although nursing has always made claims to the concept of care, rigorous research on care has been limited. Because of its broad and multicultural focus, this theory could be the means for establishing nursing as a discipline and a profession.

Chapter 20

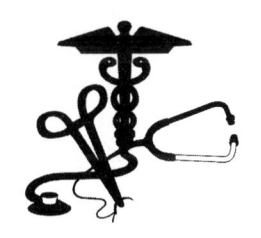

Rogers' Science of Unitary Human Beings

Martha E. Rogers was born May 12, 1914, in Dallas, Texas, the eldest of four children. She began her college education at the University of Tennessee in Knoxville, where she studied science from 1931 to 1933. She received her nursing diploma from Knoxville General Hospital School of Nursing in 19936. In 1937 she received a B.S. from George Peabody College in Nashville, Tennessee. Her other degrees in clued an M.A. in public health nursing supervision from Teacher's College, Columbia University, New York, in 1945 and an M.P.H. in 1952 and a Sc. D. in 1954, both from Johns Hopkins University in Baltimore.

For 21 years, from 1954 to 1975, she was professor and Head of the Division of Nursing at New York University. Since 1975, she has been Professor, and in 1979 she became professor Emerita.

Rogers' early nursing practice was in rural public health nursing in Michigan and in visiting nurse supervision, education, and practice in connecticut. She then established the Visiting Nurse Service of Phoenix, Arizona. Her publications include three books and over 200 articles; she continues to write and publish extensively. She has lectured in 46 states, the district of Columbia, Puerto Rico, Mexico, Holland, China, Newfoundland, Columbia, Brazil, and other countries.

Rogers has received honorary doctorates in Science, Letters, and Humane Letters from 1978 to the present from such renowned institutions as Duquesne University, University of San Diego, Iona College, Fairfield University, Emory University, Adelphi University, Mercy College, and Washburn University of Topeka. In addition, she has received numerous awards and citations for her contributions and leadership in nursing. She has received citations for "Inspiring Leadership in the Field of Intergroup Relations" by New York University, "For Distinguished Service to Nursing" by Teacher's College, and many others. She has also been honoured by the many awards, funds, and scholarships that have been established in her name.

A verbal portrait of Rogers might include such descriptive terms as stimulating, challenging, controversial, idealistic, visionary, prophetic, philosophic, academic, outspoken, humorous, blunt, and ethical. She has been widely recognized and honoured for her contributions and leadership in nursing. Her colleagues consider her one of the most original thinkers in nursing.

EVOLUTION OF THEORY

Rogers' early grounding in the liberal arts and sciences is apparent in the origin of her conceptual system and its ongoing development. Though introduced in earlier publications, the abstract system was first formally published in 1970 as *An Introduction to the Theoretical Basis of Nursing*. Rogers has continued to clarify and define her concepts in later publications and presentations such as her chapter in Explorations on *Martha Rogers' Science of Unitary Human Beings*, by Violet Malinski.

Rogers draws on a knowledge base gained from anthropology, psychology, sociology, astronomy, religion, philosophy, history, biology, physics, mathematics, literature, and other sources to create her model of unitary human beings and the environment as energy fields integral to the life process. A statement frequently repeated in her writings is, "Man is a unified whole possessing his own integrity and manifesting characteristics that are more than and different from the sum of his parts." Furthermore, human behaviour is described as synergistic, defining synergy as "the unique behaviour of whole systems, unpredicted by any behaviours of their component functions taken separately." In the prologue of *An Introduction to the Theoretical Basis of Nursing* she states, "Man's biological, physical, social, psychological, and spiritual heritages become an indivisible whole as scientific facts are merged with human warmth."

Several sources influenced Rogers' theorizations. During the mid-nineteenth century, Florence Nightingale's proposals and statistical data placed man within the framework of the natural world, and "the foundation for the scope of modern nursing was laid."

As the nineteenth century moved into the twentieth, classical physics gave way to field physics, and events of the physical world had a new unity. In 1905 Einstein's theory of relativity introduced the four coordinates of space-time.

In 1935 Burr and Northrop's "The Electro-dynamic Theory of Life" stated the concepts of the pattern and organization of the electro-dynamic field, the outcome of whose activity is wholeness, organization, and continuity. Rogers says, "An electrical field was replacing the cell as the fundamental unit of biological systems."

In the 1950s, von Bertalanffy introduced general systems theory, which presented a general science of wholeness. The term *negentropy* was brought into use to signify increasing order, complexity, and heterogeneity.

A theme of Rogers' writings and discussions may be paraphrased, "You cannot understand the whole by studying the parts, and the *whole* is more than and different from the sum of its parts."

A unitary human being is an energy field coextensive with the universe. Human-environment boundaries are only conceptually imposed and are arbitrary. The unity of human beings and environment is plausible, considering the sameness of matter and energy. Humans are more than and different from the sum of their parts, and generalities about the whole cannot be made from a study of the parts. The energy composing unitary human beings and the environmental field is characterized by four dimensions, in which a given point in time is not tenable. The four concepts—energy fields, openness, pattern and organization, and four-dimensionality–are used to derive principles that postulate how human beings develop. These principles are (i) integrality (formerly complimentarily), (ii) resonancy, and (iii) helicy. According to the principle of integrality, the human and environmental fields interact mutually and simultaneously. Resonancy postulates the nature of wave pattern changes as continuous from lower-frequency to higher-frequency patterns. Helicy asserts that field changes are innovative, probabilistic, and characterized by increasing diversity of field patterns.

Nursing seeks to care for unitary human beings in accordance with its science and art. Science is emergent and based on research and logical analysis of the principles of homeodynamics. Nursing science seeks to describe, explain, and predict. Art is the imaginative and creative use of knowledge and science. Nursing's goal is maximization of health potentials of individuals, family, and groups consistent with health's ever-changing nature. It is achieved by artfully applying emerging science, based on the principles of homeodynamics.

Martha E. Rogers draws on a knowledge base gained from anthropology, psychology, sociology, astronomy, religion, philosophy, history, biology, physics, mathematics, literature and other sources to create her model of "Unitary human being, and the environment as energy fields integral to the life process.' A statement frequently repeated in her writings is "Man is a unified whole possessing his own integrity and manifesting characteristics that are more than and different from the some of his parts." Further more, human behaviour is described as "the unique behaviour of whole systems, unpredicted by any behaviours of their component functions taken separately. In the prologue of "An Introduction to the theoretical Basis of Nursing" she states, 'Man, biological, physical, social, psychological and spiritual heritage became an indivisible whole as scientific facts are merged with human warmth."

The concept that human life is valuable did not develop until people had begun to band together into tribes, villages and towns. Such communal living allowed for sharing work and responsibility and providing mutual support. This more settled lifestyle made it possible for mothers to keep their newborns and care for more children. Thus, partly out of love and partly out of need, human beings began to develop strong feelings about and concern for fellow human beings. As culture developed, and more complex concepts in economic, political and social structures increased. Science, art and religion brought a growing awareness of one's fellow human beings. The Hebrews developed a monotheistic faith, whereas Greeks contributed philosophy, Politics and Government. Humanism was becoming strongly entrenched in culture. Following the rise of Christianity the medieval world was dominated by Christian religion whose members assumed the responsibility for nursing. With the Dark Ages came a decline in religion, cultural and political life. The end of this period led to the beginning of modern science.

As modern science evolved, new ideas mushroomed into new discoveries. The nature of universe explored. As a result of several discoveries, the rate at which society has been storing up useful knowledge, about humanity, the vast storehouse of knowledge coupled with a high degree of humanism and value of life has made advancement of nursing through scientific means and theoretical development a reality. As "a humanistic science dedicated to compassionate concern for maintaining and promoting health, preventing illness and caring for and rehabilitating the sick and disabled," nursing has meant service to humanity." Throughout nursing evolution, from the earliest ages to the present, nurturance of the human race has been an ever-preserve and central concern' over the years, the scientific extension of people's centuries long interest in life and its many manifestations has become an integral component of nursing. Rogers believed that knowledge of the past is a necessary foundation for the present understanding of nursing and for evolving the theories and principles that must guide nursing practice.

Rogers' Basic Assumptions

Nursing: Historically the term 'Nursing' most oftenly used a verb signifying 'to do.' When nursing is perceived as a science, the term 'nursing' becomes a noun signifying 'a body of abstract knowledge' Rogers describes that it is both a science and an art. "Nursing is humanistic science dedicated to compassionate concern for maintaining and promoting health, preventing illness, and caring for and rehabilitating the sick and disabled." Nursing seeks to promote symphonic interaction between the environment and man, to strengthen the coherence and integrity of human beings and to direct and redirect patterns of interaction between man and his environment for the realization of maximum health potential."

The professional practice of nursing is creative, and imaginative and exists to serve people. It is rooted in intellectual judgment abstract knowledge and human compassion. Professional nursing practice has no dependent functions but collaborative ones. Professional practitioners participate in the co-ordination of their knowledges and skills with those of professional personnel in other health disciplines. The safe practice of nursing intervention depends on the nature and amount of scientific knowledge, the individual brings to practice and the imaginative, intellectual judgment that puts such knowledge to use in the service to mankind. Nursing is a "science of unitary human being" and is therefore, unique because it is the only science that deals with the whole person."

Human being: In 1970, Rogers identified five assumptions about human beings, that are also theoretical assertions supporting her model derived from literature on man, physics, mathematics and behavioural sciences as follows:

1. Man is a unified whole possessing his own integrity and manifesting characteristics more than and different from the some of his parts (energy field).

    The distinctive properties of the whole are also significantly different from those of its parts. Extensive knowledge of the sub-systems is ineffective in enabling one to determine the properties of the living system, human being. The human being, is visible only when particular disappears

from view. Because of their wholeness, the individuals' life process is a dynamic course that is continuous, creative, evolutionary and uncertain, resulting in highly variable and constantly changing patterning.
2. Man and environment are continuously exchanging matter and energy with one another (openness).

    Environment for any individual is defined as "an irreducible, pandimensional energy field identified by pattern and integral with the human field. This constant interchange of materials and energy between the individual and the environment characterizes each of them as open systems.
3. The life process (of human being) involves irreversible and uni-directionally along the space-time continuum (Helicy)

    Rogers' view of the continuum change over time, the results continue to be the same. The undivided never go backward or be something he or she previously was. At any given point in time, then the individual is the expression of the totality of events present at the given time and influenced by preceding events.
4. Pattern and organisation identify men and reflect his innovative wholeness (Pattern and organization).

    Identifying individuals and reflecting that wholeness are life patterns. These patterns allow for self-regulation, rythmicity and dynamism. They give unity to diversity and reflect a dynamic and creative universe.
5. Man is characterised by the capacity for abstraction and imagery, language and thought, sensation and emotions (sentient, thinking being).

Of all the earth's life forms, only the human is a sentient thinking being who perceives and ponders the vastness of the cosmos.

On the basis of these five assumptions on human being, Rogers identified four building blocks, which includes energy fields openness, pattern and pandimensionality.

(a) *Energy field:* An energy field constitutes the fundamental unit of both the living and the non-living. Field is a unifying concept and energy signifies the dynamic nature of the field. Energy fields are infinite. Two fields are identified the human field and environment field. Specifically human beings and environment are energy fields.

- The unitary human being (human field) is defined as an irreducible, indivisible, pandimentional energy field identified by pattern and manifesting characteristics that are specific to the whole and which cannot be predicted from knowledge of the parts.
- The environment filed is defined as irreducible, pandimensional energy field identified by pattern and integral with the human field: Each environment field is specific in its given human field. Both change continuously and creatively.

(b) *Openness:* The concept of the universe of open systems holds that energy fields are infinite, open and integral with one another. The human and environmental field are continuous process and are open systems.

(c) *Pattern:* Pattern identifies energy fields. It is in the distinguishing characteristic of a field and is perceived as a single wave. The nature of the pattern changes continuously and innovatively. Each human field pattern is unique and is integral with its own environmental filed.

Manifestations of pattern have been described as unique and refer to behaviours, qualities and characteristics of the field; a sense of individual. The human field pattern is integral with the environmental field. The pattern is constantly changing and may manifest disease, illness or pain.

(d) *Pandimensionality:* Rogers defines Pandimensionality as a non-linear domain without spatial or temporal attributes. The term 'Pan-dimensional provides for an infinite domain without limit. It is best to express the idea of a Unitary whole.

A unifying concept for both animate and inanimate environment energy fields have no boundaries, they are indivisible, extend to infinity and are dynamic. Thus these fields are open, allowing exchange with other fields. The interchange between and among energy fields has pattern that is perceived as a single wave, these patterns are fixed but change as situations require. The interchanges occur in pan-dimensionally a nonlinear domain that is not bounded by space or time. With these building blocks as the base, unitary human being and environment being are defined (as stated in energy field). With this it is understood that there is a strong parallel between Rogers' basic assumptions and General System Theory (von Bertalanffy 1968)

According to von Bertalanffy (1968) a system is a set of interrelated elements in this abstract system are human beings and their environments. As living system and energy field, the individual is capable of taking energy and information from the environment and releasing energy and information to the environment. Because of this exchange the individual is an open system—an underlying assumption of building blocks. General system theory in a general science of wholeness. It is concerned with the problem of organization. Phenomena that are not resolvable to individual events and dynamic interaction manifested in the difference of the behaviour of the parts when isolated. As a result, order and behaviour are not understandable by investigation of respective parts in isolation. So the assumption of wholeness and the building block of pattern result. The principles of hierarchical order is applicable (von Bertalanffy). The individual as an open system attempts to move toward a higher order by a progressive differentiation. Humanbeings are higher order with two ligs with in the order of universe, i.e. human being as sentient thinking beings.

On the basis of these above stated five assumption, and building blocks, the life process in human beings becomes a phenomenon of wholeness, of continuity and of dynamic and creative change. It has its own unity. It is inseparable from the environment and occurs in pan-dimensionality. Because the individual is the recipient of nursing services, life processes of humanity are the core around which nursing revolves. The science of nursing is the study of human and environmental fields and is directed towards describing the life process of humanity and explaining and predicting the nature and directions of its developments.

ROGERS' THEORY: PRINCIPLES OF HOMEODYNAMICS

Rogers did not offer theoretical statement; but grounded her 'Principles of Homeodynamics" on the basis of Five basic assumptions and four building blocks discussed earlier. The principles of homeodynamics are composed of three separate principles—integrality, resonancy, and helicy. By combining the principles of homeodynamics with the concept of humanity from her definition of nursing, a theoretical statement can be postulated. Using the definition that a theory interrelates concepts in such a way as to create a different way of looking at a particular phenomenon, an appropriate theoretical statement might be that nursing is the use of the principles of homeodynamics for the service of humanity.

Integrality

The first principle of *integrality*. Because of the inseparability of human beings and their environment, sequential changes in the life process are continuous revisions occurring from the interactions between human beings and their environment. Between the two entities, there is a constant mutual interaction and mutual change whereby simultaneous molding is taking place in both at the same time. This molding is one of association, not causality. Thus, integrality is the continuous, mutual, simultaneous interaction process between human and environmental fields.

Resonancy

The next principle *resonancy* speaks to the nature of the change occurring between human and environmental fields. The change in the pattern of human beings and environments is propagated by waves that move from longer waves of lower frequency to shorter waves of higher frequency. The life process in human beings is a symphony of rhythmical vibrations oscillating at various frequencies. Human beings experience their environments as a resonating wave of complex symmetry uniting them with the rest of the world. Resonancy, then, is the identification of the human field and the environmental field by wave patterns manifesting continuous change from longer waves of lower frequency to shorter waves of higher frequency.

Helicy

Finally, the principle of *helicy* deals with the nature and direction of change in the human-environment field. The human-environment field is a dynamic open system in which change is continuous due to the constant interchange between the human and the environment. This change is also innovative. Because of the constant interchange, an open system is never exactly the same at any two moments; rather, the system is continually new or different. The difference cannot be predicted wince open systems have choices about the matter, energy, and information which they accept as input and send out as output; thus, the change is unpredictable. Finally, the direction of change is toward ever increasing diversity and complexity. The life process evolves through a constant series of change in a rhythmical manner. The rhythms are not repeated although they may appear to be similar over time. The changes incorporate the past and lead to new patterns. This process and these patterns are unpredictable, dynamic, and increasingly diverse. Helicy encompasses the concept of rhythmic change, evolutionary influence, and unitary human environment fields. Helicy proposes that the direction of changes which occur between human and environment fields is toward ever increasing diversity and complexity and is seen in rhythms which are not precisely repeated.

Thus, the principles of homeodynamics are a way of viewing human beings in their wholeness. Changes in the life process of humans are irreversible, non-repeatable, rhythmic and presents growing diversity of patterns. Change proceeds by continuous repatterning of both human and environmental fields by resonating oscillations of longer waves of lower frequency to shorter waves of higher frequency. Change reflects the mutual simultaneous interests between two fields as pan-dimensional.

Paradigm of Rogers' Theory

- Human beings—Rogers presents five assumptions about human beings, in relation to nursing's metaparadigm, which includes:
- Each human is assumed to be a unified being with individuality.
- The human is in continuous exchange of energy with the environment.
- The life process of a human evolves irreversibly and unpredictably in pandimensionality.
- There is a pattern of life and
- The human is capable of abstraction, imagery, language, thought, sensation and emotion.

Human being are irreducible, indivisible, pan-dimensional energy fields identified by pattern and manifesting characteristics and behaviours that are different from those of the parts and that cannot be predicted from knowledge of parts.

Environment

It consists of totality of patterns existing external to the individual. Both the individual and environment are considered to be open systems. Environment is an irreducible, indivisible, pan-dimensional energy field identified by pattern and integral with the human field.

Health

Health is not specifically addressed and indeed, is not appropriate to Rogers' theory. She viewed health as a value term. This communication confirms previous inferences that disease, pathology and health are value terms. Value terms change and, when discussed in terms of the dynamics of the behaviours manifested by the human field, need to be individually defined.

Nursing

Nursing is an art and science that is humanistic and humanitarian. It is directed toward the Unitary human and is concerned with the nature and direction of human development. The goal of nurse is to participate in the process of change so that people may benefit.

Nursing is 'Learned profession', a science and an art. A basic science, "a study of unitary, irreducible, indivisible human and environmental fields, people and their world.

Art of nursing: refers to "creative use of the science of nursing for human betterment, imaginative and creative us of nursing knowledge for human betterment.

Purposes of nursing: To promote health and wellbeing for all persons and groups wherever they are.

Uniqueness of nursing: is the focus on unitary human beings and world.

Nursing Process and Rogers' Homeodynamics

Nursing profession is viewed as concerned with unitary human beings, the principles of Homeodynamics provide guidelines for predicting the nature and direction of the individual, development as responses to health-related problems are made. Using these guidelines, the professional practice of nursing would then seek to promote symphonic integration of human beings and their environment, to strengthen the coherence and integrity of the human field, and to direct and indirect patterning of human and environmental field for the realization of maximum health. These goal would be reflected in the nursing process.

For successful use of the principles of Homeodynamics, there needs to be a consideration of the nurse and an involvement of both the nurse and the client in the nursing process. If anything or any one external to the individual is part of the environment, then the nurse would be part of the client's environment. Because of the mutual interaction of the individual and environment, it is implied that the client is a willing, integral participant in the nursing process. Consequently, individualized nursing care results, which Rogers maintains is necessary, if the client to achieve maximum potential in a positive fashion. Nursing then is working with the clients, not to or for the client. The involvement in the nursing process, by the nurse demonstrates concerns for the total person rather than one aspect, one problem or limited segments of need fulfillment.

The schematic representation of the relationship between the principles of homeodynamics and the elements of nursing process is presented in the Table 20.1. As can be seen, there is no absolute distinction between the areas covered to the various principles. Table 20.2 attempts to apply the generalities to the specific situation of Geetha who is hospitalized. In no way is either table designed to all inclusive. Rather, they offered as an attempt to make abstract ideas more concrete and operational.

The Characteristics of Theory and Research Work of Martha E Rogers

1. Theories can interrelate concepts in such a way as to create a different way of looking at a particular phenomena.

    Rogers' abstract system clearly creates an alternative view of people and their world. The theoretical statement that nursing is the use of the principles of homeodynamics for service of humanity compels one to look at nursing in a very different way. An excellent example is the principle of helicy with its emphasis on pattern and rhythmicity.

2. Theories must be logical in nature. There is definitely a logical development of the major constructs. This logical development proceeds from the identification of assumptions, through the building blocks, to the principles of homeodynamics.

3. Theories should be relatively simple yet generalizable. The theory is generalizable because it is not dependent on any given setting. It has been stated that Rogers' conception of man is elegant in its simplicity. However, the theory is far from simple in that its level of abstraction and the nature of the terminology contribute to difficulties in understanding. In addition, the theory is based on the use of open systems that are inherently complex.

Table 20.1: Relationship of the principles of homeodynamics to the nursing process

Components of the nursing process	Principles of homeodynamics		
	Integrality	*Resonancy*	*Helicy*
Nursing assessment component	Look at the interaction of the individual and the environment—how they work together rather than what they are like in isolation	Look at the variation occurring during the life process of the whole human being	Look at the rhythmic life patterns of the individual and the environment. Progression of time of necessity creates changes in the rhythmic life patterns of the whole human being. Look at life goals. Be aware of growing complexity of the whole human being
Nursing diagnosis component	Reflects integration of the individual and environmental fields	Reflects the variations in the life process of the whole individual	Reflects the rhythmic pattern of the individual and environmental fields
Nursing plan for implementation component	Intervenes in the environment as well as in the individual. Change promoted in one area will cause simultaneous change in the other simultaneous molding	Support or modify variations in the life process of the whole individual	Promote dynamic rhythmic repatterning of both the individual and the environment. Accept differences as an expression of evolutionary emergence promote dynamism and complexity rather than homeostasis and equilibrium. Support or modify life goals.
Nursing evaluation component	Evaluate changes in the integration that have occurred	Evaluate the modification made in the variation of the life process of the whole human being	Evaluate rhythmic repatterning of the individual and the environment. Evaluate goal directedness. Evaluate relationship of goal to the whole individual

4. Theories can be the bases for hypotheses that can be tested or for theory to be expanded, and
5. Theorists contribute to and assist in increasing the general body of knowledge with in the discipline through the research implemented to validate them. It is clear that the abstract level of the system leads to the generation of a plethora of research questions. Barrett (1990), Fawcett (1989), Ference (1989), Malinski (1986), Madrid and winstead-Fry (1986), and Rogers (1989) all cite numerous studies ostensibly designed to test this framework. However, research is hampered by the lack of simplicity, operation definitions, and valid instruments to measure out comes. The complex interrelationships involved in the framework contribute to these difficulties. Qualitative research approaches have been suggested as an effective method for minimizing these problems. These and other efforts designed to minimize these research problems need to be continued so that nursing can truly benefit from Roger's abstract system.
6. Theories can be used by practitioners to guide and improve their practice. Rogers' ideas can be applied to practice. When

Table 20.2: Relationship of the principles of homeodynamics to the nursing process for Geetha

Components of the nursing process	Principles of homeodynamics		
	Integrality	Resonancy	Helicy
Nursing Assessment component	1. How does Geetha see her environment? 2. What kind of differences are there between the hospital and her home? 3. How is she reacting to the changes in her environment? 4. How do her health problem and the environment affect each other?	1. What is Geetha's past history? 2. What kinds of deviations from the expected norms have there been? 3. Were these deviations individually or environmentally related? 4. What is the reason for the hospitalization? 5. How will this affect her life?	1. What are Geetha's normal behaviour patterns and routines? 2. Were the behaviour or routines undergoing a change prior to her admission? 3. What kinds of activities can she perform. 4. What kinds of past experiences has she had? 5. How might those experience influence her current situation? 6. What is Geetha's development level? 7. Will the hospital environment support or retard developmental progress? 8. What are Geetha's goals?
Nursing diagnosis component	1. What is the nature of the interactions between Geetha and the hospital	1. What is the interference this hospitalization will make in Geetha's life?	What are the rhythmic patterns that are being exhibited?
Nursing plan for implementation component	1. How can the hospital environment be modified to reduce the differences identified? 2. How can Geetha be helped to understand the difference that cannot be eliminated? 3. How can her health potential be improved by manipulating the environment	1. How can Geetha's normal development be promoted? 2. How can the effects of the interferences be minimized?	1. How can Geetha's normal behavioural patterns and routines be promoted in the hospital? 2. What kind of modifications can be made to promote her normal behavioural patterns and routines? 3. What kind of provisions can be made to promote her normal growth and development? 4. How can Geetha be helped to develop successful rhythmic behavioural patterns within the hospital environment? 5. How can Geetha be helped to reach her goals?
Nursing evaluation component	1. Has Geetha' behaviour changed as a result of environmental modification? 2. What kind of new reactions are now taking place?	1. Is Geetha developing normally based on theories? 2. Has the interference with development been minimized?	1. What kind of rhythmic repatterning has taken place? 2. Is Geetha's development being supported? 3. Is she moving towards her goals?

these ideas are applied to nursing practice, the understanding of the client's behaviour takes on new dimensions. Such dimensions include accepting diversity as the norm, empowering both nurse and client, viewing change as positive, and accepting the integral connectedness of life. This changed understanding results in alterations in the focus of nursing actions. The case study of Geetha presented in this chapter provides an example. In addition, nursing interventions such as therapeutic touch and the use of light, colour, music, and movement have been derived from Rogers' tenets. However, evidence of positive effects of nursing interventions derived from this model is needed.

7. Theories must be consistent with other validated theories, laws, and principles but will leave open unanswered questions that need to be investigated. Rogers' work is consistent with other validated theories, laws and principles. The abstract nature of the system provides great potential for generating questions for further study and deriving interventions for nursing practice. Rogers' abstract system has also been instrumental in the development of other theories, e.g. Newman (1994), Panse (1992).

EVALUATION OF THEORY

- Rogers' conceptual model is complex. She uses multiple concepts that are not easily understood. She relates these concepts in her principles of homeodynamics.
- Rogers' conceptual model is abstract and is therefore generalizable and powerful. It is usually considered a grand theory or a macro theory. It is broad in scope and attempts to explain everything.
- Many would have difficulty understanding the concepts and relationships without a strong knowledge of other fields of study. Rogers' conceptual model is deductive in logic and "the major criticism of deductive theories is the lack of empirical support." "The difficulty in understanding the principles, the lack of operational definitions, and inadequate tools for measurement are the major limitations to the effective utilization of this theory." Rogers' early model lacked empirical precision, yet empirical precision has greatly increased as Rogers' conceptual model has been further developed. The abstract system generates theories that are testable.
- Resides the previously mentioned recent studies, many other research studies have been performed. All these studies have implications for guiding nursing practice and education and suggest further research.

Rogers sees the nurse as an integral part of the client's environment. She also sees nursing as a unique science that deals with "unitary human beings" who are different from the sum of their parts. The differentiates nursing from other professions and basic sciences.

Many ideas for future study have been suggested by Rogers. Based on this, it can be said that Rogers' conceptual model is useful.

Rogers is a brilliant nursing theorist who is years ahead of her time. Understanding her concepts and principles requires a foundation in general education, a willingness to let go of the traditional, and an ability to perceive the world in a new and creative way.

Rogers has many pertinent views for the future. She states, "Only as the science of nursing takes on form and substance can the art of nursing achieve new dimensions of artistry." She continues to emphasize nursing services as indispensable to public safety and health.

The goal of health workers and of the public focuses properly on the promotion of health. In a dynamic continuously innovative world, one does not, for example, prevent disease. Rather, in the process of change there are many potentialities, only some of which will be actualised. Therapeutic modalities will increasingly emphasize the non-invasive. Diversity will be accorded high value. Human health will not be measured by adding up parameters of biological, physical, social, psychological, and like phenomena.

Again, Rogers said it well when she quoted Capra: "We are trying to apply concepts of an out-dated world view to a reality that can no longer be understood in terms of these concepts." She continued:

A science of unitary human beings basic to nursing requires a new world view and a conceptual system specific to nursing's phenomenon of concern. Seeing the world from this viewpoint requires a new synthesis, a creative leap, and the inculcation of new attitudes and values.

A science of unitary human beings identifies nursing's uniqueness and signifies the potential of nurses to fulfil their social responsibility in human service.

Chapter 21

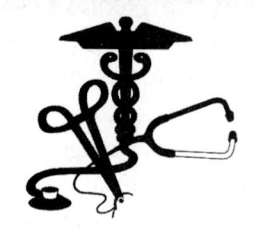

Newman's Theory of Health

Margaret A. Newman was born October 10, 1933, in Memphis, Tennessee. She earned her first bachelor's degree in Home Economics and English from Baylor University, in Waco, Texas, in 1954, and her second in nursing from the University of Tennessee in Memphis in 1962. She received her master's degree in medical-surgical nursing and teaching from the University of California at San Francisco in 1964 and her PhD in nursing science and rehabilitation nursing from New York University in New York City in 1971.

Newman progressed through the academic ranks at the University of Tennessee, New York University, The Pennsylvania State University, and since 1984 has been a professor at the University of Minnesota in Minneapolis. In addition, she has been the director of nursing for the clinical Research Center at the University of Tennessee, the acting director of the Ph.D. program in the Division of Nursing at New York University, and Professor-in-Charge of the Graduate Program and Research at The Pennsylvania State University.

Newman was admitted to the American Academy of Nursing in 1976. She received the Outstanding Alumnus Award from the University of Tennessee College of Nursing in Memphis in 1975, the Distinguished Alumnus Award from the Division of Nursing at New York University in 1984, and was admitted in 1988 to the Hall of Fame at the University of Mississippi School of Nursing. She was a Latin American Teaching Fellow in 1976-1977 and an *American Journal of Nursing* Scholar in 1979. She was Distinguished Faculty at the Seventh International Conference on Human Functioning at Wichita, Kansas, in 1983 and is listed in *Who's Who in American Women*. Newman was included in 1990 as one of the featured nursing theorists in the videotape series sponsored by Helene Fuld Health Trust.

In 1985, as a Traveling Research Fellow, Newman conducted workshops in four locations throughout New Zealand. At the University of Tampere, Finland, in 1985 Newman was the major speaker for a week-long conference on the theory of consciousness as it related to nursing. Newman has presented many papers on topics pertaining to her theory of health as expanding consciousness. She has published two books on the theory: *Health as Expanding Consciousness* in 1986 and *Theory Development in Nursing* in 1979. She has written enumerable articles in journals and book chapters. In 1986 she did a case study analysis of practice in three sites within the Minneapolis-St. Paul area in which she discussed the background of the health care system, findings within each site, and conclusions concerning the changes necessary for hospital nursing practice. Since 1986, Dr. Newman has investigated the sequential patterns of persons with heart disease and cancer.

During 1989 and 1990, Dr. Newman was the principal investigator of a project that explored the theory and structure of a professional model of nursing practice. This research was conducted at Carondelet St. Mary's Community Hospitals and Health Centers in Tucson, Arizona. In addition to her research and teaching, Dr. Newman is sought for consultation with regard to expanding her theory of health from over 40 states and Australia, Brazil, Canada, Czechoslovakia, France, Finland, Germany, Japan, New Zealand, Poland, and the United Kingdom.

Newman has served on several editorial boards, including *Nursing Research, Western Journal of Nursing Research, Nursing and Health Care, Advances in Nursing Science,* and *Nursing Science Quarterly* Essential to her theory and nursing diagnoses development was her participation as a member of the nurse theorist task force, since 1978, with the North American Nursing Diagnoses Association.

EVOLUTION OF THEORY

Central to her assumptions was the philosopher Hegel's "dialectical process of the fusion of opposites." Newman used many fields of inquiry as sources for theory development. The rationale for drawing broad conclusions from the use of a limited number of concepts came from Capra, a physicist. Capra held that many phenomena can be explained in terms of a few. Newman drew from Capra in general, and Bentov in particular, for her position on the importance of holistic health and expansion of consciousness. "Bentov has postulated that time is a measure of consciousness." Newman credited "Dorothy Johnson, during my undergraduate studies, and Martha Rogers, in a more extensive way, during my graduate study as those nurse theorists most influential on my thinking."

Bohm's theory of implicit order helped Newman put Bentov's explanation of the evolving consciousness into perspective. Newman stated she began to comprehend "the underlying, unseen pattern that manifests itself in varying forms, including disease, and the interconnectedness and omnipresence of all that there is. Young's theory of human evolution pinpointed for Newman the role of pattern recognition and "was the impetus for . . . efforts to integrate the basic concepts of my theory—movement, space, time, and consciousness—into a dynamic portrayal of life and health." Moss' experience of love as the highest level of consciousness "provided affirmation and elaboration of my intuition regarding the nature of health." Ilya Prigogine, a chemist and winner of the Nobel Prize for his theory of dissipative structures, described the pattern of harmony and disharmony as part of a rhythmic process. Newman incorporated Prigogine's concepts into her conceptualization of disease as a manifestation of the pattern of a person.

Individuals are subsumed by a greater whole and are part of multiple system levels in space. Explicit assumptions are made in relation to health, pathology, and patterns. Health can encompass pathology and disease; therefore, disease and health are not continuous variables or opposites. Pathology is manifested according to a pre-existing unitary pattern; thus disease gives clues to the pattern of a person's life, and pattern is reflected in energy exchange within humans and between humans and the environment. Personal patterns manifesting as disease are part of larger patterns, which are not altered when the disease is eliminated. Disease as a pattern manifestation may be considered health. The existence of disease may evoke tension, an important evolutionary ingredient. Disease is not advocated as a desirable state, but the significance of attending to the meaning of the disease is highlighted. Health is an expansion of consciousness, and pattern manifesting disease expands consciousness.

Consciousness, the informational capacity of the system, is reflected in both the quality and quantity of responses to stimuli. Health involves developing awareness of self and environment, coupled with increased ability to perceive and respond to alternatives. Movement is a central concept, a property of life. The concepts of consciousness, time, movement, and space are interrelated in that movement reflects consciousness and is an identifiable and specific individual characteristic. Time is an index of consciousness and a function of movement. Movement is the means by which time and space become reality, and space and time have a complimentary relationship. Without movement, time and space are not real, and there is no change at any system level. Movement reflects the organization of consciousness and therefore reflects health. The implied goal is consciousness expansion and therefore health and life. Health is not a state but an experienced process.

Evidence for the theory of Health emanated from Newman's early personal family experiences. Her mother's struggle with chronic illness and her dependency or Newman, then a young college graduate sparked an interest in nursing. Form that experience evolved the idea that "illness reflected the life patterns of the persons and that what was needed was the recognition of that pattern and acceptance of it for what it meant to that person.

Newman has stated that during her doctoral study, she was interested in theory in nursing. More specifically, as a result of her experiences during her mother's illness, she was interested in the relationship between movement, time and space, for the describes her mother as having been immobilized in time and space. She states that the did not intentionally began to develop a theory, but rather 'slid' into theory development. Her preparation to speak at a conference (1978) marked the beginning of her defined intention to explicate the temporal and spatial pattern of health. She states that at his time, she was moving toward Theory of Health. She chosen Health as a focus because she saw Disease as a meaningful aspect of health and believed health needed better definition. In developing her theory, Newman (1994) was influenced by Martha Rogers, Itzhuk Bentov, David Bohm, Richard Moss, and Arthur Young incorporate the following views of theirs.

- The Unitary of human being is open and interact with its environment (Rogers 1970).
- View of consciousness as evolving and being coexistensive with its universe supported (Bentov 1978).
- Discussion of Implicate and explicate orders supported the idea of health as pattern of the whole with normal profession towards higher levels of organisation (Bohms 1980).
- Presentation of love as the highest level of consciousness (Moss 1981).
- Importance of insight, pattern recognition, and choice provided the impetus for the interpretation of the concepts of movement, time and space into a dynamic theory of health (Young 1976).

Concepts Used in Theory of Health

Health

Health encompasses disease and non-disease. Health can be regarded as the exploitation of the underlying pattern of the person and the environment. Health is viewed as a process of "developing awareness of self and environment together with increasing ability to perceive alternatives and respond in a variety of ways." Health is viewed as including "disease as a meaningful manifestation of the pattern of the whole and is based on the premise that life is an ongoing process of expanding consciousness.

Pattern

Pattern is what identifies an individual as a particular person. Example of explicit manifestation of the underlying patter of a person would be the genetic pattern that contains information that directs our becoming the voice pattern, the movement pattern. Characteristics of pattern include movement, diversity, and rhythm. Pattern is somewhat intimately involved in energy exchange and transformation.

In health, as expanding consciousness, Newman developed pattern as a major concept that was used to understand the individual as a whole being. She described as paradigm shift that was occurring in the field of health care. The shift was from treatment of symptoms of a disease to the search for patterns. Newman stated that the patterns of interaction of person-environment constitute health. Embedded within the concept of movement, time and space is the idea that an event such as a disease occurrence is part of a larger process. " By interacting with the event, no matter how destructive the force might seem to be, its energy augments our own and enhance our power in the situation. In order to see this, it is necessary to grasp the patter of the "shole."

Pattern depicts the whole and is characterized by movement, diversity and rhythm. Movement is constant and rhythmic and the parts of diverse pattern is relatedness. The process of patterning occurs if human energy fields penetrate one another and transformation occurs. Transformation is change that occurs all-at-once rather than in gradual and lineal fashion. Patterns recognition occurs within the observer.

Consciousness

Consciousness is defined as the informational capacity of the system, the ability of the system to interact with its environment. Three correlates of consciousness (time, movement, space) serve as explanations for the changing pattern of the whole and are major concepts in the theory of health.

The life process is seen as progression toward higher levels of consciousness. The expansion of consciousness is what life and therefore health is all about. Newman referred to the time sense as a factor altered in the changing level of consciousness. Thus the perception of time is an indicator of man's health status.

Movement: " Movement is the means whereby one perceives reality and therefore, is a means of becoming aware of self." Newman emphasized that movement through space is integral to the development of a concept of time in man and is utilized by man as a measure of time. She maintained that "movement brings about change, without which there is no manifest reality." To further explain this concept, Newman used the example of the person restricted in his mobility by structural or psychological pathology (who) must adapt to an altered rate of movement.

Time and space: Time and space have a complementary relationship. The concept of space is inextricably linked to the concept of time. When one's life space is decreased, as by either physical or social immobility, one's time is increased.

Time in Newman's model includes a sense of time perspective, that is orientation to past, present and future. But it centers primarily on time as perceived duration. Perceived duration is defined as the ratio of the individual, awareness content.

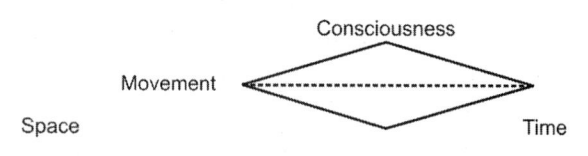

Newman Model of Health

Perceived duration is used synonymously with subjective time as defined by Bentov Factors related to the awareness component include emotional state and attention to a task, factors related to the content are external events, body movement, and metabolism.

$$\text{Subjective time} = \frac{\text{Awareness}}{\text{Content}}$$

Newman used the theories of time, perception modified by Bentov's conceptualization of time and consciousness. He calculates the index of consciousness by establishing ratio of subjective time (the number of seconds judged to have elapsed) to objective time (actual clock time). Therefore,

$$\text{Index of consciousness} = \frac{\text{Subjective time}}{\text{Objective time}}$$

Time and timing relate the rhythm of living phenomena. Examples include the variations in the effectiveness of drug and radiation-therapies throughout a 24-hour cycle. Dosages that are therapeutic at one period during the day may be fatal during another period. Timing is recognised as important in the provision of nursing care particularly in home/health.

In humans, consciousness is the information capacity includes not only all the things we normally associate with consciousness, such as thinking and feeling, but also all the information embedded in the nervous system, the endocrine system, the immune system, the genetic code and so on. As human beings develop, consciousness grows, or expands. The direction of life is ever towards higher levels of consciousness.

Newman (1994) states that she began the development of her theory with an effort to follow the demands of logical positivism. This, she identified concepts (as stated above) and assumption of her theory. Her initial assumptions were the following.

1. Health encompasses conditions heretofore described as illness or in medical terms, pathology.
2. These pathological conditions can be considered a manifestation of the total pattern of the individual.
3. The pattern of the individual that eventually manifests itself as pathology is primary and exists prior to structural or functional changes.
4. Removal of the pathology in itself will not change the pattern of the individual.
5. If becoming 'ill' is the only way an individual's pattern can manifest itself, then that is health for that person.
6. Health is expansion of consciousness.

Newman developed her central premise based on those assumptions. She stated "Health is the expansion of consciousness. The process of unfolding consciousness will occur regardless of what we as nurses do. We can however assist clients in getting touch with what is going on and in this way facilitate the process:

Newman's initial concepts were movement, time, space and consciousness. She discussed movement as an essential property of matter and the change that occurs between two states of rest, but she did not define the other concepts of initiality. She did propose relationships among the concepts on the following:

1. Time and space have a complementary relationship.
2. Movement is a means whereby space and time become a reality.
3. Movement is a reflection of consciousness.
4. Time is a function of movement.
5. Time is a measurement of consciousness.

More currently, Marchione (1993) states that Newman's implicit assumptions are that humans have the following characteristics.

- Open energy systems.
- In continual interconnectedness with a universe of the open systems (environment)
- Continuously active in evolving their own pattern of the whole (health)
- Intuitive as well as affective and cognitive beings.
- Capable of abstract thinking as well as sensation.
- More than the sum of their parts.

Paradigm and Theory of Health

Nursing's major assumptions of nursing, person, health, and environment are not addressed explicitly in the theory of health. In the following paragraphs, implicit definition of form Newman work were used to discuss the four nursing components.

Human Being

Throughout Newman's work, the terms client, patient, person individual and pattern are used interchangeably. Human beings are identified by their patterns. The patterns of individuals embedded in those of their family are, in turn, these are embedded in the patterns of the community and society.

Person is defined as "consciousness: Persons as individuals are identified by their individual patterns of consciousness. Humans are moving towards ever-increasing organisation and are capable of making their own decisions. Progression to higher level of organisation often occurs after period of disorganisation, or choice point, when the older ways no longer work. Movement and pivotal choice point is evolving consciousness and is the expression of consciousness, Restriction of movement forces are beyond space time.

Environment

Environment is not explicitly defined, but is described as being the larger whole, that which is beyond the consciousness of the individual. The pattern of consciousness that is the family and within the pattern of community interactions. A major assumption is that "consciousness is coexistensive in the universe and resides in all matter."

Health

Health is the major concept of Newman's theory of expanding consciousness. A fusion of disease and non-disease creates a synthesis that is regarded as health. Because disease and non-disease are each reflection of the larger whole a new concept is formed. Pattern of the whole. Newman stated that the "essence of the emerging paradigm of health is pattern recognition. Health and evolving pattern of consciousness are the same."

Newman states that health, disease and the pattern of the whole are consistent with Bohms (1980) theory of implicate and explicate order. Implicate order is that "unseen, multidimensional pattern that is the ground, or basis for all things." Explicate order arises out of the implicate order and includes the tangibles-those things we can identify with our senses of the world. Because we can see, touch, hear, feel the tangibles we tend to identify them as primary, which is contrary of Bohm-statement that implicate order is primary. In this sense, manifest health, encompassing disease and non-disease can be regarded as the explication of the underlying the pattern of environment.

Newman proposes that those fluctuations in pattern identified as sickness can provide the disturbance needed to reorganize the relationships of pattern more harmoniously. Illness may achieve what people have wanted but have become unable to acknowledge, it can provide or represent the disequilibrium needed to maintain the vital active exchange with the environment. We grow or evolve through experiencing diseuilibrium and learning how to attain a new sense of balance. This disease may be seen as both emergent and expanding consciousness. It is important to remember that although the individual may exhibit the emergent pattern labeled disease, that individual pattern relate to and affects the pattern of others—family, friends, community. An open system is constant instruction. Humans influence one another's pattern and evolve together.

Nursing

Nursing is seen as providing a partner in the process of expanding consciousness. The nurse can connect with the person when new rules are sought. The nurse is the facilitator who helps an individual, family and community. Focus on his or her patterns. The nursing process is one of the patterns of recognitions. She used assessment framework developed by the nurse theorist group of *NANDA* to assist the nurse in pattern identification. The dimension of assessment frame work—exchanging, communicating, relating, valuing, choosing, moving feeling and knowing are considered manifestation of unitary pattern.

Newman (1994) discusses nursing as a profession, presenting three stages in the growth of the profession as follows:
- The first stage is formative, in which nursing was in the process of becoming, of establishing its identity, and individual practitioners were responsible for their own practice.
- The second stage is normative, here nursing lost some of its authority and was more conspective and persuasive in relation to the environment. In this stage, nursing moved primarily into the hospital setting and nurses became employees.
- The third stage is integrative. In this stage, nursing will relate to the other health care provides and to clients as partners, in a cooperative, mutual manner. Newman suggests three nursing roles in the primary integration role as nurse clinician or care manager. The other roles and that of nursing team leader and staff nurse.

Newman defines nursing as " caring in the human health experience. She believes that caring is a moral imperative for nursing.

Nursing Process and Theory of Health

The nursing is the facilitator who helps an individual family or community focus on his or her pattern. The nursing process is one of pattern recognition. Newman utilized the assessment framework developed by her nurse theorist group of North American Nursing Diagnosis Association (*NANDA*) to assist nurse in pattern identification. The dimension of the assessed framework – exchanging, communicating, relating, valuing, choosing, moving, perceiving, feeling, and knowing care considered manifestation of the unitary pattern.

Pattern recognition comes from the observer. The nurse perceives the patterns of the set of data or sequence of events and the pattern of the individual changes with new information. The process of pattern recognition first involves an attempt to view the pattern of a person as "sequential pattern overtime." Data from interviews of "healthy" adults could be grouped into sequential patterns. A following interview is then conducted to share the investigations' findings with the subjects. The nurse can use this process to identify the current pattern of an individual to establish a plan of care.

The five stages of nursing process does not apply to Newman theory. The implication of the five steps process that predictive goals can be set and that outcomes should be measured against these goals is not compatible with Newman's statements that we cannot make predictions with certainty and that we do not know what form expanding consciousness will take. For Newman, the process of nursing is one of coming together as partners during a time of chaos when the client is at a choice point. The nurse is there to be with the client and to accept the unpredictable nature of life. Accepting the circumstances decreases the stress in responding to those circumstances; Although the nurse may share knowledge, provide support, or be an organizing force in the relationship, the primary function for the nurse in this caring relationship is awareness of being. Attending to silence is at least as crucial as attending to utterances and movements. When the client is ready, the nurse and client will again move apart. It is hoped that each will have reached a higher level of consciousness through the experience.

Newman's Work and the Characteristics of a Theory

1. Theories can interrelate concepts in such a way as to create a different way of looking at a particular phenomenon. For nearly three decades, Newman has challenged us to view the phenomenon of health and disease parts of the same whole, interrelated space, time, movement, and pattern in a new way. Although concepts are present within her work, they are not primary to understanding the unitary-transformative paradigm. She indicates that she has moved beyond the interrelationship of concepts to the interrelationship of the human beings.
2. Theories must be logical in nature. Newman's presentation is logical. She presents the material from which she derived her ideas as needed and discusses with clarity those works that support her theory. There are some contradictions in her work. For example, she describes disease as disequilibrium or disruption and discusses the role played by disequilibrium in growth or the expansion of consciousness. At another point, she states that disease is not necessary and may not occur if human beings can be open to and accepting of the turn of events in their lives. She also describes humans and their environment as an undivided whole and speaks eloquently to the importance of viewing them in this way. Again, in another discussion, she indicates that the whole can be seen in its parts. She does discuss the fact that the smaller the piece being viewed, is, the fuzzier the picture of the whole will be.
3. Theories should be relatively simple yet generalizable. Newman's theory of health as expanding consciousness is not limited by person or setting. It is generalizable to anybody, anywhere. Her presentation of nursing within this theory is limited to those situations in which caring occurs. She states that without caring, nursing is not present. Her statement that health is expanding consciousness, seen in the evolving pattern of the whole is relatively simple. Her ideas represent a paradigm shift in our view of health and of nursing and may be complex to those who do not comprehend the paradigm. This is true for any paradigm shift and should not be seen as a limitation of this theory.
4. Theories can be bases for hypotheses that can be tested or theory to be expanded. Newman supports the use of the theory of health as expanding consciousness as A PRIORI in research. However, she does not support the positivistic view of hypothesis development and testing. In her research methodology, the patterns that are identified through interviewing with research participants are tested against the theory. Thus, the theory of

health as expanding consciousness can be used in research and in testing. The methodology to be used does not include hypotheses, which represent a view of the world that is incongruent with the theory.

5. Theories contribute to and assist in increasing the general body of knowledge within the discipline through the research implemented to validate them. Research has been conducted by using Newman's theory. Newman has conducted studies on the needs of hospitalized patients (1966), time and movement (1972, 1976), subjective time (1982) Newman and Guadiano (1984), patterns in persons with coronary artery disease (Newman and Moch, 1991 (These studies have both added to the general body of nursing knowledge and served to refine and develop her theory. Fryback's (1993) and Moch's (1990) studies supported Newman's thesis that disease is a part of health and that the emergence of disease allows health to unfold.

6. Theories can be used by practitioners to guide and improve their practice. Newman's (1994) discussion of researches praxis makes it clear that her intention and belief is that theory must be derived from practice, reflect the realities of practice, and inform practice. She has also proposed a model for practice that is derived from the theory (Newman 1990 b) Bramlett, Gueldner, and Sowell (1990) discussed consumer-centric advocacy as accomplished through the nurse-client interpersonal relationship and supported by Newman's indication of client freedom to be the decision maker. Others have spoken of the utility of Newman's work in guiding and improving practice.

7. Theories must be consistent with other validated theories, laws and principles but will leave open unanswered questions that need to be investigated. Newman (1994) clearly documents the consistency of her theory with those of Itzhak Bentov (1978), David Bohm (1980, 1992), Richard Moss (1981), Martha Rogers (1970), and Arthur Young (1976a, 1976b). Many unanswered questions to be investigated can be derived from this evolving theory. When research is praxis, the questions arise within each nurse-client relationship and within each practice setting.

Newman reported that operationalization of the model of health as expanding consciousness has been approached in two ways: (i) by research methods designed to describe and test the relationships between the major concepts of movement, time, space, and consciousness and (ii) by attempts to describe evolving patterns of consciousness in terms of the integration of movement-space-time.

A number of studies that address research within the Newman theoretical framework have been conducted. Moch described the experiences of 20 women with breast cancer. Through pattern analyses of the person-environment interaction based on the NANDA taxonomy I dimensions, themes developed that were consistent with health as expanding consciousness.

Newman and Moch studied the life patterns of 11 clients in a cardiac rehabilitation center. The objectives of the study were to "describe the individual patterns of interaction of persons with coronary health disease, to discern similarities and differences among the individual patterns, and to interpret these findings in terms of the conceptual congruence of the overall pattern with the theory of health as expanding consciousness." The results identified similar patterns of emerging consciousness for the participants, thus supporting the theory of health.

Health patterns in 60 aging women were investigated using the theory of health as the theoretical framework. The phenomenon of powerlessness was assumed to be operative for the subjects, but was rejected in favor of high levels of perceived situational control or powerfulness. The results supported Newman's model of health as expanding consciousness.

Schorr and Schroeder studied differences in consciousness with regard to time and movement, with results supporting the concept of expanding consciousness. In another study by Schorr and Schroeder, relationships among type A behavior, temporal orientation, and death anxiety were examined as manifestations of consciousness, with mixed results.

Newman's work stresses concept of pattern recognition, of "grasping the whole in order for the parts to be meaningful." She described her attempts to identify pattern in an individual first by using the assessment framework of the NANDA. Second, by analyzing data from interviews of "healthy" (emphasis by Newman) adults into sequential patterns, Newman identified crucial experiences in which energy flow changed and patterns were elucidated. Further work in identification of patterns across the life span is recommended.

Newman's framework is developing into a fully developed theory. She used Popper's definition that a theory is a powerful, unifying idea to guide the development of her theory. However, Newman asserted that a theory must also provide for "new relationships [that] may be deducted and tested, and the date therefrom then will either strengthen or weaken the theoretical system from which the tested relationship is drawn."

Newman's concepts continue to be defined to allow for empirical testing. The interrelationships between the concepts need to be further developed, with greater focus directed toward the usefulness within applied nursing practice.

EVALUATION OF THEORY

- In Newman's *Theory Development in Nursing*, the concepts of movement, time, space, and consciousness with the five resulting relationship statements represented the evolution of the theory at that time. In *Health As Expanding Consciousness*, pattern became a major concept included for the purpose of understanding consciousness. Simplicity was sacrificed when pattern of the whole was used to describe the theory of health. Additional relationship statements are needed to incorporate pattern recognition so the theory of health can be utilized for predicting events.
- The concepts in Newman's theory are broad in scope because they all relate to health. This renders her theory generalizable. The broad scope provides a focus for future theory development.
- Aspects of the theory have been operationalized and tested within a traditional scientific mode. However,

quantitative methods are limited in capturing the dynamic, changing nature of this model. Qualitative approaches are being developed for a full explication of its meaning and application.

The model of health has little empirical adequacy because the central concepts are not consistent in their operational definitions. Completed research has operationalized time as passage of seconds on a clock and movement as walking cadence, but the operationalized concept could also be defined in other ways. However, Newman stated that each time a study is performed the concepts are operationalized. "The major concepts are meant to be summary concepts that include many more specific concepts."

The concepts of health and patterns are defined as summative units. The units are global and represent an entire complex phenomenon. A summative unit describes an entire entity in a few words, making definitions vague and overlapping. Interactions between the units are not testable, limiting their utility.

- Newman's theory is useful in nursing practice because it uses concepts already familiar to nursing, such as time and movement. It has received increased recognition regarding application to practice in recent publications and presentations at conferences.

The domain of the model of health is the nursing process. The model would be useful for guiding nursing practice and differentiating nursing's areas of concern.

Chapter 22

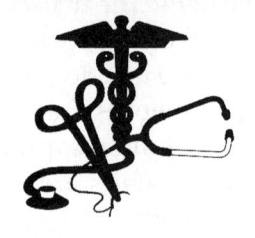

Fitzpatrick's Rhythm Model

Joyce J. Fitzpatrick was born May 4, 1944. She received her BSN in 1966 from Georgetown University in Washington, D.C., and her M.S. in Psychiatric-Mental Health from Ohio State University in Columbus in 1967. She took postmaster's courses in Community Health at Ohio State in 1971 to 1972, and achieved a Ph.D. in nursing from New York University in 1975. In 1987 she attended Harvard University's Institute for Educational Management. She is currently pursuing an Executive MBA Programme at Case Western Reserve University.

Fitzpatrick has held many positions, including staff nurse, public health nurse, instructor, and the director of training for suicide prevention, all in Columbus, Ohio. She has served as an assistant professor at New York University and Associate Professor at Wayne State University. In addition, she has also been the chairperson for the Department of Nursing Systems and the director of the Center for Health Research at Wayne State. Fitzpatrick has been Visiting Professor at Rutgers—The State University, College of Nursing. In 1982 Fitzpatrick became Professor and Dean of Nursing at case Western Reserve University in Cleveland, Ohio, and Administrative Associate at University Hospitals of Cleveland. Since 1988 she has held the Elizabeth Brooks Ford Professor of Nursing position.

Since 1974 Fitzpatrick has worked as a consultant in such areas as faculty development, research development, and development of master's and doctoral programmes in nursing with several institutions, including Indiana University, Michigan State University, The Ohio State University, Rutgers University, University of Kansas, University of Virginia, Vanderbilt University, and Wright State University.

In addition, since 1984 Fitzpatrick has worked as a consultant in such areas as doctoral programme development at University of South Carolina, conceptual framework development at University of Tennessee at Memphis, the development of a computerized nursing information system at Hospital Corporation of America, Nashville, Tennessee, consultant to nursing staff at a psychiatric hospital in Toronto, Ontario, and as consultant to Director of Nursing Affairs at American Medical Association.

Fitzpatrick has received honoraries and is affiliated with several organizations. Among numerous awards received is the 1989 Award for Excellence in Nursing Research from Sigma Theta Tau International. Fitzpatrick was awarded an honorary Doctor of Human Letters in 1990 by Georgetown University.

Professional activities have been numerous. She has presented workshops on community health, current issues in health, stress, crisis intervention, dying and death, suicidology, theory development, and research in nursing. She has been the investigator and director for several research grants, has presented numerous paper and research projects, and has published extensively. Fitzpatrick is actively involved in the building of a community of nurse scholars and delineating the field of inquiry for nursing knowledge.

EVOLUTION OF THEORY

Fitzpatrick is a well-known, published scholar among nursing professionals. She constructed her theory model based on the ideas and work of Martha Rogers. Fitzpatrick used rhythm patterns, which are operational modes specifying the pattern of person and environment that were explicated by Rogers. In addition, Fitzpatrick and Whall incorporated the peak and wave pattern ideas of E. Haus and G.G. Luce. To round out the model, she drew from G. Caplan's crisis theory.

Fitzpatrick's Life Perspective Rhythm Model is synthesized from interpretations made from Rogers' theory work. Colleagues consider Rogers one of the most original thinkers in nursing who capitalizes on knowledge from other disciplines such as anthropology, sociology, astronomy, religion, philosophy, history, and mythology. The model's concept of environment is drawn from von Bertalanffy and others who question the failure of physical laws to explain evolution of life. According to S.M. Falco and M.L. Lobo, "There is a strong parallel between Rogers' basic assumptions and general systems theory." Rogers also draws from Einstein in using the concept of four dimensionality.

Concepts Used by Theorists

The four major concepts in this model are *nursing, person, health,* and *environment.* "The ontogenetic and phylogenetic interactions among person and health are looked upon as the essence of nursing."

According to J.L. Pressler, in Fitzpatrick's rhythm model "nursing, as a noun, was described as a developing discipline whose central concern is the meaning attached to life (health). As a verb, nursing, or nursing activity, was said to be focused on enhancing the developmental process toward health so that individuals may be led to develop their potentials as human beings."

Person is seen as an open system, a unified whole characterized by a basic human rhythm. Health is viewed as a human dimension under continuous development – a heightened awareness of the meaningfulness of life. According to J. L. Pressler, Fitzpatrick mirrors Rogers' definition of environmental field.

Fitzpatrick repeats the five basic assumptions proposed by Rogers in her theory of unitary man:

1. Man is a unified whole possessing his own integrity and manifesting characteristics

that are more than and different from the sum of his parts.
2. Man and environment are open systems, continually exchanging matter and energy with each other.
3. The life process evolves irreversibly and unidirectionally along the space time continuum.
4. Pattern and organization identify man and reflect his innovative wholeness.
5. Man is characterized by the capacity for abstraction and imagery, language and thought, sensation and emotion.

According to Pressler, four implicit assumptions pertinent to understanding Fitzpatrick's model were previously identified.
1. Differences in behavioural manifestations are more easily identified during the peaks of wave patterns.
2. Identified by congruency, consistency, and integrity of rhythmic patterns, health is to the manifestations of symphonic interaction of persons and their environments.
3. Emphasized through selected research on temporality, the meaning attached to life is a central concern of nursing.
4. Nursing is a philosophy, a science, and an art.

The Life Perspective Rhythm Model is a developmental model that proposes that the process of human development is characterized by rhythms. The person is treated as an open, holistic, rhythmic system that can best be described by temporal, motion, consciousness, and perceptual patterns. It is possible to identify peaks and troughs of particular human rhythms throughout the developmental process. There are patterns within a pattern or overall life patterns. Life's pattern continues toward timelessness, becoming more dominant as one's development occurs. This process may best be described as patterns within a pattern or rhythms within an overall life rhythm. Health is viewed as a continuously developing characteristic of humans with the full life potential that may characterize the process of dying, as the heightened awareness of the meaningfulness of life, and as representing a more fully developed dimension of health. Health is seen as the interactions of persons with their environment. Nursing's central concern is focused on the person in relation to health, with the goal of enhancing the developmental process toward health so people may develop their potential as human beings. "The meaning attached to life, the basic understanding of human existence, is a central concern of nursing as science and profession." The hypothesis is that "individuals experiencing crisis had difficulty integrating the present situation within their life perspective."

A conceptual model was developed to depict the essential theoretical representation of person, environment, health, and nursing as if one were looking through a Slinky. Fitzpatrick expanded the Slinky concept to symbolize her view of person. The representation helps in picturing the relationships found in the Life Perspective Rhythm Model (Fig. 22.1).

Logical Form

Fitzpatrick developed the Life Perspective Rhythm Model using a deductive logical approach; that is, the author uses empirical

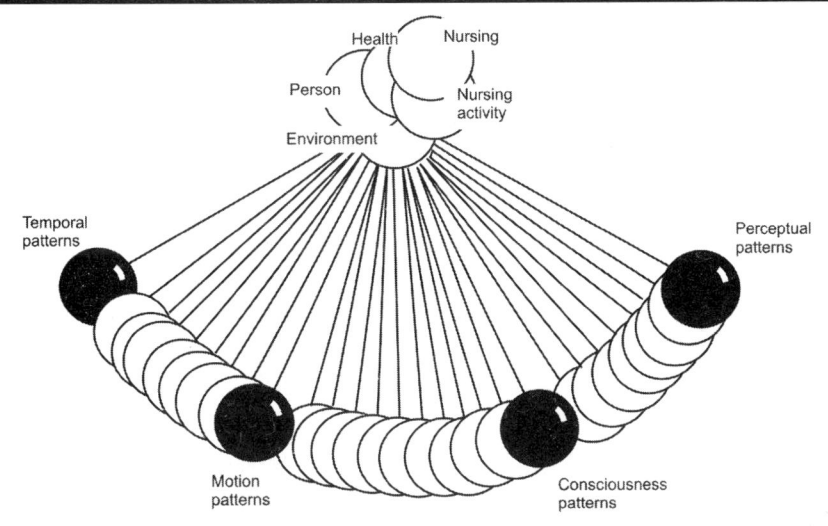

Figure 22.1: Relationships within life perspective model

findings to support a proposed developmental model. This model indicates that human development is characteristic of temporal, motion, perceptual, and consciousness rhythms. These patterns show the continuous person-environment interaction in relation to one's personal development.

An individual's progression through life contains varying high and low intervals, but the general direction represents rapidity. While explaining the broadness in life, such progression also relates life and health. In this model health represents a basic human element that is a continuous development from birth to death. Understandably, the meaning one attaches to life and health or humanness is significant in this model. Accordingly, health or potentiating health is considerably influential to one's meaning in life.

Because of Fitzpatrick's extensive work and study under Rogers, Fitzpatrick bases the Life Perspective Rhythm model on Rogers' unitary man assumptions and model concepts in addition to expanding the Slinky's representation in her own model. To add further merit to this model's development, Fitzpatrick drew from the biological rhythm theory and also from Caplan's crisis theory. Fitzpatrick also used her own personal interests and professional experience in crisis in the model's development. The model's hypothesis was derived based on these aspects. It states, "Individuals experiencing crisis had difficulty integrating the present situations within their life perspective."

The next logical step is empirical testing, which is imperative in any model's development and future. Much of the testing of this model has related to the temporal pattern with a selective population focus on the elderly in nursing homes and during hospitalization. Recent studies have dealt with terminally ill cancer patients and with suicidal individuals. Using results from the completed investigations, Fitzpatrick continues to broaden the model, such as in her meaning attached to life and death. But she acknowledges that the limitations of the empirical investigations hold back the model's developmental progress and the gathering of further logical support.

Nursing Implications

Practice

Because her model is still in the developmental stage, Fitzpatrick encourages further study and ongoing empirical testing. With more involvement by the nursing community, progress will be made. The model is apparently not being used in practice.

Education

The majority of testing has been completed by graduate students studying with Fitzpatrick. The model has not been incorporated into any nursing curriculum, but critics feel the theory is potentially adaptable for educational purposes. Fitzpatrick has incorporated her theory and conceptualization into her graduate level theory and nursing research courses.

Research

Fitzpatrick is active in current nursing research. From 1976 to 1984 she received research grants totaling more than $1 million. Her research projects have dealt with temporal experiences of the terminally ill cancer patients, the aging process, temporal experiences of the suicidal, the advancement of doctoral programs, and interpretations of life and death.

From 1985 to 1990 she received research grants totaling more than $2 million. Some of her projects include doctor of nursing evaluation, advanced nurse training in nurse-midwifery, the advancement of doctoral programs, the design and development of expert systems for decision-support in acute care nursing areas, and perinatal nurse major. Fitzpatrick's proposals are initiating new ideas and research that is useful for the advancement of nursing science.

As previously discussed, the Life Perspective Rhythm Model is in a beginning developmental stage. Fitzpatrick has not published a formal update of the model. The multiple definitions given to nursing and health in the model are problematic. The vast interrelationship between person and environment is highly complex and not easily understood. Because most of the completed research focusses on the temporal pattern, the other patterns still need to be researched. But even the completed temporal pattern research shows that operational measurement is problematic and raises other considerations for future research. Doctoral students are currently investigating rhythmic patterns of human functioning. Until significant investigation is completed in all rhythms, this model cannot be addressed holistically. Although the model's individual components may have merit and nursing support, the complete model still needs to be tested. Therefore, this model's future place in a creative nursing science, in nursing practice, and in nursing theory consideration is uncertain.

EVALUATION OF THEORY

- Fitzpatrick consistently follows theoretical form by stating a hypothesis and listing assumptions. She continues by stating relationships of concepts and displays her theory in a four dimensional Slinky's model, representing the relationship statements. Most of the empirical testing has occurred with temporal patterns, but plans are in process to develop the theory and to empirically test the conscious

rhythm, perceptual rhythms, motion rhythms, and their relationships with the meaning attached to life and life perspective.
- This model is complex in its concepts and interrelationships. Sufficiently understanding and explaining the interrelationships between health, nursing, person, environment, and nursing activity in respect to the temporal, motion, consciousness, and perceptual patterns are highly complex and involved undertakings. Such interrelationships are not easily taken from concept to operational measurement. Most of the empirical investigations relate to the elderly, terminally ill cancer patients, and suicidal individuals and contain a heavy psychosocial orientation. Fitzpatrick acknowledges that the model needs to be tested in other populations such as infants, children, and adolescents.
- Fitzpatrick and her researchers have been successful in scientifically testing and evaluating several of the relationships presented in the Life Perspective Rhythm model. However, the current literature indicates that only some educators and students are in the process of empirically testing relationships in this projected model. Interested researchers and practitioners are encouraged to become involved in the efforts to further develop the Life Perspective Rhythm model.
- The derivable consequences connect the theory with achievable nursing outcomes. Because this model is at the beginning development stage, its application and usefulness in nursing practice and science have been limited. The concepts, and some of the research, are stimulating and warrant further work and additional development. Conceivably, some concepts of the model may in the future help broaden perspectives in relation to humanness and move nursing closer to holistic nursing practice.

Chapter 23

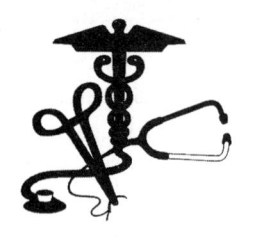

Travelbee's Human-to-Human Relationships

Joyce Travelbee was a psychiatric nurse practitioner, educator, and writer. Born in 1926, she completed her basic nursing preparation in 1946 at Charity Hospital School of Nursing in New Orleans. She earned a BS degree in nursing education from Louisiana State University in 1956 and an MS degree in nursing from Yale in 1959. In the summer of 1973, Travelbee began a doctoral programme in Florida, but was unable to complete the programme because of her untimely death later that year. She died at the age of 47 after a brief illness, leaving no survivors.

Travelbee began her career as a nursing educator in 1952, teaching psychiatric nursing at Depaul Hospital Affiliate School, New Orleans, while working on her baccalaureate degree. She also taught psychiatric nursing at Charity Hospital School of Nursing, at Louisiana State University, at New York University in New York City, and at the University of Mississippi in Jackson. In 1970 she was named Project Director at Hotel Dieu, School of Nursing in New Orleans. At the time of her death, Travelbee was the director of graduate education at Louisiana State University School of Nursing.

Travelbee began publishing articles in nursing journals in 1963. Her first book, *Interpersonal Aspects of Nursing,* was published in 1966 and 1971. A second book, *Intervention in Psychiatric Nursing,* was published in 1969.

EVOLUTION OF THEORY

Travelbee's experiences in her basic nursing education and initial practice in Catholic charity institutions greatly influenced the development of her theory. Travelbee believed the nursing care given patients in these institutions lacked compassion. She felt nursing needed "a humanistic revolution—a return to focus on the 'caring' function of the nurse—in the caring for (and) the caring about ill persons and predicted if this did not occur, consumers would demand the 'services of a new and different kind of health worker.'"

Travelbee was probably also influenced by Ida Jean Orlando, who was one of her instructors during her graduate studies at

Yale. Orlando's model possesses some similarities to the model Travelbee proposes. Orlando stated, "The nurse is responsible for helping the patient avoid and alleviate the distress of unmet needs." She also stated that the nurse and patient interact with each other. The similarities between the two models are shown by Travelbee's assertion that the nurse and patient interact with each other and by her definition of the purpose of nursing. Travelbee stated that the purpose of nursing is to assist "an individual, family, or community to prevent or cope with the experience of illness and suffering, and, if necessary, to find meaning in these experiences."

Travelbee also appears to have been influenced by Viktor Frankl, a survivor of Auschwitz and other Nazi concentration camps. As a result of his experiences, Frankl proposed the theory of logotherapy, in which a patient "is actually confronted with and reoriented toward the meaning of his life." Travelbee based the assumptions of her theory on the concepts of logotherapy.

Katharine Taylor, a former student and colleague of Travelbee, remembers Travelbee as a prolific reader whose office was often crammed with files of bibliography cards. Apparently, Travelbee's theory is based on her cumulative nursing experiences and her readings rather than the evidence of a particular research study.

Concepts Used by Travelbee

- *Human Being* "A human being is defined as a unique irreplaceable individual—a one-time being in this world—like yet unlike any person who has ever lived or ever will live."
- *Patient* The term *patient* is a stereotype useful for communicative economy. "Actually there are no patients. There are only individual human beings in need of the care, services, and assistance of other human beings, whom, it is believed, can render the assistance that is needed."
- *Nurse* The nurse is also a human being. "The nurse possesses a body of specialized knowledge and the ability to use it for the purpose of assisting other human beings to prevent illness, regain health, find meaning in illness, or to maintain the highest maximal degree of health."
- *Suffering* "Suffering is a feeling of displeasure which ranges from simple transitory mental, physical, or spiritual discomfort to extreme anguish, and to those phases beyond anguish, namely the malignant phase of despairful 'not caring,' and the terminal phase of apathetic indifference." Suffering can be placed on a continuum, which is illustrated in (Fig. 23.1).

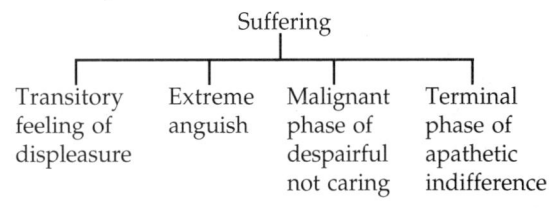

```
                         Suffering
    ┌─────────────┬──────────┬─────────────┬──────────────┐
Transitory      Extreme    Malignant      Terminal
feeling of      anguish    phase of       phase of
displeasure                despairful     apathetic
                           not caring     indifference
```

Figure 23.1: Continuum of suffering (Conceptualized by Theresa Lansinger, based on Joyce Travelbee's definition)

- *Pain* "Pain itself is not observable—only its effects are noted." Pain is a lonely experience that is difficult to communicate fully to another individual. The experience of pain is unique to each individual.

- *Hope* "Hope is a mental state characterized by the desire to gain an end or accomplish a goal combined with some degree of expectation that what is desired or sought is attainable." Hope is related to dependence on others, choice, wishing, trust and perseverance, and courage, and is future oriented.
- *Hopelessness* Hopelessness is being devoid of hope.
- *Communication* "Communication is a process which can enable the nurse to establish a human-to-human relationship and thereby fulfill the purpose of nursing, namely to assist individuals and families to prevent and to cope with the experience of illness and suffering and, if necessary, to assist them to find meaning in these experiences."
- *Interaction* "The term *interaction* refers to any contact during which two individuals have reciprocal influence on each other and communicate "verbally and/or nonverbally."
- *Nurse-patient interaction* "The term *nurse-patient interaction* refers to any contact between a nurse and an ill person and is characterized by the fact that both individuals perceive the other in a stereotyped manner."
- *Nursing need* "A nursing need is any requirement of the ill person (or family) which can be met by the professional nurse practitioner and which lies within the scope of the legal definition of nursing practice."
- *Therapeutic use of self* "The therapeutic use of self is the ability to use one's personality consciously and in full awareness in an attempt to establish relatedness and to structure nursing intervention." It "requires self-insight, self-understanding, an understanding of the dynamics of human behavior, ability to interpret one's own behavior as well as the behavior of others, and the ability to intervene effectively in nursing situations."
- *Empathy* "Empathy is a process wherein an individual is able to comprehend the psychological state of another."
- *Sympathy* Sympathy implies a desire to help an individual undergoing stress.
- *Rapport* "Rapport is a process, a happening, an experience, or series of experiences, undergone simultaneously by the nurse and the recipient of her care. It is composed of a cluster of interrelated thoughts and feelings, these thoughts, feelings and attitudes being transmitted, or communicated by one human being to another."
- *Human-to-human relationship* "A human-to-human relationship is primarily an experience or series of experiences between a nurse and the recipient of her care. The major characteristic of these experiences is that the nursing needs of the individual (or family) are met." "The human-to-human relationship, in nursing situations, is the means through which the purpose of nursing is accomplished." The human-to-human relationship is established when the nurse and the recipient of her care attained a rapport after having progressed through the stages of the original encounter, emerging identities, empathy, and sympathy (Fig. 23.2).

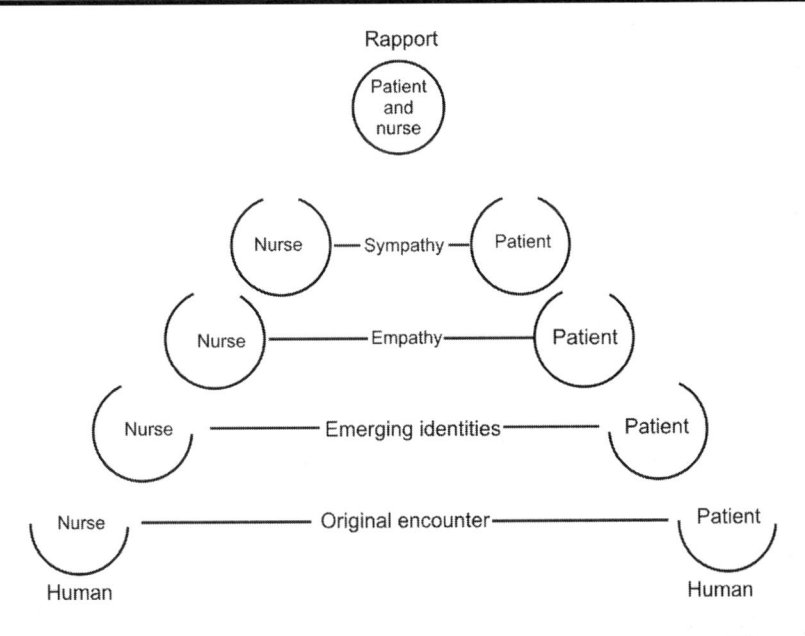

Figure 23.2: Human-to-human relationship (Conceptualised by William Hobble and Theresa Lansinger, based on Joyce Travelbee's writings)

PARADIGM OF THEORY

- *Nursing:* Travelbee defined nursing as an "interpersonal process whereby the professional nurse practitioner assists an individual, family, or community to prevent or cope with the experience of illness and suffering and, if necessary, to find meaning in these experiences." Nursing is an interpersonal process because it is an experience that occurs between the nurse and an individual or group of individuals.
- *Person:* The term *person* is defined as a human being. Both the nurse and the patient are human beings. A human being is a unique, irreplaceable individual who is in the continuous process of becoming, evolving, and changing.
- *Health:* Travelbee defined health by the criteria of subjective and objective health. A person's subjective health status is an individually defined state of well-being in accord with self-appraisal of physical-emotional-spiritual status. Objective health is "an absence of discernible disease, disability, or defect as measured by physical examination, laboratory tests, assessment by a spiritual director, or psychological counselor."
- *Environment:* Travelbee does not explicitly define environment in the theory. She does define the human condition and life experiences encountered by all human beings as suffering, hope, pain, and illness. These conditions can be equated to the environment.

Assertions of Theory

1. "The purpose of nursing is achieved through the establishment of a human-to-human relationship."

2. The human condition is shared by all human beings and is dichotomous in nature.
3. Most people, at one time or another and in varying degrees, will experience joy, contentment, happiness, and love.
4. "All persons, at some time in their lives, will be confronted by illness and pain (mental, physical, or spiritual suffering), and eventually they will encounter death."
5. The quality and quantity of nursing care delivered to an ill human being is greatly influenced by the nurse's perception of the patient.
6. The terms *patient* and *nurse* are stereotypes and only useful for communicative economy.
7. The roles of the nurse and patient must be transcended to establish a human-to-human relatedness.
8. Illness and suffering "are spiritual encounters as well as emotional-physical experiences."
9. The communication process enables "the nurse to establish a human-to-human relationship and thereby fulfill the purpose of nursing."
10. "Individuals can be assisted to find meaning in the experience of illness and suffering. The meanings can enable the individual to cope with the problems engendered by these experiences."
11. "The spiritual and ethical values of the nurse, or her philosophical beliefs about illness and suffering, will determine the extent to which she will be able to assist individuals and families to find meaning (or no meaning) in these difficult experiences."
12. "It is the responsibility of the professional nurse practitioner to assist individuals and families to find meaning in illness and suffering (if this be necessary)."

Human-to-Human Relationship

The human-to-human relationship model, shown in Figure 23.2, represents the interaction between the nurse and patient. The half circles at the point of the original encounter indicate the possibility of and need for developing the encounter into a therapeutic relationship. As the interaction process progresses toward rapport, the circles join into one full circle, representing that the potential for a therapeutic relationship has been attained.

Original Encounter

The original encounter is characterized by first impressions by the nurse of the ill person and by the ill person of the nurse. The nurse and ill person perceive each other in stereotyped roles.

Emerging Identities

The emerging identities phase is characterized by the nurse and ill person perceiving each other as unique individuals. The bond of a relationship is beginning to form.

Empathy

The empathy phase is characterized by the ability to share in the other person's experience. The result of the empathic process is the ability to predict the behavior of the individual with whom one has empathized.

Travelbee believed two qualities that enhanced the empathy process were similarities of experience and the desire to understand another person.

Sympathy

Sympathy goes beyond empathy and occurs when the nurse desires to alleviate the cause of the patient's illness or suffering. "When one sympathizes one is involved but not incapacitated by the involvement." The nurse is to create helpful nursing action as a result of reaching the phase of sympathy. "This helpful nursing action requires a combination of the disciplined intellectual approach combined with the therapeutic use of self."

Rapport

Rapport is characterized by nursing actions that alleviate an ill person's distress. The nurse and ill person are relating as human being to human being. The ill person exhibits both trust and confidence in the nurse. "A nurse is able to establish rapport because she possesses the necessary knowledge and skills required to assist ill persons, and because she is able to perceive, respond to, and appreciate the uniqueness of the ill human being."

Travelbee's theory is inductive. She has used specific nursing situations to create general ideas. Travelbee appears to follow a logical form by first defining the labels in her theory, then listing the assumptions, and finally establishing specific nursing goals.

Nursing Implications

Practice

Travelbee believed the condition of an individual exhibiting apathetic indifference is just as critical as that of an individual who is hemorrhaging. She believed that both people need emergency resuscitative measures. But an examination of patient care given by nurses today indicates the patient's physical needs still hold top priority. The acceptance and use of nursing diagnosis does appear to focus nursing care more on the total needs of the patient as compared with 25 years ago when Travelbee published her theory. However, nursing has not yet reached the humanistic revolution Travelbee proposed.

Hospice is the one area of nursing practice where the philosophy closely adheres to the tenets of Travelbee's theory. The hospice nurse attempts to develop a rapport with the patient and significant others. Most hospice nurses agree with Elisabeth Kubler-Ross "that death does not have to be a catastrophic, destructive thing; indeed, it can be viewed as one of the most constructive, positive, and creative elements of culture and life." Travelbee asserted that finding meaning in illness and suffering enables the ill individual not only to accept the illness, but also to use it as a self-actualizing life experience. An ill individual's perception of meaninglessness in his illness and suffering lead to non-acceptance of his illness and a feeling of hopelessness. One hospice nurse believes the dying person must find meaning in his death before he can ever begin to accept the actuality of his death, just as his loved ones must find meaning in his death before they can complete the grieving process.

Education

Nursing education appears to have identified the need to prepare nurses to address the emotional and spiritual needs of patients. The focus of nursing education has changed from the disease entity approach – that is, signs, symptoms, and nursing interventions – to a more holistic care approach. However, basic nursing programmes do not seem to prepare nurses adequately to help individuals find meaning in illness and suffering as Travelbee proposed. Travelbee's second book, *Intervention in Psychiatric Nursing: Process in the One-to-One Relationship,* has been used in various nursing programmes. However, this book alone does not adequately prepare nurses to help individuals find meaning in illness and suffering. Nursing programmes need to offer a much broader background in communication techniques, values clarification, and thanatology. Courses in philosophy and religion would also be helpful in preparing nurses adequately to fulfill the purpose of nursing as stated in Travelbee's theory.

Research

Some aspects of the one-to-one relationship proposed by Travelbee have been cited by several sources in research studies. One study by O'Connor *et al*, which is closely related to some of Travelbee's ideas, explored how individuals who were recently diagnosed with cancer described their personal search for meaning. Six major themes, which were (i) seeking an understanding of' the personal significance of the cancer diagnosis, (ii) looking at the consequences of the cancer diagnosis, (iii) review of life, (iv) change in outlook toward self, life, others, (v) living with cancer, and (vi) hope, were identified, and two major sources of support were found—faith and social support. The findings of this study revealed that the search for meaning seems to be both a spiritual and psychosocial process. Nursing interventions that would support this process were identified. No other major research studies generated by Travelbee's specific theory, which could stimulate further development, were found.

The advent of diagnostic-related groups (DRGs) has created the need to produce the highest quality nursing care by the most economical method. Tools such as patient acuity systems have been devised to determine nursing staffing patterns in accordance with the nursing needs of patients. Although this type of tool can account for the emotional needs of patients, emotional needs are not weighed as heavily as patients' physical needs. DRGs may shift the nursing focus back to meeting only the patient's physical needs. If nurses are to prevent this shift, they must prove to health care administrators and health care consumers that the time taken by the nurse to meet a patient's emotional and spiritual needs is a valuable investment. Travelbee's theory could be used to provide the research data to justify this time investment. However, Travelbee's theory does not currently contain the empirical precision to support such research data. To be more readily accepted, the theory's major assumptions must be assigned operational definitions. Then the theory could perhaps generate the data needed to facilitate further acceptance.

- All concepts are defined in the Travelbee theory, but definitions are not consistent with regard to origin and explicitness. Some are the author's own definitions, whereas others were adopted from Webster's dictionary. Some of the definitions are explicitly presented, but others are derived from contextual usage. None of the concepts is operationally defined. Travelbee also uses different terms for the same definition. The terms *rapport*, *human-to-human relationship*, and *human-to-human relatedness* all had the same definition.

The goal or purpose of nursing, as stated in Travelbee's definition of nursing, is inconsistent with the emphasis of her presentation. Travelbee focussed on adult individuals who are ill and the nurse's role in assisting them in finding meaning in their illness and suffering. She addressed families and their needs minimally, and communities were not included at all.

- Travelbee's theory does not possess simplicity because there are many variables. The theory is designed to help nurses appreciate not only the patient's humanness, but also the nurse's humanness. To be human is to be unique; so the variables present in each phase of the human to-human relationship will be numerous.
- Travelbee's theory has a wide scope of application. It was primarily generated as a result of Travelbee's experience with psychiatric patients, but is not limited to use in this setting. It is applicable whenever the nurse encounters ill persons in distress. It would seem to be most useful when working with those who are chronically ill, those who are undergoing long-term rehabilitation, or those who are terminally ill.
- Travelbee's theory appears to have a low degree of empirical validity. Most of the lack of empirical validity can be traced to the lack of simplicity in the theory. Concepts have been theoretically defined, but they have not been operationally defined. Because the model has not been tested, there is no empirical support.
- The usefulness of a theory is related to its ability to describe, explain, predict, and control phenomena. Travelbee's theory does describe some variables that may affect the establishment of a therapeutic relationship between nurse and patient. However, the lack of empirical precision also creates a lack of derivable consequences. Travelbee's theory focuses on the development of the attribute of caring. In this respect, the theory can be useful, because caring is a major characteristic of the nursing profession.

Nursing is an interpersonal process aimed at assisting individuals, families, or communities to prevent or cope with the process of illness and suffering and, if necessary, to find meaning in the experience. Nursing's purpose is achieved through human-to-human relationships, which are established by a disciplined intellectual approach to problems, combined with therapeutic use of self. Human-to-human relationships require transcending roles of nurse and patient to establish relatedness and rapport and respond to the humanness of others. Nursing activities are a means to establishing relatedness and rapport and achieving nursing's purpose. Nurses values and beliefs determine the quality of nursing care provided and thus the extent to which nurses are able to help the ill find meaning in their situation.

Illness and suffering are spiritual, emotional, and physical experiences. The nurse assists the ill patient to experience hope as a means of coping with illness and suffering. Communication, a central concept for Travelbee, implies guiding, planning, and purposely directing interaction to fulfil nursing's purpose. Communication is instrumental in establishing relatedness and rapport (knowing persons), ascertaining and meeting nursing needs, and fulfilling nursing's purpose. Communication also implies that exchanged messages are understood. Communication techniques should enable the nurse to explore and understand the meaning of the person's communication. Establishment of the human-to-human relationship is phasic. The phases are (i) the original encounter, (ii) emerging identities, (iii) empathy, and (iv) sympathy. In such a relationship the needs of the person are met. Achievement of a human-to-human relationship requires openness to experiences and freedom to use personal and experiential background to appreciate and understand the experiences of others.

Health and illness may be defined subjectively and objectively. Objective criteria depend on cultural and societal norms, whereas subjective criteria are peculiar to the human being. The meaning of the symptoms of illness (or criteria for health) for the person is more significant than affixing a label of health or illness to its results.

Chapter 24

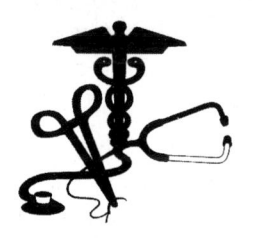

Benner's Excellence and Power in Clinical Nursing Practice

Patricia Benner was born in Hampton, Virginia, and spent her childhood in California, where she received her early and professional education. Majoring in nursing, she obtained a bachelor of arts degree from Pasadena College in 1964. In 1970, she earned a Master's Degree in Nursing, with her major emphasis in medical-surgical nursing from the University of California, San Francisco School of Nursing. She worked as a research assistant to Richard Lazarus at the University of California, Berkeley, while working on her Ph.D. in stress, coping, and health, which was conferred in 1982.

Benner has a wide range of clinical experience including acute medical-surgical, critical care, and home health care. She has held staff and head nurse positions.

Benner has a rich background in research and began this part of her career in 1970 as a postgraduate nurse researcher in the school of nursing at the University of California, San Francisco. In 1982, Benner achieved the position of associate professor in the Department of Physiological Nursing at the University of California, San Francisco, and in 1989 was tenured to professor, a position she currently holds. She teaches primarily at the doctoral and master's level and serves on 8 to 10 dissertation committees per year. Benner acknowledges that her thinking in nursing has been greatly influenced by Virginia Henderson. Henderson writes that Benner's *From Novice to Expert* as clinically focussed research might materially affect practice and the preparation of nurses for practice. The foreword to Benner's work *The Primary of Caring Stress and Coping in Health and Illness* has been written by Virginia Henderson. Hubert Dreyfus, a philosophy professor at Berkeley introduced her to phenomenology, Stuart Dreyfus, in operations research, and Herbert Dreyfus, in philosophy, developed the Dreyfus Model of Skill Acquisition, which Benner applied in her work *From Novice to Expert*. She credits Jane Rubin's scholarship, teaching, and colleaguesh ip as sources of inspiration and influence, especially in relationship to the works of Heidegger and Kierkegaard. R.S. Lazarus, with whom she worked at Berkeley, has involved her in the field of stress and coping.

Judith Wrubel has been a participant and co-author with Benner over the last 16 years, collaborating on the ontology of caring and caring practices.

Benner has published extensively and has been the recipient of numerous honors and awards including the 1984 and 1988 *American Journal of Nursing* Book of the Year awards for *From Novice to Expert* and *The Primacy of Caring*, respectively. In 1985 she was inducted into the American Academy of Nurses; in 1989 she received the National League for Nursing's Linda Richards Award for Leadership in Education. She is invited worldwide to lecture and lead workshops on her research findings.

Benner expressed that nursing is a cultural paradox in a highly technical society and that we are slow to value and articulate caring practices. She feels that the value of extreme individualism makes it difficult to perceive the brilliance of caring in expert nursing practice.

EVOLUTION OF THEORY

Benner studied clinical nursing practice in an attempt to discover and describe the knowledge embedded in nursing practice, that is, that knowledge that accrues over time in a practice discipline, and to describe the difference between practical and theoretical knowledge. One of the first theoretical distinctions Benner made was related to theory itself. Benner stated that knowledge development in a practice discipline "consists of extending practical knowledge (know-how) through theory-based scientific investigations and through the charting of the existent `know-how' developed through clinical experience in the practice of that discipline.

She believes that nurses have been delinquent in documenting their clinical learning and "this lack of charting of our practices and clinical observations deprives nursing theory of the uniqueness and richness of the knowledge embedded in expert clinical practice." It is the description of the know-how of nursing practice that Benner has contributed.

Scientists have long distinguished interactional causal relationships as "knowing that" from "knowing how." Citing philosophers of science Kuhn and Polanyi, Benner emphasized the difference in "knowing how," a practical knowledge that may elude formulations, and "knowing that," or theoretical explanations. "Knowing that" is the way one comes to know by establishing causal relationships between events. "Knowing how" is that skill acquisition that may defy the "knowing that," that is, one may know how prior to the development of a theoretical explanation. Benner stated that practical knowledge may extend theory or be developed ahead of scientific formulas. Clinical situations are always more varied and complicated than theoretical accounts and therefore clinical practice is an arena of inquiry and knowledge development. Clinical practice embodies the notion of excellence; by studying it we can uncover new knowledge. Nursing must develop the knowledge base of its practice (know-how) and through scientific investigation and observation begin to record and develop the know-how of clinical expertise. In an ideal world, practice and theory set up a dialogue that creates new possibilities. Theory is derived from practice and then practice is altered or extended by theory.

Dreyfus and Dreyfus' (180, 1986) model of skill acquisition and skill development was adapted by Benner to clinical nursing practice. The Dreyfus model was developed by Stuart and Hubert Dreyfus, both professors at the University California at Berkeley. The model is situational and describes five levels of skill requisition and development: novice, advanced beginner, competent, proficient, and expert. The model posits that in movement through the levels of skill acquisition changes in four aspects of performance occur: (i) movement from a reliance on abstract principles and rules to use of past, concrete experiences; (ii) shift from reliance on analytical, rule-based thinking to intuition; (iii) change in the learner's perception of the situation from one in which it is viewed as a compilation of equally relevant bits to an increasingly complex whole in which certain parts are relevant; and (iv) passage from detached observer, standing outside the situation, to one of a position of involvement, fully engaged in the situation." "The performance level can be determined only by consensual validation of expert judges and the assessment of the outcomes of the situation."

In subsequent research further explicating the Dreyfus model, Benner identified two interrelated aspects of practice that also distinguish the levels of practice from advanced beginner to expert. First, clinicians at different levels of practice live in different clinical worlds, recognizing and responding to different guides for action. Second, clinicians develop what Benner terms agency or the sense of responsibility towards the patient and evolve into becoming a member of the health care team.

Benner attempted to highlight the growing edges of clinical knowledge, rather than to describe a typical nurse's day. Benner's explanation of nursing practice goes beyond the rigid application of rules and theories and instead is based on "reasonable behavior that responds to the demands of a given situation." The skills acquired through nursing experience and the perceptual awareness expert nurses develop a decision makers from the "gestalt of the situation" lead them to follow their hunches as they search for evidence to confirm the subtle changes by observe in patients.

The concept of experience defined as the outcome when preconceived notions are challenged, refine, or refuted in the situation in based on Heidegger and Gadamer. As the nurse gains experience, clinical knowledge becomes a blend of practical and theoretical knowledge. Expertise develops as the clinician tests and modifies principle-based expectations in the actual situation. Heidegger's influence in evident in this and in Benner's subsequent writings on the primary of caring. Benner refutes the dualistic cartesian descriptions of mind-body person and espouses Heidegger's phenomenological description of person as a self-interpreting being who is defined by concerns, practices, and life experiences. Persons are always situated, that is, engaged meaningfully in the context of where they are. Persons come to situations with an understand of the self in the world. Heidegger called the kind of knowing that occurs when one is involved in the situation *practical knowledges*. Persons share background meanings, skills, and habits derived from their cultural practices. Benner and Wrubel state "skilled activity, which is made possible by our embodied intelligence, has been long regarded as 'lower' than intellectual, reflective activity" but argue that intellectual, reflective capacities are dependent on embodied knowing. Embodied knowing and the meaning of being are premises for the capacity to care; things matter to us and "cause us to be involved in and defined by our concerns.

While doing her doctoral studies at Berkeley, Benner was a research assistant to Richard S. Lazarus, who is known for his development of stress and coping theory. As part of Lazarus' larger study, Benner conducted a study of mid-career men's meaning of work and coping, which was published as *Stress and Satisfaction on the Job. Work Meanings and Coping of Mid-Career Men*. In this study coping is defined as a form of practical knowledge, and it was determined that work meanings influence what is experienced as stress and what coping options are available to the individual.

Lazarus' theory of stress and coping is described as phenomenological, that is, the person is understood to constitute and be constituted by meanings. Stress is described as the disruption of meanings, and coping is what the person does about the disruption. Both doing something and refraining from doing anything about the stressful situation are ways of copying. Copying is bounded by the meanings inherent in what the person counts as stressful. The person must be understood as a "participant self" in a situation, which is shaped by reflective and nonreflective meanings and concerns. "The way the person is in the situation sets up different possibilities." Benner uses this key concept to describe clinical nursing practice in terms of nurses making a positive difference by being in the situation in a caring way.

Benner's early work focussed on the anticipatory socialization of nurses. Benner and Kramer studied the differences between nurses who worked in special care units and those who worked in regular hospital units. She was a research consultant for a nursing activity study to determine the use and productivity of nursing personnel in 1974 and 1975. Concurrently, she was a consultant on a study of new nurse work-entry. Benner and Benner conducted a systematic evaluation of the competencies, the job-finding, and work-entry problems of new graduate nurses. Benner also studied methods of increasing teacher competencies through the use of a mobile micro-teaching laboratory.

From 1978 to 1981 she was the author and project director of a federally funded grant, "Achieving Methods of Intraprofessional Consensus, Assessment and Evaluation, "known as the AMICAE Project. This research led to the publication of *From Novice to Expert* and numerous articles. Benner and Wrubel have further explained and developed the background to this study in *The Primacy of Caring: Stress and Copying in Health and Illness*, "an interpretive theory of nursing practice as it is concerned with helping patients cope with the stress of illness. The primacy of caring is three-pronged" as the producer of both stress and copying in the lived experience of health and illness, . . . as the enabling condition of nursing practice (indeed any practice), and the ways that nursing practice based in such caring can positively affect the outcome of an illness."

Benner continues to conduct research focusing on practical knowledge or skilled clinical knowledge developed by practicing nurses and the stress and copying techniques of patients experiencing chronic illness. Currently, she is investigating the expert clinical knowledge as a form of practical knowledge in critical care settings, as well as the stress, copying and self-care practice that develop during the first 6 months from diagnosis in patients with major curative-intent cancer therapies.

Benner directed the AMICAE Project to develop evaluation methods of participating schools of nursing and hospitals in the San Francisco area. It was an interpretive descriptive study that led to the use of Dreyfus' five levels of competency to describe skill acquisition in clinical nursing practice. In describing the interpretive approach, Benner stated that a rich description of nursing practice from observation and narrative accounts of actual nursing practice provide the test for interpretation (hermeneutics). The nurses' descriptions of patient care situations in which they made a positive difference "present the uniqueness of nursing as a discipline and an art." Over 1200 nurse participants completed questionnaires and interviews and were observed by trained researchers. Twenty-one paired preceptor-preceptee interviews about patient care situations they had in common were conducted with beginning nurses and nurses who were recognized for their expertise. "The research was aimed at discovering if there were distinguishable, characteristic differences in the novice's and expert's descriptions of the same clinical incident." Further interviews and participant observations were conducted with 51 nurse clinicians and other newly graduated nurses and senior nursing students to "describe characteristics of nurse performance at different stages of skill acquisition." The purpose "of the inquiry has been to uncover meanings and knowledge embedded in skilled practice. By bringing these meanings, skills, and knowledge into public discourse new knowledge and understandings are constituted."

The Dreyfus model of skill acquisition was developed as a result of studying the performance of pilots in emergency situations and chess players. In applying the model to nursing, Benner noted that skilled nursing requires a sound educational base that allows for a safer and quicker experience-based skill acquisition. Skill and skilled practice, as defined by Benner, means skilled nursing interventions and clinical judgment skills in actual clinical situations. In no case does this refer to context-free psychomotor skills or other demonstrable enabling skills outside the context of nursing practice.

Thirty-one competencies emerged from analysis of the transcripts of interviews with nurses' detailed-descriptions of patient care episodes, including their intentions and interpretations of the events. From these competencies identified from actual practice situations, the following seven domains were inductively derived on the basis of similarity of function and intent:

- The helping role
- The teaching-coaching function
- The diagnostic and patient-monitoring function
- Effective management of rapidly changing situations

- Administering and monitoring therapeutic interventions and regimens
- Monitoring and ensuring the quality of health care practices
- Organizational work-role competencies

Each of the domains was described with the related competencies from the exemplars describing nursing practice.

Concepts Used by Benner

Novice

In the novice stage of skill acquisition from the Dreyfus model, one has no background experience of the situation in which one is involved. Context-free rules and objective attributes must be given to guide performance. There is difficulty discerning between relevant and irrelevant aspects of a situation. Generally, this level applies to students of nursing, but Benner has suggested that nurses at higher levels of skill in one area of practice could be classified at the novice level if placed in an unfamiliar area of situation.

Advanced Beginner

The advanced beginner stage in the Dreyfus model develops when one can demonstrate marginally acceptable performance, having coped with enough real situations to note, or to have pointed out by a mentor, the recurring meaningful components of the situation The advanced beginner has enough experience to grasp aspects of the situation. Unlike attributes and features, aspects cannot be completely objectified because they require experience based on recognition in the context of the situation.

Nurses functioning at this level are rule-guided and task-completion oriented and have difficulty grasping the current patient situation in terms of the larger perspective. Clinical situations are viewed as a test of the nurses' abilities and the demands it places on them rather than in terms of the patient needs and responses. Advanced beginners feel highly responsible for managing patient care yet still largely rely on the help of those more experienced. Benner places most newly graduated nurses at this level.

Competent

Through learning from actual practice situations and following the actions of others, the advanced beginner moves to the competent level. The competent stage of the Dreyfus model is typified by considerable conscious and deliberate planning that determines which aspects of the current and future situations are important and which can be ignored.

"Consistency, predictability, and time management are important, and gaining a sense of mastery through planning and predictability is the accomplishment." There is an increased level of efficiency but "the focus is on the management and the nurse's organization of the task world rather than on timing in relation to the patient's needs." The competent nurse may display hyperresponsibility for their patients, often more than is realistic and exhibit an ever present and critical view of the self.

Proficient

At the proficient stage of the Dreyfus model, the performer perceives the situation as a whole (the total picture) rather than in terms of aspects, and the performance is guided by maxims. The proficient level is a qualitative leap beyond the competent. Now the performer recognizes the most salient aspects and has an intuitive grasp of the situation based on background understand.

Nurses at this level demonstrate a new ability to see changing relevance in a situation including the recognition and the implementation of skilled responses to the situation as it evolves. They no longer rely on preset goals to organize and they demonstrate an increased confidence in their own knowledge and abilities.

Expert

The fifth stage of the Dreyfus model is achieved when "the expert performer no longer relies on an analytical principle (rule, guidelines, maxim) to connect her or his or his understanding of the situation to an appropriate action. Benner described the expert nurse as having an intuitive grasp of the situation and as being able to identify the region of the problem without wasting consideration on a range of alternative diagnoses and solutions.

The expert nurse has this ability of pattern recognition based on deep experiential background. For the expert nurse, meeting the patient's actual concerns and needs is of utmost importance, even if it means planning and negotiating for a change in the plan of case. There is almost transparent view of the self.

- *Aspects of a situation* The characteristics of the situation recognized and understood in context because of prior experience.

- *Attribute of a situation* Measurable properties of a situation that can be explained without previous experience in the situation.

- *Competency* Competency is "an interpretively defined area of skilled performance identified and described by its intent, functions, and meanings." This team is unrelated to the competent stage of the Dreyfus model.

- *Domain* An area of practice having a number of competencies with similar intents, functions, and meanings.

- *Exemplar* An example of a clinical situation that conveys one or more intents, meanings, functions, or outcomes easily translated to other clinical situations.

- *Experience* Now a mere passage of time but an active process of refining and changing preconceived theories, notions, and ideas when confronted with actual situations; implies there is a dialogue between what is found in practice and what is expected.

- *Maxim* A cryptic description of skilled performance that requires a certain level of experience to recognize the implications of the instructions.

- *Paradigm case* A clinical experience that stands out and alters the way one perceives and understands future clinical situations. Paradigm cases create new clinical understanding and open new clinical perspectives and alternatives.

- *Salience* A perceptual stance of embodied knowledge whereby aspects of a situation stand out as more or less importance.

Paradigm of Benners' Theory

Benner incorporated assumptions from the Dreyfus model, "that with experience and mastery the skill is transformed." This model assumes that all practical situations are far more complex than can be described by formal models, theories and textbook descriptions."

In her subsequent writing Benner explicated the themes of nursing, person, situation and health.

Nursing

Nursing is described as a caring relationship, an "enabling condition of connection and concern." "Caring is primary because caring sets up the possibility of giving help and receiving help." Nursing is viewed as a caring practice whose science is guided by the moral art and ethics of care and responsibility." Benner understands nursing practice as the care and study of the lived experience of health, illness, and the disease and the relationships between these three

Person

Benner has used Heidegger's phenomenological description of person. "A person is a self-interpreting being, that is, the person does not come into the world predefined but gets defined in the course of living a life. A person also has . . . an effortless and nonreflective understanding of the self in the world." "The person is viewed as a participant in common meanings."

Finally, the person is embodied. Benner and Wrubel have conceptualized the major aspects of understanding the person must deal with as the role of the situation, the role of the body, the role of personal concerns, and the role of temporality. Together these aspects of the person make up the person in the world. This view of the person is based on the works of Heidgger, Merleau-Ponty, and Dreyfus. Their goal is to overcome cartesian dualism, namely, the view that the mind and body are distinct, separate entities. Benner and Wrubel give a central place to embodiment in their theory and defined *embodiment* as the capacity of the body to respond to meaningful situations. Based upon the work of Merleau-Ponty and Dreyfus (1979), they outline five dimensions of the body: (i) the unborn complex, the unacculturated body of the fetus and newborn baby; (ii) the habitual skilled body, the social learned postures, gestures, customs, and skills evident in bodily skills such as seeing, and "body language" that are "learned over time through identification, imitation, and trial and error;" (iii) the projective body, the way the body is set (predisposed) to act in specific situations, for example, opening a door or walking; (iv) the actual projected body, one's current bodily orientation or projection in a situation that is flexible and varied to fit the situation, such as when one is skillful in using a keyboard; and (v) the phenomenal body, the body aware of itself, that ability to imagine and describe kinesthetic sensations. Benner and Wrubel point out that nurses attend to the body and the role of embodiment in health, illness and recovery.

Health

Based on Heidegger and Merleau-Ponty, Benner "focusses on the lived experience of being healthy and being ill." *Health* is defined as what can be assessed, whereas well-being is the human experience of health or wholeness. Well-being or being ill are understood as distinct ways of being in the world. Health is described as not just the absence of disease and illness. Also a person may have a disease and not experience themselves as ill because illness is the human experience of loss or dysfunction, whereas disease is what can be assessed at the physical level.

Situation

Benner used the term *situation* rather than *environment* because *situation* conveys a peopled environment, with social definition and meaningfullness. She used the phenomenological terms of being *situated* and *situated meaning*, which are defined by the person's engaged interaction, interpretation, and understanding of the situation. "To be situated implies that one has a past, present, and future and that all of these aspects. . . influence the current situation." Persons "enter into situations with their own sets of meanings, habits, and perspectives." "Personal interpretation of the situation is bounded by the way the individual is in it."

Assertions of Theory

Benner stated that theory is crucial in order to form the right questions to ask in a clinical situation; theory directs the practitioner in looking for problems and anticipating care needs. There is always more to any situation than theory predicts. The skilled practice of nursing exceeds the bounds of formal theory. Concrete experience provides the learning about the exceptions and shades of meaning in a situation. The knowledge embedded in practice discovers and interprets theory, precedes or extends theory, and synthesizes and adapts theory in caring nursing practice. Some of the relationship statements included in Benner's work follow.

Discovering assumptions, expectations, and sets can uncover an unexamined area of practical knowledge that can then be systematically studied and extended or refuted.

The clinician's knowledge is embedded in perceptions rather than precepts.

Perceptual awareness is central to good nursing judgement and . . . begins with vague hunches and global assessments that initially bypass critical analysis; conceptual clarity follows more often than it precedes.

Formal rules are limited and discretionary judgment is used in actual clinical situations.

Knowledge . . . accrues over time in the practice of an applied discipline.

Expertise develops when the clinician tests and refines propositions, hypotheses, and principle-based expectations in actual practice situations.

Through qualitative descriptive research, Benner applied the Dreyfus model of skill acquisition to clinical nursing practice. Following the logical sequence developed by Dreyfus, Benner was able to identify the performance characteristics and teaching-learning needs in-he rent at each level of skill. From her research, Benner identified 31 competencies of expert practice, which she classified inductively into seven domains of nursing practice. In reporting her research, Benner used exemplars taken directly from interviews and observation of expert practice to help the reader form a clear picture of such practice. Benner accomplished the goal of her research which she stated to be "to uncover meanings and knowledge embedded in skilled practice . . . by bringing these meanings, skills, and knowledge into public discourse, new knowledge and understanding are constituted."

Nursing Implications

Practice

Benner has described clinical; nursing practice by using an interpretive approach. Included in *From Novice to Expert* are several examples of application of her work in practice settings. The model has been used to aid in the development of clinical ladders of promotion, new graduate orientation programmes, and clinical knowledge development seminars. Symposiums focusing on excellence in nursing practice have been held for staff development, recognition, and reward and as way of demonstrating clinical knowledge development in practice.

Fenton reported the use of Benner's approach in an ethnographic study of the performance of clinical nurse specialists. She found that the nurse were functioning at an advanced level of preparation, but that "we have not yet developed accurate written and verbal descriptions of that advanced practice." Balasco and Black and Silver used Benner's model as a basis for differentiating clinical knowledge development and career progression in nursing.

Neverveld used Benner's rationale and format in her development of basic and advanced preceptor workshops.

Crissman and Jelsma applied Benner's findings when developing a cross-training programmes to aid in staffing imbalances. "Cross-training delineates specific performance objectives for the nurse in her novice role and provides a preceptor in the setting for the clinical area unfamiliar to her. There, as a novice, she aims to become and advanced beginner able to function independently with an experienced nurse available as a resource.

Benner has been cited extensively in nursing literature regarding nursing practice concerns and the role of caring in such practice. She continues to publish applications of the model to clinical situations. Currently, Benner authors a bi-monthly column in the *American Journal of Nursing* in which she provides interpretive commentary on submitted narrative accounts of clinical situations by practising nurses. Benner believes "this column has the potential to become a data source for a systematic study of the practical moral reasoning of nurses as well as extend the work on expert clinical nursing knowledge. . . serves to raise consciousness about the level and nature of the caring practices of nurses, which the currently threatened by lack of societal recognition and valuing.

Education

Benner has critiqued the concept of competency-based testing by contrasting it with the complexity of the proficiency and expert stages described in the Dreyfus model of skill acquisition and the 31 competencies. In summary, she stated, competency-based testing seems limited to the less situational, less interact ional areas of patient care where the behavior can be well defined and patient and nurse variation do not alter the performance criteria.

Fenton described the application of the domains of expert practice as the basis for studying the skilled performance of master's-prepared nurses. The analysis verified the performance skills of expert nurses reported in the AMICAE project and identified new areas of skilled performance and five preliminary categories relevant for curriculum evaluation in the graduate programme.

According to Barnum, surprisingly it is not Benner's development of the seven domains of nursing practice that has had the greatest impact on nursing education but rather the "appreciation of the utility of the Dreyfus model in describing learning and thinking in our discipline." Nursing educators have realized that learning needs at the early stages of clinical knowledge development are different from those required at later stages. These differences must be acknowledged and valued when educators develop teaching curriculums.

Research

The preceding example by Fenton presented an application of educational research. Lock and Gordon, a medical anthropologist who has been a research assistant on the AMICAE project, extended the inquiry to study the formal models used in nursing practice and medicine. She concluded that formal models may serve as maps directing and can substitute for knowledge and result in conformity. She cautions that a misuse of formal models occurs when nurses apply models without using judgment, use them to exert control, and use language from them that can cover up meanings, or not really know what they mean. Finally "formal models should be used with discretion" as tools and so as not to eclipse the relational, holistic, intuitive aspects of nursing.

Benner and Wrubel have extended the basis and interpretation of the study of clinical nursing practice in *The Primary of Caring: Stress and Coping in Health and Illness*. This work explores the philosophies affecting our thinking and practice. Benner and Wrubel suggest that the adoption of a phenomenological view of person with shared meanings in the situation gives the potential for an understanding of caring and expert nursing practice and stress and coping. "Theory must be informed by real-world experience and experiments, which are in turn subject to theoretical interpretation. . . . A theory is needed that describes, interprets, and explains not an imagined ideal of nursing, but actual expert nursing as it is practiced day by day."

Benner's application of the Dreyfus model in clinical nursing practice has provided rich descriptions of nursing as it is practiced. In the interpretation of the five levels of practice, Benner provided suggestions for matching competency to nursing practice and for the development of each staged based on experience. It is better to place a new graduate with a competent nurse preceptor who can explain nursing practice in ways that the beginner comprehends. The intuitive knowledge of the expert will elude beginners who do not have the experienced know-how to grasp the situation.

To date, the model provides concept definitions and in-depth descriptions of each from nursing practice. From these situated descriptions, 31 competencies in seven domains have been derived from actual nursing practice. By maintaining the context of these situated performances, the descriptions are holistic or synthetic, rather than procedural and elemental. "The competencies within each domain, [are] in no way intended as an exhaustive list." "A situation-based interpretive approach to describing nursing practice overcomes some of the problems of reductionism . . . and overcomes the problem of global and overly general descriptions based on nursing process categories."

In recent research, Benner examined the role of narrative accounts in understanding the notion of good or ethical caring in expert clinical nursing practice. "The narrative memory of the actual concrete event is taken up in embodied know-how and comportment, complete with emotional responses to situations." The narrative memory can evoke perceptual or sensory memories that enhance pattern recognition.

Dunlop explored the nursing literature related to the science of caring. She draws a distinction between a science for caring and a science of caring. "A science of caring implies that caring can be operationalized is some way as a set of behaviors which can be observed, counted or measured. Benner has taken ha hermeneutical form to uncover the knowledge embedded in clinical nursing practice. "As she does this, she is also uncovering the nursing-caring with which it is deeply intertwined." Although useful, Dunlop noted that it does not provide us with any universal truths about caring in general or about nursing-caring in particular-indeed it does not make any such pretension.

EVALUATION OF THEORY

- Benner has developed an interpretive descriptive account of clinical nursing practice. The concepts are the levels of skilled practice from the Dreyfus model, including novice, advanced beginner, competent, proficient, and expert. She uses the five concepts to describe nursing practice from interviews, observations, and the analysis of transcripts of exemplars provided by the nurses. From these descriptions, 31 competencies were identified, and these were grouped into seven domains of nursing practice based on common intentions and meanings. The model is relatively simple with regard to the five stages of skill acquisition and provides a comparative guide for identifying levels of nursing practice from individual nurse descriptions and observations of actual nursing practice. The interpretations are validated by consensus. A degree of complexity is encountered in the subconcepts for differentiation between the levels of competency and the need to identify meanings and intentions. This interpretive approach is designed to overcome the constraints of the rational-technical approach to the study and description of practice. Although providing a decontextualized (i.e. object) description of the novice level of performance is possible, the limits of objectification are encountered as soon as an understanding of the situation is required for expert performance. Clinical knowledge is relational and contextual and often deals with local, specific, historical issues. To capture the contextual and relational aspects of practice, Benner uses narrative accounts of actual clinical situations and maintains that the exemplar enables the reader to recognize similar intents and meanings, even though the "objective" circumstances may be quite different.
- The descriptive model of nursing practice has the potential for universal application as a framework, but the descriptions are limited by dependence on the actual clinical nursing situations from which they must be derived. Its use depends on the

understanding of the five levels of competency and the ability to identify the characteristic intentions and meanings inherent at each level of practice. The model has universal characteristics in that it is not restricted by age, illness, health, or location of nursing practice. The characteristics of theoretical universality, however imply properties of operationalization for prediction that are nor a part of this perspective. Indeed, this phenomenological perspective critiques the limits of "universality" in studies of human practices.

- The model was empirically tested using qualitative methodologies, and 31 competencies and seven domains of nursing practice were derived inductively. Subsequent research suggests that the framework is applicable and useful in providing knowledge of the descriptions of nursing practice. Benner stated that "if we choose only scientific, technical and organizational strategies for legitimizing expert nursing care, we will miss the primacy of caring and the central ethic of care and responsibility embedded in expert nursing practice." It is precisely the use of alternative models of discovering nursing knowledge that makes it difficult to address the work of *From Novice to Expert* within a rational-empirical framework for critique. Utilizing the scientific approach, one would look for lawlike relational statements to predict practice. Nevertheless, using the qualitative methods in an interpretive approach, Benner describes expert nursing practice in many exemplars. Positivistic science takes an alternative approach by seeking formulas and models to apply. Her work seems to be hypotheses generating rather than hypotheses testing. Benner provides no universal "how to" for nursing practice, but rather provides a methodology for uncovering and entering into the situated meaning of expert nursing care. The interpretation of the meaning and level of nursing practice will no doubt frustrate "objective" researches who seek precision and control. The strength of the Benner model is that it is data-based research that contributes to the science of nursing.
- Benner's *From Novice to Expert* model provides a general framework for identifying, defining, and describing clinical nursing practice. Benner uses a phenomenological approach to describe persons and derives meaning and abilities from interactions in life-situations. The significance of Benner's research findings lies in her conclusion that "a nurse's clinical knowledge is relevant to the extent to which its manifestation in nursing skills makes a difference in patient care and patient outcomes.

Nursing is the involved interaction with persons in a caring mode. *The Primacy of Caring* further develops these themes. Benner described her work as description of the knowledge embedded in actual nursing practice. The five levels of competencies are descriptions of the practical nursing knowledge of each level in the context of the situations described. The approach to generalization is through common meanings, skills, practices, and embodied capacities rather than through general a historical laws. The knowledge embedded in clinical nursing practice should no longer be ignored but brought forth as public knowledge so that a greater understanding of nursing practice can occur. Benner believes the scope and complexity of nursing practice are too extensive simply to rely on idealized, decontextualized views of practice. or experiments. "The platonic quest to get to the general so that we can get beyond the vagaries of experience was a misguided turn. we can redeem the turn if we subject out theories to our unedited, concrete, moral-experience and acknowledge that skilful ethical comportment calls us not to be beyond experience but tempered and taught by it.

The generalizations are depicted through exemplars that demonstrate relational and contextually relevant intents and aspects of clinical knowledge. This approach takes issue with the common approaches used for universality or generalization in physics and the natural sciences and claims that the basis for generalization in clinical knowledge cannot be structural or mechanistic but rather must be based on common meaning and practices. The strategies for generalization are not based on abstraction through removing the situation or content (objectification) but rather by showing how the skilled knowledge, the intent, content, and notion of good in clinical knowledge must be depicted by exemplars that illustrate the role of the situation. Benner claims that this is not a privativistic or subjectivistic approach, but rather an attempt to overcome the limits of subject-object descriptions. Benner's call is to "increase public storytelling to validate nursing as an ethical caring practice and "to extend, alter, and preserve ethical distinctions and concerns." Benner's work is useful in that it has framed nursing practice from the context of what nursing actually is and does, rather than from idealized theoretical descriptors that are context-free.

Chapter 25

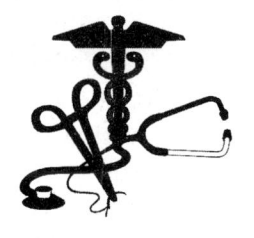

Mercer's Theory in Maternal Role Attainment

Ramona T. Mercer began her nursing career in 1950, when she was graduated from St. Margaret's School of Nursing, Montgomery, Alabama. She was graduated with the LL Hill Award for Highest Scholastic Standing. In the 10 years that followed, she worked as a nurse, head nurse, and instructor in the areas of pediatrics, obstetrics, and contagious diseases before returning to school in 1960. She completed a Bachelor of Science degree in Nursing in 1962, graduating with distinction, from the University of New Mexico, Albuquerque. She went on to earn an MSN in maternal child health nursing from Emory University in 1964 and a PhD in Maternity Nursing from the University of Pittsburgh in 1973.

From 1961 through 1963, while pursuing studies in nursing, Mercer worked as a clinical instructor. In 1964 she was awarded the HEW Public Health Service Nurse Trainee Award and was inducted into Sigma Theta Tau. From 1964 to 1971, she was an assistant professor of Maternal Child Health Nursing to Emory University. During this time she was again awarded an HEW Public Health Service Nurse Trainee Award and also the Bixler Scholarship for Nursing Education and Research, Southern Regional Board.

Mercer moved to California in 1973 and accepted the position of Assistant Professor, Department of Family Health Care Nursing, at the University of California, San Francisco. She held that position until 1977, when she was promoted to associate professor. In 1983 she accepted a position as a professor in the same department and remained in that role until her retirement in 1987. Mercer remains active in writing, speaking engagements, and consultations.

In early research efforts, Mercer focussed on the behaviors and needs of breastfeeding mothers, mothers with postpartum illness, and mothers bearing infants with defects. The results were published in several articles and led to the writing of *Nursing Care for Parents at Risk*, which was published in 1977 and received an *American Journal of Nursing* Book of the Year Award in 1978. This prior research led Mercer to study mothers of various ages, family relationships, and antepartal stress as related to familial relationships and the maternal role. A portion of that work, concerning teenage mothers over the first year of motherhood, resulted in the book *Perspectives on Adolescent Health Care,* which in 1980 also received an *American Journal of Nursing* Book of the Year Award. In 1986, Mercer's work on mothers at various ages was drawn together in *First-time Motherhood: Experiences From Teens to Forties.*

Mercer's fifth book, *Parents at Risk,* published in 1990, also received an *American Journal of Nursing* Book of the Year Award. *Parents at Risk* focusses on strategies for facilitating early parent-infant interactions and promoting parental competence in relation to specific risk situations. In the 25 years since her first publication in 1968, she has published five books, articles in both nursing and non-nursing journals, six book s, and many abstracts, forewords, editorials, and book reviews.

As of 1992, Mercer maintained membership in seven professional organizations, including the American Nurses Association and the American Academy of Nursing and has been an active member on many national committees. From 1983 to 1990 she was the associate editor of *Health Care for Women International.* She serves on the review panel for *Nursing Research* and *Western Journal of Nursing Research,* and is on the executive advisory board of *California Nursing* and *Nurse Week.* She has also served as a reviewer for numerous grant proposals. Additionally, she has been actively involved with regional, national, and international scientific and professional meetings and workshops.

Other honors with awards she has received include Maternal Child Health Nurse of the Year Award by the National Foundation March of Dimes and American Nurses Association, Division of Maternal Child Health Practice in 1982; Fourth Annual Helen Nahm Lecturer, University of California, San Francisco, School of Nursing in 1984; ASPO/Lamaze National Research Award in 1987; in 1988 the Distinguished Research Lectureship Award, Western Institute of Nursing; Western Society for Research in Nursing; and in 1990 the American Nurses Foundation's Distinguished Contribution to Nursing Science Award.

EVOLUTION OF THEORY

Mercer received her Ph.D. from the University of Pittsburgh where her mentor Reva Rubin was a professor and director of graduate programmes in maternity nursing.

Early in Mercer's research, she drew from Mead's interactionist theory of self and Von Bertalanffy's general systems theory. As her research developed into attainment of the maternal role, she also combined the work of Werner and Erikson with Burr and associates' theory to develop a theoretical framework of role theory from an interactionist approach. Reva Rubin's research on maternal role attainment and Mercer's own research conducted on the different variables affecting the maternal role were also major theoretical sources.

Mercer used many measurement tools to test the variables under investigation in her maternal role research: To measure early postpartum and the first-month attachment, she used E.R. Broussard and Hartner's prediction of neonatal outcomes and perceptions work, and later she used the Degree of Bothersome Inventory to measure stress related to infant behavior. Samko and Schoenfeld's measurement tool was adapted by Mercer and Marut to a 29-item questionnaire to assess the effect of the perception of the birth experience. Leifer's How I Feel About My Baby questionnaire was used to measure attachment at 1, 4, 8, and 12 months. She also used Leifer's Child-Trait Checklist at 1 month because of its representation of the claiming behaviors described by Gottlieb (1978), Robson and Moss (1970), and Rubin (1961, 1972). Gratification of the maternal role was measured by an adaptation of Russell's (1974) Gratification Checklist. Maternal behavior was measured by Disbrow and associates (1977, 1982). Ways Parents Handle Irritating Behavior Scale was originally used for discriminating between abusive and nonabusive parents. Maternal behavior in Mercer's studies, as observed by the raters, was measured by an adaptation from Blank's (1974) scale.

To measure social stress, Mercer used the Life Experience Survey constructed by Sarason, Johnson, and Siegel (1978). She also used the Checklist of Bothersome Factors to reflect infant stress in the transition to parenthood developed by Hobbs (1965), who revised it for a replicated study (Hobbs and Cole, 1976). A seven-item subscale, derived from the Hobbs Checklist, relating to change in the mate relationship, was utilized during the eight-month test period. An adaptation of Burr and associates' (1979) Scale of Role Strain was used as a reflection of stress in the role of parenting at 4, 8, and 12 months. Mercer also used a 12-item empathy scale from Scotland's 96-item scale by Disproof's Child Abuse prediction project.

To measure maternal rigidity, she used a 15-item scale constructed by Larsen (1966). Maternal temperament was measured by using Thomas, Mittelman, and Chess's (1982) 140-item Early Adult Life Temperament Questionnaire. This questionnaire was chosen because of "its high isomorphism with the Carey Infant Temperament Questionnaire that was used to measure infant temperament" (Carey 1970, Carey and McDevitt, 1978). The Tennessee Self Concept Scale (TSCS) was selected by Mercer to measure maternal self-concept, personality integration, and personality disorders in her research subjects. Two measures, the Parent Child-Rearing Attitude Scales developed by Disbrow and associates (1977) and the Maternal Attitude Scale (MAS) developed by Cohler and associates (1970), were used for those variables.

In her research on the effects of antepartum stress on mothers' and fathers' health status, mate relationships, attachment to their infants, and family functioning, a family developmental approach was used to study change from pregnancy over 8 months postpartum within the family system and subsystems. Measures used in this study were Feetham's Family Function Scale; Locke and Wallace's Marital Adjustment Test; Cranley's Fetal Attachment Scale; Leifer's How I Feel About My Baby Scale; Davies and Ware's General Health Index; Revisions of Hobel's Pregnancy, Intrapartal, and Newborn Risk Scores; Norbeck's revision of the Life Experiences Survey; Rosenburg's Self-Esteem Scale; Barerra's Inventory of Socially Supportive Behaviors (received support); McMillan and Wandersman's Feelings of Support (perceived support); Checklist of Supportive Persons (network support); Pearlin's Sense of Mastery; Spielberger and associates: Trait and State Anxiety Scales; Radloff's Center for Epidemiologic Studies Depression Scale; and Gibaud-Wallston and

Wandersman's Parental Sense of Competence Scale.

Mercer's theory is based on the evidence of her research spanning 25 years. Many other researchers' findings were also used in the formulation of the Maternal Role Attainment theory. The work of Reva Rubin on maternal role attainment stimulated Mercer's initial interest. The focus of Mercer's work, however, went beyond the "traditional" mother to encompass adolescents, older mothers, ill mothers, mothers with defective children, families experiencing antepartal stress, parents at high risk, and mothers who had cesarean deliveries. Rubin also dealt with role attainment from the point of the acceptance of the pregnancy to 1 month postpartum; Mercer looked beyond that period to 12 months postpartum.

Concepts Used by Mercer

Mercer bases her theory for maternal role attainment on the following factors:

- *Maternal role attainment* An interactional and developmental process occurring over a period of time, during which the mother becomes attached to her infant, acquires competence in the care-taking tasks involved in the role, and expresses pleasure and gratification in the role. "The movement to the personal state in which the mother experiences a sense of harmony, confidence and competence in how she performs the role is the end point of maternal role attainment–maternal identity."
- *Maternal age* Chronological and developmental.
- *Perception of birth experience* A woman's perception of her performance during labor and birth.
- *Early maternal-infant separation* Separation from the mother after birth due to illness and/or prematurity.
- *Self-esteem* "An individual's perception of how others view one and self-acceptance of the perception."
- *Self-concept (self-regard)* "The overall perception of self that includes self-satisfaction, self-acceptance, self-esteem, and congruence or discrepancy between self and ideal itself."
- *Flexibility* Roles are not rigidly fixed; therefore, who fills the roles is not important.

  "Flexibility of childrearing attitudes increases with increased development older mothers have the potential to respond less rigidly to their infants and to view each situation in respect to the unique nuances."
- *Childrearing attitudes* Maternal attitudes or beliefs about childrearing.
- *Health status* "The mother's and father's perception of their prior health, current health, health outlook, resistance-susceptibility to illness, health worry concern, sickness orientation and rejection of the sick role."
- *Anxiety* "A trait in which there is specific proneness to perceive stressful situations as dangerous or threatening, and as situation-specific state."
- *Depression* "Having a group of depressive symptoms, and in particular the affective component of the depressed mood."
- *Role strain* The conflict and difficulty felt by the women in fulfilling the maternal role obligation.

- *Gratification* "The satisfaction, enjoyment, reward, or pleasure that a woman experiences in interacting with her infant, and in fulfilling the usual tasks inherent in mothering."
- *Attachment* A component of the parental role and identity. Attachment is viewed as a process in which an enduring affectional and emotional commitment to an individual is formed.
- *Infant temperament* An easy versus a difficult temperament, it is related to whether the infant sends hard-to-read cues, leading to feelings of incompetence and frustration in the mother.
- *Infant health status* Illness causing maternal-infant separation, interfering with the attachment process.
- *Infant characteristics* Temperament, appearance, and health status.
- *Family* "A dynamic system which includes subsystems-individuals (mother, father, fetus/infant) and dyads (mother-father, mother-fetus/infant, and father-fetus/infant) within the overall family system."
- *Family functioning* The individual's view of the activities and relationships between the family and its subsystems and broader social units.
- *Stress* Positively and negatively perceived life events and environmental variables.
- *Social support* "The amount of help actually received, satisfaction with that help, and the persons (network) providing that help.

Four areas of social support are the following:

Emotional support "Feeling loved, cared for, trusted, and understood."

Informational support "Helps the individual help herself by providing information that is useful in dealing with the problem and/or situation."

Physical support A direct kind of help.

Appraisal support "A support that tells the role taker how she is performing in the role; it enables the individual to evaluate herself in relationship to others' performance in the role."

- *Mother-father relationship* Perception of the mate relationship that includes intended and actual values, goals, and agreements between the two.
- *Culture* The total way of life learned and passed on from generation to generation.

For maternal role attainment, Mercer stated the following assumptions:

1. A relatively stable "core self," acquired through lifelong socialization, determines how a mother defines and perceives events; her perceptions of her infant's and others' responses to her mothering, along with her life situation, are the real world to which she responds.
2. In addition to the mother's socialization, her developmental level and innate personality characteristics also influence her behavioral responses.
3. The mother's role partner, her infant, will reflect the mother's competence in the mothering role via growth and development.
4. The infant is considered an active partner in the maternal role-taking process, affecting and being affected by the role enactment:
5. Maternal identity develops along with maternal attachment and each depends on the other.

PARADIGM OF MERCEBS THEORY

Nursing

Mercer does not define *nursing* but refers to nursing as a science emerging from a "turbulent adolescence to adulthood." Nurses are the health professionals having the most "sustained and intense interaction with women in the maternity cycle." Nurses are responsible for "promoting the health" of families and children; nurses are "pioneers" in developing and sharing assessment strategies for these clients.

Obstetrical nursing, according to Mercer, is the diagnosis and treatment of women's and men's responses to actual or potential health problems during pregnancy, childbirth, and the postpartum period.

Person

Mercer does not specifically define *person* but refers to the "self" or "core-self." She views the self as separate from the roles that are played. Through maternal individuation, a woman may regain her own "personhood" as she extrapolates her "self" from the mother-infant dyad. The core self evolves from a culture context and determines how situations are defined and shaped.

Health

In her theory Mercer defines *health status* as the mother's and father's perception of their prior health, current health, health outlook, resistance-susceptibility to illness, health worry concern, sickness orientation, and rejection of the sick role. Health status of the newborn is the extent of pathology present and infant health status by parental rating of overall health. The health status of a family is negatively affected by antepartum stress. Health status is an important indirect influence on satisfaction with relationships in childbearing families.

Environment

Mercer does not define *environment*. She does, however, address the individual's culture, mate, family and/or support network, and size of that network as it relates to maternal role attainment. A mate's love, support, and nurturance were important factors in enabling a woman to mother her child. The responses of mates, parents, other relatives, and friends are closely evaluated by the role taker. Supportive responses provided sanction for their mothering role and seemed to communicate confidence in their ability to mother. The mate, parents, family, and friends were also identified as sources of coping and help for the new mother

Assertions of Theory/Model

Mercer's model of Maternal Role Attainment is placed within Bronfenbrenner's (1979) nested circles of the macrosystem, exosystem, and macrosystem (Figure 25.1).

1. The immediate environment in which the maternal role attainment occurs is the microsystem, which includes the family, and factors such as family functioning, mother-father relationship, social support, and stress. The variables contained within the microsystem interact with one or more of the other variables in affecting maternal role. The infant as an individual is embedded within the family system. The family is viewed as a semiclosed system maintaining boundaries and control over interchange between the family system and other social systems.

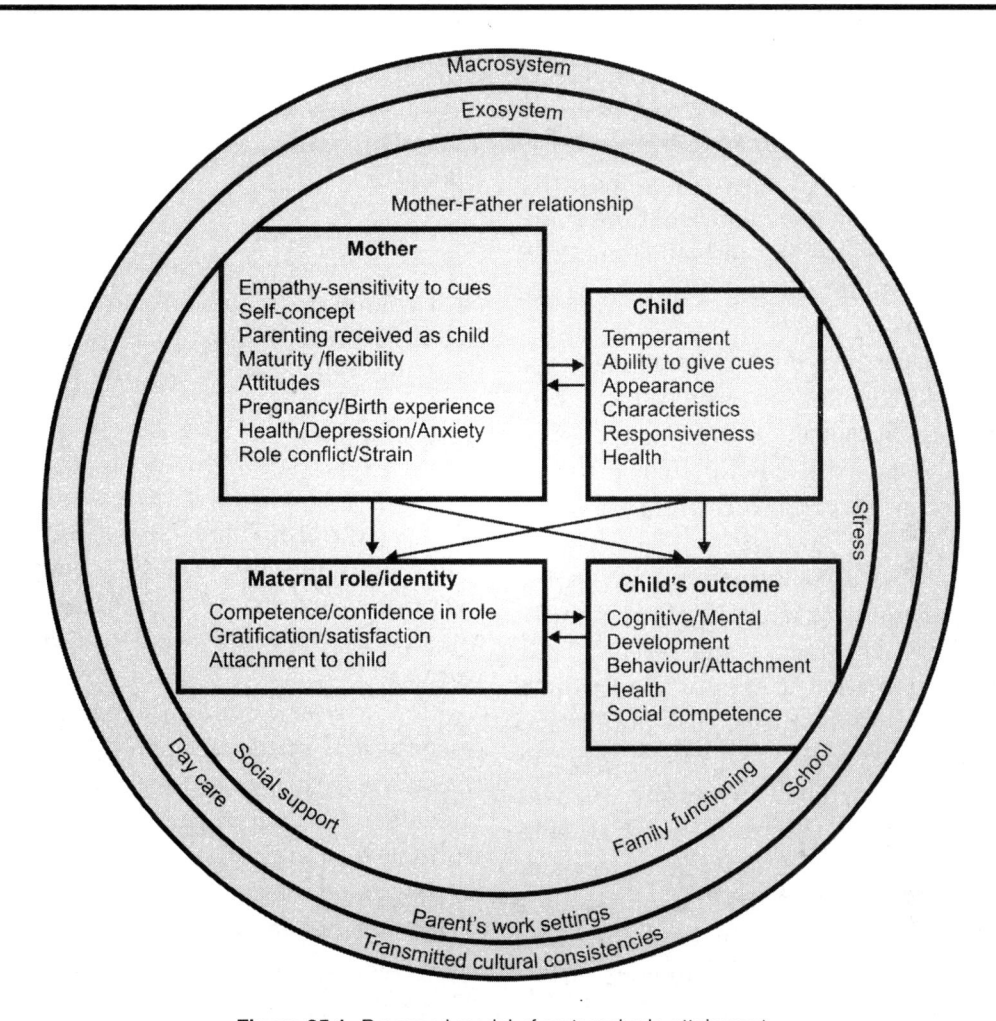

Figure 25.1: Proposed model of maternal role attainment

2. The exosystem encompasses, influences, and delimits the microsystem. The mother-infant unit is not contained within the exosystem, but the exosystem may determine in part what happens to the developing maternal role and the child.
3. The macrosystem refers to the general prototypes existing in a particular culture or transmitted cultural consistencies.

Maternal role attainment is a process that follows four stages of role acquisition (adapted from Thornton and Nardi, 1975):

1. *Anticipatory*—Begins social and psychological adjustment to the role by learning the expectations of the role. The mother fantasizes about the role, relates to the fetus *in utero*, and begins role play.
2. *Formal*—Begins with assumption of the role at birth; role behaviours are guided by formal, consensual expectations of others in the mother's social system.
3. *Informal*—Begins as mother develops unique ways of dealing with the role not conveyed by the social system.

4. *Personal*—The mother experiences a sense of harmony, confidence, and competence in the way she performs the role; maternal role is achieved.

Mercer used both deductive and inductive logic in developing the theoretical framework for studying factors that influence maternal role attainment in the first year of motherhood.

Deductive logic is demonstrated in her use of works from other researchers and disciplines. Both role and developmental theories and the work of R. Rubin on maternal role attainment provided a base for the framework.

Mercer also used inductive logic in the development of her maternal role attainment theory. Through practice and research, she observed adaptation to motherhood from a variety of circumstances. She noted that differences existed in adaptation to motherhood when maternal illness complicated the postpartum, when a child with a defect was born, and when a teenager became a mother. These observations directed the research about those situations and subsequently the development of her theoretical framework.

Nursing Implications

Practice

When considering practice using Mercer's framework, a clinical practice was set up using part of the concepts in the research conducted by Neeson, Patterson, Mercer, and May, "Pregnancy Outcomes for Adolescents Receiving Prenatal Care by Nurse Practitioners in Extended Roles."

The concepts theorized by Mercer have been used by nursing in multiple obstetrical textbooks. She is often cited as taking the work by Rubin and expanding its use. Her theory is extremely practice oriented.

Education

As previously stated, Mercer's work has appeared extensively in nursing texts, not just as it relates to maternal role attainment, Rather, each individual piece of research is used and valued.

Research

Mercer has tested factors that she theorized and/or hypothesized have a impact on maternal attainment. She has reviewed the literature extensively and formulated questions and models that guide future research.

Mercer has written articles on nursing research and stated her belief that nursing research is the bridge to excellence in practice. She also advocates the involvement of students in faculty research, with faculty serving as mentors.

During her tenure at the University of California, she chaired committees and was a committee member for numerous graduate theses and/or dissertations. Her work was used as the basis for at least eight graduate students' topics of research.

The theoretical framework for the correlational study exploring differences between three age groups for first-time mothers (ages 15 to 19, 20 to 29, and 30 to 42) has been tested in part by others, including Lorraine Walker and associates, University of Texas, Austin, and reported in *Nursing Research*. Angela B. McBride wrote, "Maternal role attainment has been a fundamental concern of nursing since the pioneering work of Mercer's mentor, Rubin, almost two decades ago. It is now becoming the research-based, theoretically sound construct that nurse researchers have been searching for in their analysis of the experience of new mothers."

Collaborative research with a graduate student and a junior faculty member in 1977 and 1978 led to the development of a highly reliable, valid instrument that measured attitudes about the labor experience. Over 80 researchers have requested permission to use the instrument.

Mercer believes that areas in need of further development and research are the mate relationship, that is, finding a tool that accurately reflects the dyadic relationship; investigating maternal role attainment among younger adolescents; developing more reliable and valid measurements of social support; and extending measurements into pregnancy, especially with the adolescent population. She also believes that further investigation into family dynamics and situational events that occur simultaneously with maternal role attainment is necessary.

In her book *First-Time Motherhood: Experiences from Teens to Forties*, she presents a model of four phases occurring in the process of maternal role attainment during the first year of motherhood. The four phases are labeled as follows: the physical recovery phase, occurring from birth to 1 month; the achievement phase from 2 to 4 or 5 months; the disruption phase occurring from 6 to 8 months; and finally the reorganization phase from after the eighth month and still in process at 1 year. Additionally, adaptation to the maternal role is proposed to occur at three levels—biological, psychological, and social—which are interacting and interdependent throughout the phases. These phases and levels of adaptation are briefly described and applied to her research on maternal role attainment. This model appears very logical and useful but is in need of further explanation, exposure, and development.

Additionally, research could investigate the application of this framework to multigravidas and extend the time frame beyond the first year. An interesting study would be to investigate whether differences exist in maternal role attainment among mothers conceiving and rearing children from multiple gestations (i.e. twins, triplets) compared with mothers rearing only one child. More explicit definitions of concepts and a greater consistency in labeling some concepts would benefit the reader. Mercer continues to develop her theory. She is collecting published research to review the state of the art in maternal role attainment for a new book and is reviewing instruments used to measure facets of maternal role attainment and researchers using the instruments, and reporting research to date.

EVALUATION OF THEORY

- The concepts, variables, and relationships are nor explicitly defined but rather are described and implied. They are, however, theoretically defined and operationalized. The operational and theoretical definitions are consistent. Some interchanging of terms and labels used to identify concepts (e.g. adaptation and attainment, social support and support network) can create some confusion for the reader. Additionally, *maternal role attainment* is not consistently defined and thus obstructs clarity. Overall, the

- concepts, assumptions, and goals are organized into a logical and coherent whole, and understanding the interrelationships among the concepts is relatively easy.
- In spite of numerous concepts and relationships, the theoretical framework for Maternal Role Attainment organizes a rather complex phenomenon into an easily understood and useful form. The theory is predictive in nature and thus readily lends itself to guide practice. Concepts are not specific to time and place, and so are abstract, but are described and operational-ized to the extent that meanings are not easily misinterpreted. It should be noted, however, that the research completed to define and support the theoretical relationships was very complex, largely due to the great number of concepts.
- Maternal role attainment is a theory specific to parent-child nursing. The theory can be generalized to all women during pregnancy through the first year after birth, regardless of age, parity, or environment. Mercer has also respecified her theory for a study to predict parental attachment to include the pregnant woman's partner.
- Mercer's work has done much to broaden the range of application of previously existing theories on maternal role attainment, as her studies have spanned various developmental levels and situational contexts, a quality that other studies do not share.
- Mercer's work was derived from extensive research efforts. The concepts, assumptions, and relationships are grounded predominantly in empirical observations and are congruent. The degree of concreteness and the completeness of operational definitions further increase the empirical precision.
- The theoretical framework for exploring differences between age groups of first-time mothers lends itself well to further testing and is being used by others, as previously discussed in the acceptance section of this The theoretical framework for maternal role attainment in the first year has proven to be useful, practical, and valuable to nursing. Mercer's work is repeatedly utilized in research, practice, and education. The framework is also readily applicable to any discipline that works with mothers and children in the first year of motherhood McBride wrote, "Dr. Mercer is the one who developed the most complete theoretical framework for studying one aspect of parental experience, namely, the factors that influence the attainment of the maternal role in the first year of motherhood."

According to Chinn and Jacobs, nursing theory should "differentiate the focus of nursing from other service professions." By combining the social, psychological, and biological sciences, Mercer achieves his criteria.

Throughout her career, Mercer has consistently linked research to practice. Implications for nursing and/or nursing interventions are addressed and provide the bond between research and practice in most of her works. She believes that nursing research is the "bridge to excellence" in nursing practice.

Chapter 26

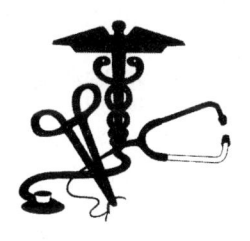

Adam's Conceptual Model on Nursing

Evelyn Adam was born April 9, 1929, in Lanark, Ontario, Canada. She graduated from Hotel Dieu Hospital in Kingston, Ontario, in 1950 with a Diploma in Nursing. She received a B.Sc. degree in 1966 from the University of Montreal and an MN degree from the University of California at Los Angeles in 1971. At UCLA she met Dorothy Johnson, who she feels has "definitely been the most important influence" on her professional life.

In 1979 she published her first book *Etre Infirmiere* (3rd edition, 1991) and in 1980 wrote the English version of *To Be a Nurse* (2nd edition, 1991). Since then, her book has been translated into Dutch (1981), Spanish (1982), Italian (1989), and Portuguese (1993). Adam has also written numerous articles on conceptual models for nursing and has coauthored several others. Professional journals publishing her articles include *Infirmiere Canadienne, Canadian Nurse, Journal of Advanced Nursing, Nursing Papers: Perspectives in Nursing*, and *Journal of Nursing Education*.

Adam has been a visiting professor at several universities. She has functioned as a resource person and speaker for various professional corporations, clinical and educational settings, and national and international conventions. From 1983 and 1989 she was a member of the review board for *Nursing Papers*. She taught at both undergraduate and graduate levels at the Faculty of Nursing of the University of Montreal. She was faculty secretary from 1982 until her retirement in 1989, at which time the University named her professor emeritus. She is in *Who's Who in the World* since its eighth edition (1987/1988). In 1992, Laval University (Quebec City) awarded her an honorary doctorate. She continues to write and also does consulting work.

Whereas nursing care of the elderly is a recent professional interest, promoting conceptual models for nursing has predominated since 1970. She strongly feels that "nursing practice, education, and research must be based on an explicit frame of reference specific to nursing."

Adam's work makes an important distinction between a conceptual model and a theory. "A (conceptual) model is usually based on, or derives from, a theory... A model, emerging from a theory, may become the basis for a new theory." "A conceptual model, for whatever discipline, is not reality; it is a mental image of reality or a way of conceptualising reality. A conceptual model for nursing is therefore a conception of nursing."

Adam accepts Roy and Roberts' definition of a theory as "a system of interrelated propositions used to describe, predict, explain, understand, and control a part of the empirical world."

Therefore a theory is useful to more than one discipline. A conceptual model for a discipline is useful only to that particular discipline. Adam believes "The day may come when nursing theory will be as useful to related disciplines as existing theories, developed in other fields, are today useful to nursing."

Adam writes that "a conceptual model is an abstraction, a way of looking at something, an invention of the mind."

A conceptual model for a discipline is a very broad perspective, a global way of looking at a discipline. Most of the conceptual models for nursing that we know have come from two sources: one, a theory, chosen by the author, and the other, her professional experience.

A conceptual model is the precursor of a theory. The model specifies the discipline's focus of inquiry, identifies those phenomena of particular interest to nursing, and provides a broad perspective for nursing research, practice, and education. The study of phenomena that concern nursing, that is, nursing research, may lead to theories that will describe, explain, or predict those phenomena. Such theories will not be theories of nursing but theories of phenomena that are nursing's focus of inquiry.

Many nurses are unable to communicate clearly and explicitly their conception of the service they offer to society. Adam contends this is not because they do not have a conception of nursing but because they do not have a conception of nursing but because their conceptual base is not clear. If the nurse's mental image of nursing is vague or blurred, it will therefore be difficult to put into words. The nurse will then be unable to articulate her particular role in health care and may well find that her professional activities are based on a perspective borrowed from another discipline.

Adam states that "a model indicates the goal of our (nursing) profession–an ideal and limited goal, because it gives us direction for nursing practice, nursing education, and nursing research." Nurses who have a clear, concise conceptual base specific to nursing will be able to identify areas for theory development, prepare future practitioners of nursing, and demonstrate in their own practice nursing's contribution to health care. In this way health care will improve and the nursing profession will grow.

Although it is not necessary for every nurse to adopt the same conceptual model, it is essential that every nurse have a concise and explicit framework on which to base her work. The conceptual model is "the conceptual departure point" for her teaching, research or nursing care. Speaking figuratively, Adam places the conceptual model in the nurse's occipital lobe, known also as her visual lobe. The nurse uses a great deal of scientific knowledge as well as her experience, intuition, and creativity. In drawing on this knowledge, she is guided by her conceptual model, that is, her mental image of nursing.

The abstraction that is the conceptual model is linked to the reality that is nursing practice through the nursing process. The data we collect depend on our conceptual base. The way we interpret the data, the plan we develop, the nursing action we choose, and the evaluation of our intervention also depend on our model. The number of steps in the nursing process is not significant because the difference is the conceptual base.

In addition to the conceptual model and the nursing process, the nurse must also establish with the client what will be perceived to be a helping relationship. Adam considers this perhaps the most important component of being a nurse. It is the climate of empathy, warmth, mutual respect, caring, and acceptance that determines the effectiveness of nursing care.

Adam feels that three components constitute nursing practice: the client, the nurse (with her conceptual model as a base for the nursing process), and the relationship between the client and nurse. She has created a pictorial representation of nursing practice in her books (Fig. 26.1).

Adam insists that the helping relationship and the systematic process (which nurses have, perhaps wrongly, labelled the "nursing" process) are important to all health professionals. Nursing fits into the whole of health care as an integral component of the interdisciplinary health team. Each discipline makes a unique contribution to the promotion and preservation of health and to the prevention of health problems. Although some services overlap within this interdisciplinary health team, each discipline is

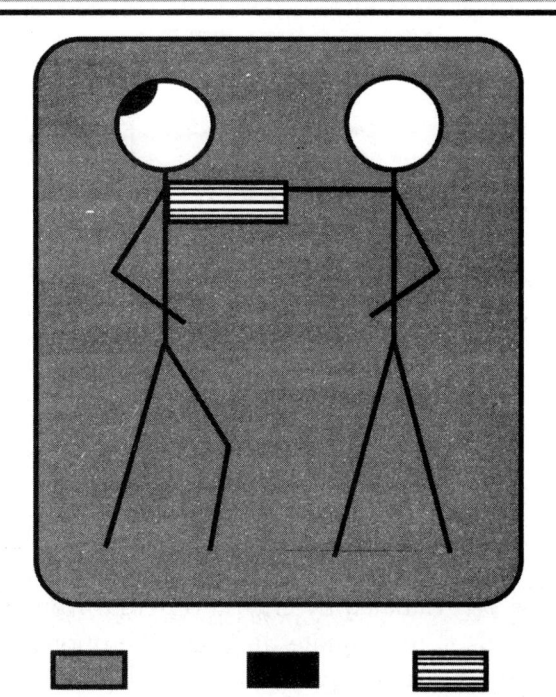

Figure 26.1: Pictorial representation of nursing practice

present because of its distinct and specific contribution to health.

This relationship can be illustrated with a schematic flower (Fig. 26.2). Each petal represents a distinct health discipline: nursing, medicine, physical therapy, speech therapy, or nutrition, for example. The center of the flower indicates the shared functions. A part of each petal is separate and distinct from the others, and the largest part of each petal represents the unique contribution of each discipline. Our conceptual model clarifies and makes explicit nursing's "petal."

Nurses currently have several conceptual models from which to choose. The decision to adopt one of the conceptual models for (not of) nursing is often made by considering the eventual evaluation of that particular model. Adam insists that conceptual models

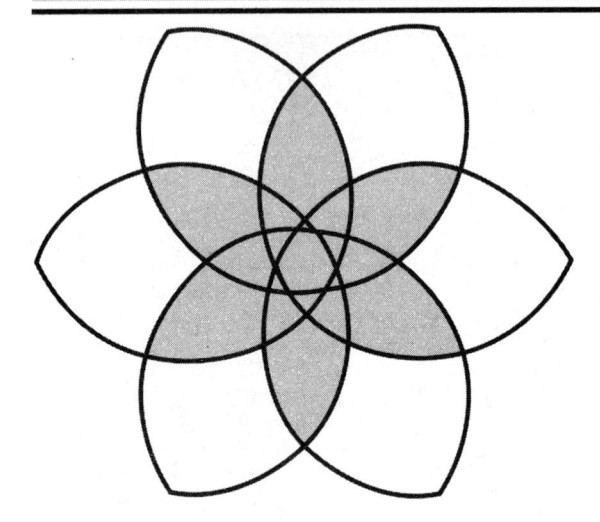

Figure 26.2: Interdisciplinary health team

must be evaluated by criteria different from these used to evaluate theories. She quotes the three criteria established by Dorothy Johnson:

1. *Social significance.* Clients would be asked if the service (nursing) was significant to their health.

2. *Social congruence.* Clients would be asked if the service (nursing) was congruent with their expectations.

3. *Social utility.* Nurses would be asked if the conceptual model provided useful direction for education, practice, and research.

Such criteria are extrinsic to the model itself. However, in order to use these criteria the conceptual model in question must already have been adopted in practice, education, and research settings. A vicious cycle may develop because some nurses may hesitate to adopt a model until it has been evaluated, and it cannot be evaluated until it has been adopted. Adam recognizes a model can be evaluated intrinsically for content, logic, and other criteria that will help nurses choose one model rather than another. However, the social decisions (extrinsic criteria) constitute the definitive evaluation of the conceptual base of a service profession.

Adam's conviction that every nurse should have a conceptual base specific to nursing rather than one borrowed from another discipline has led her to publish many articles and books, to speak at professional meetings, and to teach courses on this subject. She feels that the existing models are often viewed as being too abstract or too complex and therefore beyond the understanding of many nurses. Adam published *Etre Infirmiere* and *To Be a Nurse* to help nurses understand the writings of Virginia Henderson. She accomplished this by placing Henderson's concept of nursing within the structure of a conceptual model and by developing and refining the subconcepts identified by Henderson.

This model Adam developed in her book, is not a theory, but it does suggest areas for theory development. In this *To Be a Nurse*, Adam explains the essential elements of a conceptual model as presented by Dorothy Johnson. She then develops Virginia Henderson's concepts model.

EVOLUTION OF THEORY

Adam says she chose to work with Henderson's concept of nursing for two reasons. First, she felt that Henderson's was "partly known but badly known," that is, incompletely known or understood, even though many nurses were acquainted with it. She hoped that her own publications would contribute to the recognition of Henderson's work as a useful conceptual base for nursing practice, research, and education. In addition, she felt that Henderson's work was more immediately accessible than other works, because the language was already familiar to nurses. Adam "is not saying that Henderson's frame of reference is any better, or more useful, or more significant or more congruent than others. Such an evaluation has not yet been done . . . but it seems more immediately accessible."

Adam's concern for the need for an explicit conceptual model for nursing was developed when she was a student of Dorothy Johnson. It was also through Johnson that Adam became familiar with the structure of a conceptual model: assumptions, values, and major units. Adam believes Johnson was the first nurse to avail herself of that structure, which was already being used in fields such as sociology, psychology, and mathematics.

In choosing Virginia Henderson's writings as the basis of her conceptual model, Adam accepted the scientific principles on which Henderson based her work. The chapter on Virginia Henderson discusses the contribution of Claude Bernard's principle of physiological balance and Abraham Maslow's hierarchy of needs. Because Adam did not change the basic content but merely developed it further, this empirical foundation also is unchanged.

In the previous section of this chapter the source of the structure (assumptions, values, and six major units) was identified as sociology, mathematics, and other sciences. This structure has been extensively used in several sciences so it has good reliability.

Concepts Used by Adam

- *Assessment tool* Instrument that the professional uses in collecting information about the beneficiary; the nursing history tool; the data collection tool.
- *Assumption* The theoretical or scientific basis of a conceptual model; the premises which support.
- *Beneficiary* The second major unit of a conceptual model; the person or group of persons, toward whom the professional directs her activities; the client; the patient.
- *Change* A substitution of one thing in place of another; an alteration.
- *Collection of data* The first step of the nursing process; the collecting of information about the client; the client's nursing history.
- *Concept* An idea; a mental image; a generalization formed and developed in the mind.
- *Conception* A way of conceptualising a reality; an invention of the mind; a mental image. Depending on its level of abstraction, a conception may be a philosophy, a theory or a conceptual model.
- *Conceptual model* An abstraction or a way of conceptualising a reality; a theoretical frame of reference sufficiently explicit so as to provide direction for a particular discipline; a conception made up of assumptions, values, and major units.
- *Conceptual model for nursing* A mental representation, concept, or conception of nursing that is sufficiently complete and explicit so as to provide direction for all fields of activity of the nursing profession.
- *Consequences* The sixth major unit of a conceptual model; the results of the professional's efforts to attain the ideal and limited goal.
- *Goal of the profession* The first major unit of a conceptual model; the end that the members of the profession strive to achieve.

- *Helping relationship* The interaction between the beneficiary (the helpee) and the professional (the helper) that aids the helpee to live more fully; the interpersonal exchange in which the helper illustrates such facilitating qualities as empathy, respect, and others.
- *Intervention* The fifth major unit of a conceptual model; the focus and modes of the professional's intervention [In the context of the nursing process, the intervention is the fourth step (implementation of the plan of action or the nursing action itself).]
- *Intervention focus* part of the fifth major unit of a model; the focus, or center, of the professional's attention at the moment he intervenes with a client.
- *Intervention modes* part of the fifth major unit; the means or ways of intervening at the professional's disposal.
- *Major units* The six essential components of a complete and explicit conception.
- *Need* A requirement; a necessity.
- *Need, fundamental* A requirement common to all human beings, well or ill.
- *Need, individual* A specific, particular, or personal requirement that derives from a fundamental need.
- *Nursing care plan* A written plan of action; the written communication that comes from the second and third steps of the nursing process; a plan to be followed; a projection of what is to be done.
- *Nursing process* A methodical, systematic way of proceeding toward an action; a dynamic and logical method; a five-step process.
- *Practice* One of the three fields of activity of a service profession (the other two being education and research); the field of activity of the administrator and the practitioner of the service.
- *Problem* A difficulty to be reduced or removed.
- *Problem-solving method* The scientific process of solving problems; the systematic manner of proceeding used to solve problems.
- *Role* The third major unit of a conceptual model; the part played by the professional; the societal function of the professional.
- *Source of difficulty* The fourth major unit of a conceptual model; the probable origin of the client difficulty with which the professional is prepared to cope.
- *Values* The value system underlying a conceptual model.

In developing Henderson's work into a conceptual model, Adam described the goal of nursing as maintaining or restoring the client's independence in the satisfaction of his 14 fundamental needs. The nurse plays a complementary-supplementary role, complementing and supplementing the client's strength, knowledge, and will.

The nurse has a unique province, although she shares certain functions with other health professionals. Society wants and expects the nurse to provide her unique service.

In this model the person is portrayed as a complex whole, made up of 14 fundamental needs. Each need has biological, physiological, and psychosociocultural dimensions. When a need is not satisfied, the person is not complete, whole, or independent. The nurse's client may also be a family or a group. The concept of environment is specifically addressed in only one of the fundamental needs. However, environment is implicit in all the fundamental needs because the sociocultural dimension is integral to each need.

Health is not defined separately in *To Be a Nurse*. But Adam uses this term in discussing the goal of nursing. She says, "The goal of nursing is to maintain or to restore the client's independence in the satisfaction of his fundamental needs. This goal, congruent with the goal common to the entire health team, makes clear the nurse's specific contribution to the preservation and improvement of health." Since an entirely satisfactory definition of health is still a subject of debate, it behooves each health discipline to make explicit its particular contribution to health.

Assertions of this Model

In the description of the conceptual model's major units, the relationships among the basic concepts can be seen in the elements Adam has labelled beliefs and values. She feels these constitute the why of the model and must be shared by all who use the model. Values are not subject to the criteria of truths, but must reflect the values of the larger society nursing wishes to serve.

1. "The nurse has a unique function, although she shares certain functions with other professionals." The nurse must have a conceptual model in order to have a distinct professional identity and to assert herself as a colleague of the other health team members.
2. "When the nurse takes over the physician's role, she delegates her primary function to inadequately prepared personnel." The nurse who strives to assume the physician's role will relinquish the nurse's role to some other care provider who may not have the skills and the knowledge base required for nursing.
3. "Society wants and expects this service (nursing) from the nurse and no other worker is as able, or willing to give it." Nursing owes its existence to the fact that it fulfils a societal need, as does any service profession.

Nursing Implications

Practice

Basing her practice on this conceptual model, the nurse is seen in a complementary-supplementary role, and her goal is client independence in the satisfaction of his needs. The model serves as a guide for using the nursing process and the problem-solving method. Guided by the 14 fundamental needs, the practitioner, in whatever setting, will assess the independence of the client in need satisfaction. She will then identify his specific needs; determine the source of difficulty; and plan the intervention to complement client strength, will, or knowledge. After the care is given, it is evaluated in reference to the client's objectives–have the specific needs been satisfied and has the client's independence been increased? A *nursing problem*—a client's health problem requiring a nurse's intervention—is a dependency problem in need satisfaction. A *nursing diagnosis* is a specific need that is unsatisfied because of insufficient strength, will, or knowledge. Criteria for identifying specific needs have been developed. According to Adam, the nurse "carried out the social mission of contributing to the public's improved health by working toward greater client independence."

Education

Adam discusses the educational objectives and goals and the programme content in *To Be a Nurse*. She states, "Following Henderson's concept of nursing, the nursing curriculum is planned to prepare a health worker capable of maintaining and restoring the client's independence in the satisfaction of his fundamental needs." With this concept, a student learns the complementary-supplementary role. Adam divides the programme into official and unofficial content, both of equal importance. Unofficial content "covers everything that is learned in an educational programme without being taught." Official content "is formally recognized and actually taught." Official content is further divided into nursing and nonnursing.

According to Henderson's frame of reference, nursing content includes:
1. The goal of nursing, which is to preserve or re-establish the client's independence in the satisfaction of his basic needs.
2. The detailed description of the 14 fundamental needs, each with its biological, physiological, psychological, social, and cultural dimensions.
3. The individual variations in fundamental needs.
4. The various problems of dependence originating from a lack of strength, will, or knowledge.
5. The explanation of the complementary-supplementary role.
6. The description of the various needs of intervention.
7. The study of the desired consequences: continued or increased independence and, in certain circumstances, a peaceful death.
8. The study of the systematic process and the problem-solving method as applied to nursing.

Essential subject matters, regardless of the conceptual model for nursing, are "the helping relationship, the concept of health and the history of nursing."

The theoretical courses, in the nonnursing content, include anatomy, physiology, pathology, psychology, sociology, and anthropology. In relation to Henderson's model, the first three relate to the biophysiological dimension and the last three to the psychosociocultural aspect of the fundamental needs.

Subject matter derived from the conceptual model's assumptions is "the concepts of independence and dependence; the concepts of universal and individual human needs, hierarchy of human needs, and need satisfaction; and the concept of wholeness."

The practical aspect of nursing content consists of technical procedures and clinical experiences. Techniques are important in the complementary-supplementary role because the nurse is assisting the client in those activities that cannot be completed because of insufficient strength, will, or knowledge. Techniques help pursue the goal of client independence in the satisfaction of his needs. Adam feels that the student with opportunities to help a client recover his independence in the satisfaction of his basic needs."

Although the level of education may increase, the model remains the conceptual base. The baccalaureate student's formal education will help her identify complex and subtle specific needs, find new ways of complementing and supplementing, and form and continue a helping relationship. Master's level students learn to be specialists in independence nursing or in the teaching and administration of independence nursing. Doctoral students may use the concept of independence in need satisfaction as a basis of research for theory development.

Research

Adam posed 12 questions from the conceptual model for research development. These include:
1. How can client independence be measured?
2. How can his degree of dependence be qualified?
3. What dependency problems are solved by what nursing interventions?
4. At what point must the intervention be discontinued if independence is to be promoted?
5. How can certain interventions be made more easily acceptable?
6. How can the nurse determine how much intervention is enough?
7. What dependency problems are most often encountered among selected groups, e.g. cancer patients, the aged, the mentally confused?
8. How does pain, anxiety, etc. affect independence?
9. How can linguistic barriers be overcome?
10. How can the nurse help certain ethnic or socio-economic groups to be independent?
11. How can the nurse increase client participation in health care?
12. Is the conceptual model socially useful, significant, and congruent?

Adam, states that various clinical and educational settings in Canada are at varying stages of basing nursing care and teaching on her model and research for a small number of master's theses has been based on it. Correspondence received from Canada, the United States and abroad indicates her books have received very favourable reviews.

Adam has used the structure of a conceptual model that was useful in various other sciences before being introduced into nursing. The essential elements of a model for a helping or service profession follow.

Assumptions The assumptions are "the suppositions that are taken for granted by those who wish to use the model; they are the 'how' of the model, its foundation."

Beliefs and Values The beliefs and values "constitute the 'why' of the model and are not subject to the criteria of truth." They must "reflect the value system of the larger society that the profession wishes to serve" and "be shared by the members of the profession who wish to use the model."

Major Units The major units "are the 'what' of the conceptual model." They "make clear what nursing is in any setting and at any time."

Ideal and Limited Goal The ideal and limited goal of the profession is "*ideal* because it represents the ideal that all members of the profession would like to achieve and *limited* because it delineates the parameters of the profession."

Beneficiary The beneficiary of the professional service is "that person or group of persons toward whom the professional directs his attention." "The nurse must have a clear mental image of her client – whether he is well or ill."

Role of the Professional The role of the professional is "the role in society played by the members of the discipline."

Source of Difficulty of the Beneficiary The source of difficulty of the beneficiary "refers to the probable origin of the client's difficulty; one with professional, because of his education and experience, is prepared to cope." "The probable origin of those client problems which the nurse is prepared to solve must be made explicit."

Intervention

- *Intervention focus* The focus or center of the intervention is "the focus of the professional's attention at the moment he intervenes with the client. The patient or beneficiary is perceived as an extremely complex individual; however, within that complexity only one aspect can receive all the professional's attention at any given moment. . . No one person can do everything at the same time."
- *Intervention modes* The modes of intervention "are the means the professional has at his disposal to intervene. . . A conceptual model for nursing will indicate what means are at the nurse's disposal when she intervenes as a health professional."

Consequences

The consequences "are the desired results of the professional activities and must be congruent with the ideal goal."

Adam has developed Henderson's concept of nursing into a conceptual model for nursing by placing Henderson's writings in the structure of a model. She has supplied the logical form that was less apparent in Henderson's work. Through the logical form of the resulting conceptual model, clear direction is provided to nursing practitioners, educators, and researchers.

Through the use of the structure that comprises a conceptual model and Henderson's writings, it may be said that Adam used the deductive form of logical reasoning.

Although no empirical evidence has been collected for theories deriving from this model, Adam feels it could be the basis for theory development. As with other conceptual models for nursing, this one specifies nursing's focus of inquiry. From Henderson's conceptual departure point of independence in need satisfaction, descriptive and experimental studies could be carried out to result in the identification of descriptive terms peculiar to the concept under scrutiny. The identification of descriptive terms is the first step in theory development. Possible developments might be a theory of need satisfaction or a theory of complementing knowledge or of supplementing motivation in specific client populations. Such theories would not be theories of nursing, but theories of the phenomena that concern nursing.

"Nurse theorist will of course look at phenomena that interest other disciplines as well. They must, however, study them from a nursing perspective if they want to develop nursing theory." "For example, if pain were studied from Henderson's perspective, it would be examined as a phenomenon that interferes with client independence in need satisfaction."

In a letter of February 16, 1988, Evelyn Adam states, "Some Ontario colleges and clinical settings are showing increasing interest in basing their practice and teaching on Henderson's model as I presented it. It is still popular in Quebec and in the Atlantic provinces. Graduate students often quote it as their conceptual departure point, i.e., to justify their research project. They seldom seek to develop it."

EVALUATION OF THEORY

- The essential elements listed by Adam give the appearance of a simple conceptual model. However, on closer inspection, we find that the number of subconcepts produces a complex picture. The interrelatedness of the components necessary for the care of the whole client also adds to the complexity of the model. The concepts presented are clearly defined and easy to follow.
- The assumptions, values, and major units involve nursing and clients in all aspects of society. They are not limited to age, medical diagnosis, or health care setting. Each of the 14 basic needs has biophysiological and psychosociocultural aspects.
- Although testing of the model is unavailable at this time, it appears to have the potential for a high degree of empirical precision. This is related to its reality base and designated subconcepts.
- Because of the empirically based concepts and broad scope, the model is potentially applicable to nursing practice, education, and research.
- Adam's work in developing the conceptual model is unique in that she has taken Henderson's previously existing concept of nursing and presented it within the previously existing structure of a model. The result is something more than the sum of the two. It is a complete, concise, explicit conceptual model. Adam then clarified the interrelatedness of the model, the process, and the client-nurse relationship. Making a clear distinction between model and theory, Adam explained the impact of the model on nursing research, practice, and education.

Adam states that "the adoption of a conceptual will not solve all of nursing's problems." A conceptual model makes explicit nursing's particular contribution to health care and provides nurses a professional identity and a conceptual point of departure.

It would seem that every nurse who adopts a concise and explicit conceptual model is a potential nursing theorist. A nurse who is able to articulate the scope of nursing practice would be more likely to identify areas for nursing theory development and nursing research. Imagine that the majority of nurses have an explicit conceptual model, that is, a conceptual departure point for theory development, and are able and willing to provide written documentation that would become the basis for empirical evidence. This opens the door to a marked increase in nursing theory and knowledge.

Chapter 27

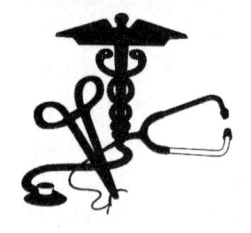

Parse's Man-Living-Health Theory

Our lives are comprised of situations diverse in richness and magnitude. Much of what adds colour to our daily existence slides by us almost unperceived. Other happenings stand out much more sharply and mark our passage through life-educational achievements, employment, close relationships, defining experiences, professional networks, academic networks.

The unfolding of **Rosemarie Rizzo Parse's** Man-Living-Health theory is inseparable from the lesser and greater situations that comprise her life. The idea for Man-Living-Health, Parse recalled, "began many years ago when I began to wonder and wander and ask way not? The theory itself surfaced in me in Janusian fashion over the years in interrelationship with others primarily through my lived experience in nursing. Numerous "predecessors, contemporaries, and successors" helped Parse see her idea more clearly. "Yet the theory has only begun to be viewed and enhanced by those who take up the challenge to evolve nursing science to a higher level of complexity and specificity."

Parse received her nursing education in Pittsburgh. Her master's and doctorate in nursing and higher education were earned at the University of Pittsburgh. At the time she was developing her theory, Parse was Dean of the School of Nursing at Duquesne University the Pittsburgh. At about this same time-during the 1960s and 1970s-Duquesne was regarded as the center of the existential-phenomenological movement in the United States. Dialogues she had with those in this school of thought stimulated and focussed her thinking.

Currently, Parse is president of Discovery International, Inc., an organization she founded to promote excellence in nursing science. This firm provides consultation services, seminars, and health guidance to individuals, families, and communities. She is also Professor or Graduate Nursing and Coordinator of the Center for Nursing Research at Hunter College, City University of New York, as well as editor of the scholarly journal *Nursing Science Quarterly*.

Her research activities and interests are wide-ranging. A partial listing includes lived experiences of hope, laughter, health, aging, and quality of life

EVOLUTION OF THEORY

Parse's theoretical sources are a major reason her theory is regarded as unique for nursing. By synthesizing the Science of Unitary Human Beings, as developed by Martha E. Rogers, and existential-phenomenological thought, as articulated by Martin Heidegger, Jean-Paul Sartre, and Maurice Merleau-Ponty, Parse pushes nursing toward an unfragemented view of man. Man cannot be reduced to constituent systems of parts and still be understood, she declares. Man is "a living unity."

Moreover, Parse challenges the traditional view of nursing as an emerging natural science. Rightly understood, nursing is a human science. The thrust of her approach is clear:

A theory of nursing rooted in the human sciences is a system of interrelated concepts describing unitary man's interrelating with the environment while cocreating health. Essential to the theory is the man-environment interrelationship, coconstitution of health, the meaning unitary man gives to being and becoming, and man's freedom in each situation to choose alternative ways of becoming.

In developing her theory, Parse used Rogers' major principles of helicy, complimentarity (now called *integrality*), and resonancy, and her corresponding concepts of energy field, openness, pattern, and organization (Rogers has recently deleted organization) and four-dimensionality.

From existential-phenomenological thought, Parse drew the tenets of intentionality and human subjectivity and the corresponding concepts of coconstitution, coexistence, and situated freedom. *Intentionality* "means that in being human man is open, knows, and is present to the world. To be man, then, is to be intentional and to be involved with the world through a fundamental nature of knowing, being present and open. Human subjectivity indicates that "Man encounters the world and is present to it in a dialectical relationship. Man grows through this relationship, giving meaning to the projects that emerge in the process of becoming. Man coparticipates in the emergence of projects through choosing to live certain values." *Coconstitution* "refers to the idea that the meaning emerging in any situation is related to the particular constituents of that situation. Man interrelates with the various views of the world and others and indeed cocreates these views by a personal presence." *Coexistence* means that "man, an emerging being, is in the world with others. Man knows self in the comprehension of dispersed concrete achievements and through the perceptions of others. Without others one would not know that one is. *Situated freedom* indicates that "one participates in choosing the situations in which one finds oneself as well as one's attitude toward the situations. Man, therefore, is always choosing. This choosing occurs on two levels: prereflectively and tacitly, and reflectively and explicitly. "In choosing ways of being with situations, one expresses value priorities. Our choices, however, "are made without full knowledge of the outcomes yet with full responsibility for the consequences.

"Nursing does not have practice and research traditions of its own," observed Parse. "Quantitative and qualitative methods of research used to enhance nursing science presently flow from the natural sciences and from the human sciences, respectively, Because parse sees nursing as a human science, she has sought to enhance her theory by using descriptive research methodologies borrowed from the human sciences. One such methodology, phenomenology, has become increasingly important in recent years in nursing, psychology, and sociology. Because of its philosophical base, this research methodology fits well with Parse's theory. It is also congruent with the importance other nurse theorists (e.g., Leininger, Orlando, Patterson and Zderad, Peplau, Travelbee, Watson) have placed on understanding patients' unique perspectives in providing nursing care. But phenomenology broadens and deepens the notion of what it means to talk about and study an individual's unique point of view.

Parse creatively blended principles, tenets, and concepts from Rogers's Science of Unitary Human Beings and existential-phenomenological thought to craft the assumptions under-pinning Man-Living-Health. Each assumption "connects three specific concepts in a unique way." The three concepts Parse units in each assumption were drawn both from Rogers and from existential phenomenology. This underscores just how firmly Parse's theoretical sources undergird her theory. "To draw upon the work of these theorists, of course, is to build upon a solid foundation and to maintain a bridge to the past necessary in the establishment of any scientific theory."

Nursing

By proposing that nursing is a human science, Parse rejects the traditional view of nursing as an emerging natural science. She contends that nursing has paralleled medicine's development, echoing its themes. Man's participative experience with health situations has been virtually ignored," she declared. "Nursing, rooted in human sciences, focusses on Man as a living unity and Man's qualitative participation with health experiences." For nursing to evolve as a distinct discipline, it must move away from its medical model orientation.

Parse strongly affirms nursing's responsibility to society. "The responsibility to society relative to nursing practice is guiding the choosing of possibilities in the changing health process. Specifically, "Nursing practice is directed toward illuminating and mobilizing family interrelationships in light of the meaning assigned to health and its possibilities as languaged in the cocreated patterns of relating. *Family,* it should be noted, is used by Parse to signify those persons with whom we have close relationships.

Man

Man is a major reason for nursing's existence. (Another major reason, of course, is health). This has been the case since the time of Nightingale and the publication of her *Notes on Nursing.* In keeping with this tradition, Parse explicitly discussed Man in her assumptions. Man is integral to her theory's concepts principles, theoretical structures, and practice propositions-all of which flow directly from Man-Living-Health's assumptions. Parse hails Rogers as the first nurse theorist to reject the traditional "totality" paradigm and embrace the "simultaneity" paradigm. The totality paradigm views the human being "as a total, summative, organism whose nature is a combination of bio-psycho-social-spiritual features." In constant, the simultaneity patadignet views the human being "as more than and different from the sum of parts, changing mutually and simultaneously with the environment." For Parse, human beings evidence "a pattern of patterns of relating." Because we exist in the world with others, we cannot not relate. "When one person encounters another person, rhythmical patterns of relating unfold as words become sentences and are shared with a certain volume at a particular tempo with unique intonation, simultaneously with a certain gaze, gesture, touch, and posture. In this way, our perceptions of ourselves, others, and our situations emerge. As we live our own life stories and the historical story of our species, we grow more complex and diverse. Living simultaneously in all spheres of time-past, present, and future-we are influenced by our "ancestors, successors, and contemporaries through personal interrelationships, ideas, and future planning. They sharpen our sensitivity to life's rhythms-its joys and sorrows, aspirations and disappointments, births and deaths. We become aware of our mortality and the possible extermination of our species. Art and music heighten our awareness of death: through them we celebrate life and the mystery it holds for us. Human beings, then, experience life as an all-at-once multidimensional experience.

Health

For Parse, health is a lived experience. It is not the absence of disease or a sate of well-being, nor can it be placed on a continuum. "Man's health, then, is not a linear entity that can be interrupted or qualified by terms such as good, bad, more, or less. It is not man adapting to or coping with the environment. Such a description of health dichotomizes and denies man's unitary nature. Unitary man's health is a synthesis of values, a way of living." Health occurs as Man "structures meaning in Situations." It is a process of being and becoming.

Environment

"Man as a pattern and organization is distinct from the pattern and organization of the environment." But man and environment are inseparable. Interchanging energy, unfolding together towards greater complexity and diversity, influencing one another's rhythmical patterns of relating, they are a construct: Man-Environment. "Man and environment, then, interchange energy to create what is in the world, and man chooses the meaning given to the situations he creates.

Concepts Used by Parse

From the assumptions underpinning her theory, Parse drew three thematic elements: meaning, rhythmicity, and cotranscendence. She then deduced the three principles of Man-Living-Health.

Principle 1

Structuring meaning multidimensionally is cocreating reality through the language of valuing and imaging. The essential concepts of this principle are imaging, valuing, and languaging.

Meaning, the thematic element of Parse's first principle, "arises from Man's interrelationship with the world. It refers to both ultimate meaning and the meaning moments of everyday life. Ultimate meaning is our view of life's absolute purpose. It is usually expressed in religious or philosophical language. The meaning moments of everyday life are those common happenings to which we attach varying degrees of significance. We do so through the process of imaging, "the cocreating of reality that, by its very nature, structures the meaning of an experience.

Our worldview provides the framework for cocreating reality. Valuing "is Man's process of confirming cherished beliefs and is reflective of one's worldview. This confirming of beliefs is choosing from imaged options and owning the choices. Languaging is expressing valued images. It encompasses all modes of self-presentation, including the rhythmical patterns of speech and movement. Our rhythmical patterns of speech and movement reflect our cultural heritage as well.

Principle 2

Cocreating rhythmical patterns of relating is living the paradoxical unity of revealing-concealing, enabling-limiting while connecting-separating. The essential concepts are revealing-concealing, enabling-limiting, and connecting-separating.

This principle's thematic element, rhythmicity "is revealed as man and environment move toward greater diversity. Rhythmical patterns are cocreated in the man-environment interrelationship and are paradoxes lived all at once." Revealing-concealing "is the simultaneous disclosing of some aspects of self and hiding of others." When we disclose ourselves to another person, we gain knowledge about ourselves. Yet by moving in one direction, we are limited in another. This is the rhythmical pattern of enabling-limiting. "Man cannot be all possibilities at once, and, in choosing, one is both enabled and limited." To move in one direction and not in another involves reordering relationships. "Connecting-separating can be recognized as man is connecting with one phenomenon and simultaneously separating from others. In separating from one phenomenon and dwelling with another, a person integrates thought, becomes more complex, and seeks new unions."

Principle 3

Cotranscending with the possibles is powering unique ways of originating in the process of transforming. The essential concepts of this principle are powering, originating and transforming.

Cotranscendence, the thematic element of Parse's third principle, "is the process of reaching out beyond self to the not-yet." This process "is powered through origination in transforming." Powering "is a continuous rhythmical process incarnating one's intentions and actions in moving toward the possibilities." Its rhythm is pushing-resisting, creating a tension, which, when changed, sometimes conflicts. When conflict surfaces, one is faced with new possibilities from which to choose in moving toward the future. Creating unique ways of living is originating. Man originates in mutual energy interchange with the environment. "Powering ways of originating is man distinguishing self from others." Transforming is man moving towards greater diversity through living new imaged possibilities and transcending the present. Parse calls transforming "the changing of change, coconstituting anew in a deliberate way." Sarter views of principles as representing the three aspects of consciousness: knowing, feeling, and willing.

Assertions of Theory

Parse's theoretical structures flow directly from Man-Living-Health's assumptions and principles. Each structure interrelates three concepts (Fig. 27.1). As the purpose of the theoretical structures is to guide nursing practice and research, Parse invites their validation in these areas. Man-Living-Health's theoretical structures are:

1. Powering is a way of revealing and concealing imaging.
2. Originating is a manifestation of enabling and limiting valuing.
3. Transforming unfolds in the languaging of connecting and separating.

Other theoretical structures may be derived, Parse noted.

In 1987, Parse expressed her theoretical structures as practice propositions at the next lower level of abstraction. As a practice proposition, the first theoretical structure "can be stated as *struggling to live goals discloses the significance of the situation*"; the second as "*creating a new shows one's cherished beliefs and leads in a directional movement*"; and the third as

The person is unitary—that is, an indivisible being who interrelates with the environments while cocreating health. Theoretic assumptions synthesize the concepts of energy filed, openness, pattern and organization, four dimensionality helicy, integrality, coconstitution, coexistence, and situated freedom with tenets of human subjectivity and intentionality. Assumptions (nine in the 1981 book were reduced to three in the 1987 article) state that man is a recognizable pattern who evolves simultaneously with environment. Man environment relationships are such that a continuity of what was and what will be unfolds in the now. Man chooses the meaning given to cocreated situations and is responsible for choices made. Unitary man is recognized by individual patterns of relating, which are cocreated in man-environment interchange. There is mutual man-environment interrelatedness as man chooses to move towards irreversible possibilities.

Principle 1: Structuring meaning multidimensionally is co-creating reality through the languaging of valuing and imaging

Principle 2: Cocreating rhythmical patterns of relating is living the paradoxical unity of revealing-concealing and enabling-limiting while connecting separating

Principle 3: Cotranscending with the possibles is powering unique ways of originating in the process of transforming

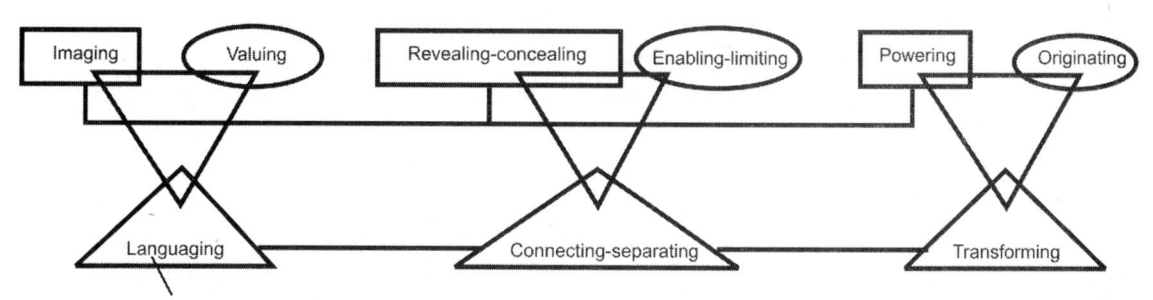

Relationship of the concepts in the squares:
Relationship of the concepts in the Ovals:
Relationship of the concepts in the triangles:

Powering is a way of revealing and concealing imaging
Originating is a manifestation of enabling and limiting valuing
Transforming unfolds in the languaging of connecting and separating

Figure 27.1: Relationship of principles, concepts, and theoretical structures of man-living-health

Man experiences in multiple dimensions simultaneously and relatively. The negentropic interchange of man-environment both enables and limits becoming.

Health is an open process of becoming, an incarnation of man's choosings. As man and environment connect and separate, health is cocreated. Thus health is a synthesis of values cocreated in open interchange with environment. Health is a continuous process of transcending with the possibles—that is, reaching beyond the actual. Health is an emergent: a negentropic unfolding. The theory of man-living -health emerges from the stated assumptions, and three principles are notable: (i) structuring meaning multidimensionally is cocreating reality through the languaging of valuing and imaging, (ii) cocreating rhythmic patterns of relating is living the paradoxical unity of revealing-concealing and enabling-limiting while connecting-separating, and (iii) cotranscending with the possibles is powering unique ways or originating in the process of transforming.

Principle 1 asserts that reality is continually cocreated by assigning meaning to all-at-once experiences occurring multidimensionally. Imaging, valuing, and languaging serve to structure meaning multidimensionally. *Principle 2* asserts that there is an unfolding cadence of coconstituting ways of being. Ways of being are recognized in the man-environment interchange and are lived rhythmically. Rhythms of revealing-concealing, enabling-limiting, and connecting-separating are integral in the principles. The final principle asserts that concepts of cotranscending with the possibles—powering, originating, and transforming—are man's ways of aspiring toward the "not-yet." Three theoretic structures are posited: (i) powering is a way of revealing and concealing imaging, (ii) originating is a manifestation of enabling and limiting valuing, and (iii) transforming unfolds in the languaging of connecting and separating.

Parse's theoretic sources are a major reason, her theory is regarded as unique for nursing. Her unique theory of Nursing titled "Man-Living-Health" (1981), which synthesized principles and concepts from Rogers' (1970/84) and concepts and tenets from existential phenomenology. She said that man refers to 'Homosapiens,' a generic term for all human beings. Parse challenged the traditional view of nursing as an emerging natural science. Rightly understood, nursing as a human science. The trust of her approach is clear.

"A theory of nursing rooted in the human science is a system of interrelated concepts describing unitary man's interrelation with the environment while cocreating health. Essential to the theory is the man-environment interrelationship, coconstitutions of health, the meaning of unitary man gives to being and becoming and man's freedom in each situation to choose alternative ways of becoming."

In developing her theory, parse used Rogers major principles of helicy, complimentary (now called integrality) and resonancy, and her corresponding concepts of energy filed, openness, pattern and organization. From existential phenomenological through Parse drew the tenets of intentionality and human subjectivity and corresponding concepts of coconstitution, coexistence and situated freedom.

- Intentionality means that in being human man is open, knows, and is presented to

he world. To be man, then, is to be intentional, and to be involved with the world through a fundamental nature of knowing, being present and open.
- Human subjectivity indicates that "Man encounters the world and is present to it in a dialectical relationship. Man grows through this relationship, giving meaning to the projects that emerge in process of becoming. Man coparticipates in the emergence of projects through choosing to live certain values.
- Coconstitution refers to this idea that meaning emerging in any situation is related to the particular constituents of the situation. Man inter-relates with the various views of the world with others, and indeed cocreates these views by a personal presence.
- Coexistence means that man an emerging being, is in the world with others. Without other, one would not know that one is.
- Situated freedom indicated that one participates in choosing the situations in which one finds oneself as well as one's attitude toward the situation. This choosing occurs on two levels. i.e. prereflectively and tacitly and reflectively and explicitly.

Assumptions of Theory

Parse treats man, environment and health as constructs, her assumptions defy classification (Nursing is not a concept per se; it is the scientific endeavour described by the concepts; it is the discipline itself). Accordingly, parse (1981) original nine assumptions with relatedness are the following:
1. Man is coexisting while coconstituting rhythmical patterns with the environment (concepts of coconstitution, coexistence and pattern and organization.
2. Man is an open being, freely choosing meaning in situations and bearing responsibility for decisions (concepts of situated freedom, openness and energy filed).
3. Man is living unity continuously coconstituting patterns of relating (concepts of energy filed, coconstitution, and pattern and organization).
4. Man is transcending multidimensionally with possible (concepts of openness, coconstitution and situated freedom).
5. Health is an open process of becoming, experienced people (concepts of openness, coconstitution, and situated freedom).
6. Health is a rhythmically coconstituting process of the man-environment inter-relationship (concepts of coconstitution, pattern and organization, and four dimensionality).
7. Health is man's pattern of relating value priorities (concepts of pattern and organization, openness, and situated freedom).
8. Health is an intersubjective process of transcending with the possibles (concepts of coexistence, openness, and situated freedom).
9. Health is unitary man's negentrophic unfolding (concepts of coexistence energy filed, and four dimensionality).

The original assumption now (1992) reads as four assumptions concerning to human and five assumptions concerning becoming. They are:

Human Assumptions

1. The human is coexisting while coconstituting rhythmical patterns with the universe.

2. The human is open being, freely choosing meaning in situation, bearing responsibility for decisions.
3. The human is a living unity continuously coconstituting pattern of relating.
4. The human is transcending multidimensionally with the possibles.

Becoming Assumptions

1. Becoming is a open process experienced by the human.
2. Becoming is a rhythmically coconstituting process of human-universe interrelationship.
3. Becoming is the human pattern of relating value priorities.
4. Becoming is an intersubjective process of transcending with possibilities.
5. Becoming is human unfolding.

Subsequently, Parse (1985) synthesized these nine assumptions into the three assumptions about Man-Living-Health. These three assumptions have also been revised to reflect Human becoming as follows:
1. Human Becoming (Man-Living-Health) is freely choosing personal meaning in situations in the intersubjective process of relating values priorities.
2. Human becoming (Man-Living-Health) is cocreating rhythmical patterns of relating in open interchange with the universe (environment)
3. Human-Becoming (Man-Living-Health is cotranscending multidimensionally with the unfolding possibles.

The first assumption states that Human-Becoming is a subject-to-subject, subject-to-universe interchange where the meanings assigned to the experience reflects one's personal values. This assumption appears to be a synthesis of number. Two, five, and seven of her original nine, which are based on the concept of energy field, openness, situated freedom, coconstitution and pattern and organization.

The second assumption states that Human Becoming is an open interchange with the universe and that together, the human being and the environment create rhythmical patterns. This assumption appears to be a synthesis of original assumption one, three, and six, which are based on the concept of energy field, openness, situated freedom, pattern and organization and cocostitution.

The third assumption states that Human becoming is moving beyond the self at all levels of the universe as a dream becoming realities. Parse defines cotranscending as a moving beyond with others and the universe multidimensionally. Multidimensionally refers to the various levels of the universe that human experience "all at once" and choose possibles from the various situations. This assumption appears to be a synthesis of original assumption four, eight, and nine, which are based on the concepts of openness, four dimensionality, situated freedom, coexistence and energy field.

Principles

As already stated earlier three main themes can be identified in Parse's (1987) assumptions: meaning, rhythmicity, and cotranscendence. She then deduced to the three principles of Man-Living-Health. Each leads to a principle of Human-Becoming.

Principle I

Structuring meaning multidimentionally is cocreating reality through the languaging of valuing and imaging.

The essential concept of the principle are imaging, valuing, and languaging. Imaging refers to knowing and includes both explicit and tacit knowledge; valuing is the process of living cherished beliefs while adding to one's personal world view. Languaging reflects images and values through speaking and movements using this principle. Nurses identify and guide individuals and families to relate the meaning of a situation by making the meaning more explicit.

Principle II

Cocreating rhythmical patterns of relating is living the paradoxical unity of revealing-concealing, enabling-limiting while connecting-separating.

The essential concepts are revealing-concealing, enabling-limiting, and connecting-separating. In interpersonal relationships, one reveals parts of the self but also conceals other parts. While making choices or decisions enables an individual in some ways but limits in others. Connecting-separating is a rhythmical process of moving together and moving part. The nurse does not try to calm or balance rhythms or attempts to help the family adapt, but integrates or synchronises the rhythms.

Principle III

Cotranscending with the possibles is powering unique ways of originating in the process of transforming.

The essential concepts of principles of powering, originating rhythm of which is the pushing-resisting of inter-human encounters. Transforming is defined as the changing of change. Nurse guides individuals and / or families to plan for the changing of lived health patterns.

Structures

The theoretical structures of the theory of human becoming are non-causal in nature and consistent with the assumptions and principles. They are designed to guide nursing practice and research. The three theoretical structures identified are:
1. Powering is a way of revealing and concealing imaging.
2. Originating is a manifestation of enabling-limiting, valuing.
3. Transforming unfolds in the languaging of connecting-separating.

In 1983 Parse expressed her theoretical structures at a less abstract level in order for them to be used to guide nursing practice. As a practice, proposition, the first theoretical structure "can be stated as struggling to live goals, discloses the significance of the situation" the second as "creating new show one's cherished beliefs and lead in a directional movement," and third, "changing views emerge in speaking and moving with others. Parse cautions however, that "details of nursing practice can only be specified in the context of particular nurse person and nurse group situations.

In the first theoretical structure, the nursing practice focus "is on illuminating the process of revealing-concealing unique ways a person or family can mobilize transcendence in considering new dreams, to image new possibilities." Parse describes a nurse-family situations in which members share their thought and feelings about a situation, which both reveals and conceals all they know about their struggle to personal goals. In disclosing the significance of the situation, the meaning of the situation changes for the family members and therefore the meaning changes for the favour.

In the second theoretical structures, the nursing practice focus with a person or family would be on illuminating ways of being alike and different from others in changing values. By synchronizing rhythms, the members discover opportunities and limitations created by the decisions made in choosing ways to be together. New ways of choices being together, mobilize transcendence.

In the third theoretical structures the nursing focus would be on illuminating the meaning of relating ways of being together as various changing perspectives shed different lighten the familiar, which gives rise to new possibles, synchronizing rhythm. In nurse-family situation, members relate their value through speech and movement which helps to mobilize transcend.

Paradigm and Parse Theory

Human Being

For Parse, human being evidences "a pattern of patterns of relating. Because we exist in the world with others, we cannot relate." When one person encounters another person, rhythmical patterns of relating unfold as words become sentences and are shared with a certain volume at a particular tempo with unique intonation, simultaneously with certain gaze, gesture, touch and posture. In this way, we perceive self and others. Parse's first four assumptions specifying the human being in mutual process with the universe, cocreating patterns of relating others." She states that the human being "lives at multidimensional realms of the universe all at once, freely choosing ways of becoming a meaning is given to situation.

Health

Parse describes health as a process of becoming that is experienced by the person, coconstituted through the human-universe experience, and incarnated as patterns of relating value priorities. Health is viewed by Parse "as a process of changing life's meanings, a personal power emerging from the individual collective relationships with others and the universe."

Nursing

Parse defines nursing as a scientific discipline, the practice of which is a performing art. She places nursing in the company of drama, music, and dance in each of which, the artist creates something unique. The knowledge base of the discipline is the science of the art, and the performance is the art creatively lived (1992). She states that nursing responsibility to society is in the guiding of individuals and families in choosing possibilities in changing the health process, which is accomplished by inter-subjective participation with people. She further states that nursing practice involves innovation and creativity which are not encumbered by prescriptive rules.

In Parse's theory, the nurse is an interpersonal guide, who acts in true presence, an active, energetic way of being with authority, responsibility and the consequences of decisions are accorded to the client. The traditional nursing roles of caregiver, advocate, counselor and leader to not appear to be congruent with Parse's views of nursing. Teaching however, is reflected in the dimension of illuminating meaning by explicating, and acting as a change agent is reflected in the dimension of mobilizing transcendence by moving beyond the meaning to what is not yet.

Parse (1989) proposes a set of fundamental essentials for fully practicing the art of nursing, which include the following.

- Know and use nursing frameworks and theories
- Be available to others
- Value the other as a human presence
- Respect difference in view
- Own what you believe and be accountable for your actions
- Move on the new and untested
- Connect with others
- Take pride in what you do
- Like what you do
- Recognize the moments of joy in the struggles of living
- Appreciate the mystery and be open to new discoveries
- Be competent in your chosen area
- Rest and begging new

She defines the contextual situation of nursing practice as being nurse-person or nurse-group participation. She does not define specific practice setting, but advises the nurse to approach the person/family as nurturing gardener, not as fix-it machinist.

Nursing process and theory of Parse does not tally directly.

PARSE'S WORK AND CHARACTERISTICS OF THEORY

1. Theories can interrelate concepts in such a way as to create a different way of looking at particular phenomena. Parse's theory of Human Becoming creates a new way of looking at human beings, health, environment, and nursing. Parse has synthesized Rogers' principles of helicy, complementarity (now called integrality), and resonancy, and her four concepts of openness, energy filed, pattern and organization, and four dimensionality (now called pan-dimensionality) with the tenets of existential-phenomenological thought. This synthesis created the nine assumptions upon which the theory is based.

    Parse's (1987) synthesis creates a theory in which humans are open beings who, with their universe, cocreate health. She views nursings as being rooted in the human sciences and having the goal of quality of life from the perspective of the person. In this worldview, the health-illness continuum is irrelevant as are care plans based on health problems. The authority, responsibility, and consequences of decision making reside with the person, not with the nurse. The nurse is presented as a guide who focusses on illuminating meaning, synchronizing rhythms, and mobilizing transcendence with the person or family relative to changing health patterns.

2. Theories must be logical in nature. Parse's theory of Human Becoming describes a logical sequence of events. Parse (1981) presents Rogers's principle and concepts as well as tenets and concepts from existential phenomenological thought. She then synthesizes these tenets, principles, and concepts to create her nine assumptions. Each assumption is based on three concepts. Six of the assumptions are based on two concepts from Rogers and one concept from existential-phenomenology: the other three assumptions are based on two concepts from existential-phenomenology and one concept from Rogers (Philips, 1987).

    Parse presented three assumptions about Human Becoming (formerly Man-Living-Health) (Parse, Coyne, and Smith, 1985) that are derived from the nine assumptions of the theory and flow from them with logical precision. The principles of the theory of Human becoming are derived from the assumptions, with each principles relating three concepts to each other.

Parse then derived three theoretical structures, each of which uses three concepts, one from each principles. She defines theoretical structure as a statement that interrelates concepts in a way that can be verified (Parse, 1992b). Philips (1987) points out that the stem of each theoretical structure is taken from the third principle. He speculates that greater importance might be attached to this principle but qualifies this thought by saying that Parse makes it clear that other theoretical structures may be generated from her principles.

Levine (1988), Philips (1987), and Winkler (1983) speak to the difficulty of Parse's terminology for those unfamiliar with existential phenomenology. They concur, however, that there is consistency in meaning at each level of discourse.

3. Theories should be relatively simple yet generalizable. Although Parse's theory can be generalized to any lived experience, it is far from simple. Bringing the theory from an abstract level to a practical level is complicated. Terminology that is difficult and unfamiliar to nurses is used and may be a cause of confusion. The range of possibilities that exists in the lived experiences of open, interrelating beings makes this theory inherently complex.

4. Theories can be bases for hypotheses that can be tested or for theory to be expanded. Because Parse's theory is rooted in the human sciences rather than the natural sciences, qualitative rather than quantitative research methodologies are used to expand it. Qualitative research methodologies do not pose hypothesis in the cause-effect or associative relationship tradition of quantitative research methods. Instead, qualitative research methods focus on entities for study that are lived experiences. (Parse, 1987).

Parse (1987) describes the theory of Human Becoming research methodology that includes the identification of major entities for study, the scientific processes of investigation, and the details of the processes appropriate for enquiry. She states that the two aspects of lived experience to consider in selecting an entity for study are nature and structure. The aspect of nature refers to common lived experiences that surface in the human-universe interrelationship and are health related; examples include "being-becoming, value priorities, negentropic unfolding, and quality of life." Parse cited the example of "waiting" as being consistent with her definition of a common lived experience.

The second aspect of lived experience to consider in selecting an entity for study is structure. Parse (1987) defines structure as "the paradoxical living of the remembered, the now moment, and the not-yet all at once." Thus, the research question could be: "What is the structure of the lived experience of waiting?." The researcher would then proceed to uncover the structure of this lived experience.

Whereas quantitative research methods test hypotheses or tentative assumptions about phenomena, the theory of Human Becoming research methodology explores questions about the lived experience.

5. Theories contribute to and assist in increasing the general body of knowledge within the discipline through the research implemented to validate them. The book *Nursing Research: Qualitative Methods* by Parse, Coyne, and Smith (1985) reports support of the theory of Human Becoming theory, through phenomenological, descriptive, and ethnographic methods. Five major qualitative studies are reported in this book. They focus on such topics as the phenomenology of health, persisting in change, the lived experience of being exposed to toxic chemicals, aging, and retirement. Parse states that these five studies demonstrate similar findings that are supportive of Human Becoming. She reports that meaning, rhythmicity, and transcendence, the major themes in her theory, can be seen in varying ways in all the studies.

    Published research studies guided by this theory have generated descriptive and theoretical structures about the lived experience of hope, the meaning of living with AIDS (Nokes and Carver, 1991), the drive to be ever thinner (Santopinto, 1989 b), recovering from addiction (Benonis, 1989), and living through unemployment (Smith 1990).

6. Theories can be used by practitioners to guide and improve their practice. As previously discussed, the theory of Human Becoming is not congruent with the traditional use of the nursing process. The theory of Human Becoming guides practice through its own practice methodology, which is composed of dimensions and processes. The dimensions are *Illuminating Meaning, Synchronizing Rhythms, and Mobilizing Transcendence* and the processes are *Explicating, Dwelling with and Moving Beyond* (Parse, 1987). A cardinal rule of this practice methodology is that the authority and responsibility for decision making lies with the person (client), not with the nurse.

    There is little doubt that use of Parse's theory would individualize nursing care. Critical care situations and situations where the client is unconscious require that the nurse have a deep understanding of the concept of true presence.

    Frik and Polluck (1993) report use of Parse's theory by graduate students practicing in chronic illness settings, a community mental health setting, and an emergency department. The theory was used in promoting compliance in adults with diabetes, implementing hypertensive screening in the emergency room, promoting effective coping skills related to drug abuse, and improving the nutrition of neurologically impaired adults.

    Mitchell (1991) reports successful use of Parse's theory on an acute medical-surgical unit. Cody and Mitchell (1992) report successful use of this theory by Jonas (1989) in an outpatient settings and by Santopinto (1989 a) in a long-term care setting. Cody and Mitchell report that nurses in all these studies reported initial difficulties in changing their approach to being with person and giving up the urge to apply the nursing process in the traditional manner. However, increased professional satisfaction convinced them of the validity of the new approach.

7. Theories must be consistent with other validated theories, laws and principles but will leave open unanswered questions that

need to be investigated. Parse's theory of Human Becoming is consistent with Roger's principles and concepts and with the tenets and a concept of existential-phenomenological thought. However, as Philips (1987) points out, Parse has synthesized these concepts and created a new product, which does not speak the same language as that of her sources.

Consistent with other nurse theories, Parse addresses the phenomena of human beings health, environment, and nursing. Although Parse's (1981) definition of human beings as an open being who cocreates health multidimensionally is unique, it is similar to that of other nurse theorists. Fitzpatrick (1989). Newman (1986), and Rogers (1992) speak to man and environment interacting to manifest health. Parse's view of the importance of the lived experience and quality of life is congruent with Paterson and Zderad (1976/1988), and Newman. As the theory of Human Becoming focusses on lived experiences, innumerable research questions can be posed for further investigation.

A strength of Parse's theory is the logical flow from construction of her assumptions to the deductive derivation of principles, theoretical structures.

Nursing Implications

Practice

Man-Living-Health presents an implicit guide for practice. Parse feels that nursing based on Man-Living-Health is quite unlike nursing based on other models. Winkler observed, "Basing care planning on the client's perspective of health and her/his care would encourage innovation in activities designated nursing, and acceptance of unique self-care activities."

In the original presentation of her theory, Parse discussed in detail a family situation and its implications from the perspective of her theory. In the example, she viewed nursing practice as an "intersubjective participation in guiding [the family] in the choosing of possibles in the changing health process."

Unlike some more established models, Man-Living-Health has not been used extensively in practice. Its practice methodology is evolving. Butler used the theory to change the health situation of a family facing the loss of its central figure following major neurosurgery. Papers on the theory's applicability to practice have been resented in the United States and Canada. Mitchell used Parse's theory to guide care for an elderly woman. In a replication of a study done by Parse in 1987, Santopinto is studying the difference Parse's theory makes in a practice setting.

Education

Parse writes for an audience composed of graduate students in nursing, faculty in schools of nursing, and nursing administrators in university and major health care settings. Her unwavering focus, however, is on master's and doctoral students-nursing's emerging scholars. They will be the ones most likely to share or adopt her perspective and conduct much of the research needed to develop her theory further. They will also use her model for curriculum development as they gain faculty rank.

In *Man-Living-Health: A Theory of Nursing*, Parse presented a sample masters'-in-nursing curriculum that incorporated the assumptions, principles, concepts, and theoretical structures of Man-Living-Health. She outlined in detail this process-based curriculum, including course descriptions and course sequencing.

Two courses in nursing theory are listed as focal courses in the curriculum, indicating the importance Parse attaches to theory and its development.

Research

Man-Living-Health has been validated by research. Six studies using qualitative methodologies-descriptive, phenomenological, and ethnographic-have been published. In addition to validating Parse's theory, these studies complemented each other. The authors explained the complementarity thusly.

The qualitative approach offers the researcher the opportunity to study the emergence of patterns in the whole configuration of Man's lived experiences. It is an approach in which the researcher explicitly participates in uncovering the meaning of these experiences as humanly lived.

Man-Living-Health has embedded in it countless research questions. A research methodology specifically designed to investigate these questions is evolving. The advantage of this theory-derived research methodology is the congruence of the approach with the belief system. Any theory-including this one-must be learned in detail before it can be used in research. This takes time. The qualitative research studies needed to develop the theory are another time-consuming process. Once completed, research may take up to 2 years before it is published. To broaden the theory's "circle of contagiousness," Parse has conducted several programmes in which results of research studies related to her theory have been presented. A number of master's theses have been completed using Parse's theory. Doctoral dissertations are beginning to be written using Man-Living-Health. For instance, Beauchamp is investigating the concept of power, specifically the decision by those who test positive for the HIV antibody to seek treatment. He is being assisted in this research by Marchette. Postdoctoral studies are in progress as well. Smith is investigating the lived experience of struggling through the difficulty of unemployment. Liehr and Flores are studying the human experience of "living on the edge." Participants in the study are persons who have suffered at least one cardiac arrest. To understand cocreating living on the edge, the study has been expanded to include participants' spouses. These studies are an important indication that more research related to Man-Living-Health will be forthcoming.

We can anticipate Man-Living-Health's continuing evolution. Ongoing research is expected to refine concepts, clarify interrelationships, and lead to higher levels of theory development. As schools of nursing adopt and teach Man-Living-Health, nurses can be expected to use it more in practice. As nurses use the theory in practice to guide patients through the changing health process, its usefulness will be more fully appreciated by society.

Unfortunately, many nurses avoid exploring this theory because of its very abstract language and philosophical base. Those who shun attempting to learn it forget that effort and discipline are required to move from "a state of understanding less to one of understanding more." Parse, Coyne, and Smith reframed this belief specifically for nursing when they wrote:

Learning the theory in scientific disciplines requires formal study, a reverence for quite contemplation, and creative synthesis. Neither Man-Living-Health nor the methodologies presented in this work can be learned quickly. The nature of the content compels the learner to abide with the conceptualizations and study the movements in discourse required by scholars who aspire to research and theory development in nursing.

EVALUATION OF THEORY

Man-Living-Health is an abstract and complex theory. It is a theory-and not a model-because its concepts and interrelationships have received empirical validation

- In keeping with theoretical discourse, Man-Living-Health's major concepts are defined by Parse in highly abstract and philosophical terms. Parse's use of quotations and references in *Man-Living-Health: A Theory of Nursing* rounded out the concepts and rendered them more understandable. The examples Parse cited were clear and simple. However, a first-time reader might be tempted to dismiss them as too simple to convey the complexity inherent in her theory. To do so, though, would be a mistake; lingering with her examples and drawing them out are more beneficial. Parse's principles, theoretical structures, and practice propositions clearly set for the interrelationships she sees, operating in the world. Consistent with the expectations we have of any scientific theory, Man-Living-Health has the potential to describe, explain, and predict.
- Man-Living-Health's conceptualization is broad in scope and applicable to individuals, families, or communities in change or crisis. To say, as Winkler did, that Parse ignores biological manifestations is to miss her point: Man-Living-Health is about the unity of man's lived experience. It is facile to talk about the biological manifestations of a physical condition and not talk about it phenomenologically. For example, when discussing chronic pain, Turk, Holzman, and Kerns stated that "a psychologically based treatment, or any treatment, must consider the patient's perspective and the phenomenology of chronic pain in developing and implementing a therapeutic regimen." The same can be said about diabetes, asthma, or cardiovascular disease-in children and adults. Because Man-Living-Health addresses the lived experience of health, it is at the cutting edge of health care.
- Parse defines Man-Living-Health's concepts denotatively and at the philosophical level of discourse. Although the concepts are highly abstract and theoretical, they can be observed in situations nurses encounter daily. But without study many nurses will not see what is going on around them. For this reason Parse's theory is exciting: It fires the imagination because it enables us to see anew. Linking it and research and practice will help us "better understand how Man chooses and bears responsibility for the rhythmical patterns of personal health."
- Parse allies nursing and the human sciences. This is in sharp contrast to most theories of nursing, which mirror medical science. With consumers more aware of strategies for promoting their health and

demanding a greater voice in is management, Parse's emphasis on Man's participation in and responsibility for health is timely. Societal questions about the quality of life in chronic, terminal, and marginal conditions suggest the potential Parse's theory has for meeting nursing's responsibility to society by addressing these questions. "Parse's model" predicted Phillips, "will contribute to a transformation of the knowledge base of nursing and the practice of nursing from a unitary perspective. The Man-Living-Health model provides new hope that there will be greater focus in the future of [sic] the meaning and quality of life and health that transcends the disease orientation; it will deal with improved quality of life for all people as perceived by them."

The future of Man-Living-Health lies in demystifying the language, developing middle-range testable theory and most important, in convincing nurses to replace the scientific method with the humanistic method.

Chapter 28

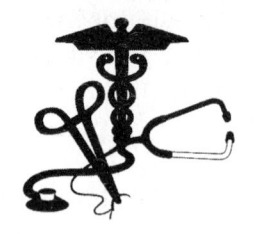

Joan Riehl's Symbolic Interactionism

Joan Riehl was born in Davenport, Iowa, she spent most of her childhood and young adult life in a Chicago suburb. She attended the University of Illinois in Urbana and Chicago where she obtained her BSN. After graduation she worked as a clinical instructor, a supervisor, and an in-service director in Texas and in California before returning to college for her masters's degree in nursing. After receiving her MSN from UCLA, Riehl taught pediatric nursing at California State University for three years before joining the faculty at the University of California in Los Angeles. There she began teaching theoretical concepts and their application. Two major professional events resulted from this instruction. First, she began writing nursing textbooks on conceptual models to use for teaching graduate students, and she began to identify her own theoretical framework. Her interest resulted in doctoral study at UCLA in sociology, which afforded the opportunity to pursue the knowledge base needed to develop the particulars of her model. Symbolic interactionism is the foundation upon which this model is built.

Role theory and self-concept are components of the theory. They constituted her dissertational investigation for her Ph.D., which she received in 1980.

Like many nurses who attend graduate school, Riehl worked part-time to maintain her clinical and research skills. The positions she held during this period included being a staff nurse in medical-surgical and psychiatric nursing and in the ICU-CCU, and being a supervisor in a gerontological hospital in Southern California. She also worked as a research assistant and coordinator in several research projects at the University of California at Los Angeles.

After graduation, Riehl moved to San Antonio, Texas. While there she taught sociology, psychiatric, nursing, and mental health concepts as a lecturer in the Department of Social Science at the University of Texas and as an associate professor in the Division of Nursing at Incarnate Word College. She also served as a research evaluator on a government grant that examined numerous variables regarding the RN to BSN student. When the three-year grant in Texas was completed, Riehl was named Chairperson of the Department of Nursing at the Harrisburg Area Community College in Harrisburg, Pennsylvania.

In 1985, Riehl became an associate professor at the graduate level in the Department of Nursing at Indiana University of Pennsylvania. She served as the graduate coordinator for the MSN programme and was responsible for teaching master's-prepared students theoretical foundations, research, curriculum theory and practice, ethical, legal and political dimensions of health care, family theory and practice, and administration theory and practicum. Riehl is currently residing in California and is working on a state-supported research project to determine if it is possible to reduce hospitalization of the mentally ill and in what manner the reduction can be accomplished. She is writing a paper about one part of the project. Riehl continues to receive national and international recognition as a pioneer and leader for publishing in the field of nursing theory.

Riehl is a member of numerous professional organizations. They include the National League of Nursing, American Nurses' Association, the ANA Council of Nurse Researchers, Sigma Theta Tau, the American Sociological Association, and the American Association for the Advancement of Science.

EVOLUTION OF THEORY

Riehl's theory is derived from symbolic interactionism (SI). In SI theory, interaction occurs between human beings who interpret or define each others' actions instead of merely reacting to them. The response is based on the meaning which the individual attaches to the action. Human interaction is mediated by the use of symbols, by interpretation, or by ascertaining the meaning of one another's action. This mediation is equivalent to inserting a process of interpretation between the stimulus and the response the case of human behavior.

"Communication is a key component of symbolic interactionism. While verbal communication is usually the major source of exchange between human beings, nonverbal communication is often considered equally important. This certainly applies in nursing. Consequently, Riehl claims several theoretical sources from sociology and social psychology, including George Mead, Herbert Blumer, Arnold Rose, L. Edward Wells, Gerald Marwell, and Robert E.L. Faris.

During the past 50 years, the SI theory has been supported by numerous empirical studies. Many theoretical sources, including those mentioned earlier, have illustrated the utility of this theory and have contributed to further refinement and clarification of its components. Blumer eloquently states, "It is my conviction that an empirical science necessarily has to respect the nature of the empirical world that is its object of study. In my judgment symbolic interactionism shows that respect for the nature of human group life and conduct."

Concepts Used by Riehl

Riehl's theory and model adapt four key concepts from the SI theory described by Blumer. In addition, Riehl uses the "me" and "I" concepts developed by Mead. Finally, she identifies role reversal and sick role as examples of the concept.

- *People:* "People, individually and collectively, are prepared to act on the basis of the meaning of the objects that comprise their world. In the Riehl model, the term *people* includes the patient, the nurse, other health care professionals, and the patient's family and friends. Riehl and Roy describe the nurse as one who knows her capabilities, is self-directed, and assumes more than one role in a given period.

- *Association:* "The association of people is necessarily in the form of a process in which they are making indications to one another and interpreting each other's indications. Riehl summarizes this as the defining process of rile taking, a social-psychological concept instituted by Mead. Role taking occurs when in individual cognitively internalizes another person's perceptions of reality in varied situations. Hence, the formative meanings of actions arise from this reciprocal interaction. The nurse-patient interface is an example of this interaction.
- *Social acts:* "Social acts, whether individual or collective, are constructed through a process in which the actors note, interpret, and assess the situations confronting them. Riehl states, "Their interpretation of these situations influence their social acts toward each other. "She expounds on the interpretive phase as described by Faris, in which is delayed response promotes clear thought, reduced frustration, and prospective learning. This concept correlates to Riehl's method of process recordings, which allows the nurse to assess and respond more appropriately to a patient's behavior.
- *Interlinkages:* "The complex interlinkages of acts that comprise organizations, institutions, division of labor, and networks, of interdependency are moving and not static affairs." From this concept Riehl derives that patient assessment is a dynamic process that often necessitates the use of several resources in meeting patient's needs, particularly in long-term care.
- *Me:* Riehl defines *me* synonymously with a role taker in a given situation. In other words, the me learns and assumes the attitudes of others. This is a concept used in the development of one's behavior as well as a method of understanding another's actions.
- *I (Self-concept):* Riehl defines *I*, of *self-concept,* as the individual's total behavioral perceptions, reflecting the summation of roles. She states, "The self-concept refers to a global, relatively constant self-perception that an individual holds and it changes only gradually.
- *Role reversal:* Role reversal is an example of a potential consequence resulting during the interaction between nurse and patient. Riehl defines role reversal as an inadvertent situation in which "the patient assumes the therapeutic role while the nurse becomes the recipient of the care." Rectification of this situation may require assistance from a third person.
- *Sick role:* Riehl defines the *sick role* "as the position one assumes when one perceives himself as ill. There may be a problem "when a patient is reluctant to part with the sick role." As with roie reversal, this situation suggests the need of additional resources for the patients rehabilitation.

Assumptions Made by Riehl

Riehl relates Arnold Rose's genetic and analytic assumptions to nursing and uses them in her derived theory. Rose divides his assumptions into two categories. The first, genetic assumptions, deals with only the child. The second is the analytic assumptions, which focus on all ages of man other than the child.

Genetic Assumptions

Rose cites the following four genetic assumptions applicable to the SI theory:
1. "Society-a network of interacting individuals-with its culture-the related meanings and values by means of which individuals interact-precedes any existing individual."
2. "The process by which socialization takes place can be thought of as occurring in three stages." These stages are:
   a. "The infant is habituated to a certain sequence of behaviors and events through a psychogenic process such as trial and error."
   b. "When the habit is blocked, the image of the incomplete act arises in the infant's mind and the thus learns to differentiate the object in that act by a symbol.
   c. " As the infant acquires a number of meanings he uses them to designate to others, and to himself, what he is thinking."
3. "The individual is socialized into the general culture and also into various subcultures."
4. "While some groups and personal meanings and values may be dropped and become lower on the reference-relationship scale, they are not lost or forgotten."

Analytic Assumptions

The five analytical assumptions pertaining to the SI theory according to Rose follow.

1. "Man lives in a symbolic as well as in a physical environment and can be stimulated to act by symbols as well as by physical stimuli."
2. "Through symbols, man has the capacity to stimulate others in ways other than those in which he himself is stimulated." Riehl states that role taking, a concept included under this assumption, is important in nursing.
3. "Through communication of symbols, man can learn huge numbers of meanings and values-and hence ways of acting-from other men." Riehl summarizes that as a result of this assumption man's behavior is not learned through trial and error or through conditioning, but rather through symbolic communication.

    "According to the SI theory, an individual's perception of how others evaluate him is more important in forming his self-concept than the actual evaluation that others hold." Riehl explains that it can be deduced from this assumption that "through the learning of a culture, or subculture, men are able to predict each other's behaviour and gauge their own behaviour accordingly."
4. "The symbols-and the meanings and values to which they refer-do not occur in isolated bits, but in large and complex clusters." This assumption refers to man's role. As defined in the discussion of concepts, the "me" is the role-taker and the "I," of self-concept, is the perception of a person as a whole. "Since the 'me' is made up of the attitudes of others, these others can take this role and predict an individual's behavior in a given capacity." Consequently, a person is able to gain insight into another's problem by taking

the other's role, anticipating how he will act, and implementing a plan of action to help him accomplish his goal.

5. "Thinking is the process by which possible symbolic solutions and others future courses of action are examined, assessed for their relative advantages and disadvantages in terms of the values of the individual, and chosen for action or rejected." Riehl discusses two major points involving this assumption. First, the assumption encompasses the four steps of the nursing process: "nursing assessment, diagnosis, planned intervention, and evaluation of action." Second, the points out, "Since meaning arises in the process of interaction between two persons, and individuals differ, even the most carefully thought out plan may go awry."

Assertions of Theory/Model

Riehl has identified several theoretical assertions in her model. These include:

1. "The premise that social action is built up by the acting unit through the process of noting, interpreting, etc. implies how social action should be studied." Riehl identifies the acting unit as the individual.
2. "According to Blumer (1969), in order to treat and analyze social action, one must observe the process by which it is constructed." Riehl identifies "one" as the nurse, who must view the social action as the individual sees it.
3. "Since the self-concept is an integral part of this model, the nurse must continue to develop self-insight through self-evaluation regarding his/her own actions to understand end results of interactions with others."
4. "The goal of action is to guide the patient in maintaining and regaining a higher level of wellness to improve the quality of life and to gain insight during life's journey regardless of the health problem." "The goal of action is bases upon a key factor of SI, which is taking the role of the others." Riehl identifies three methodological approaches the nurse uses to achieve this goal. The first approach, role taking, allows the nurse to understand why the patient does what he does. The second method entails interpretation of these actions. The third involves the use of process recordings. Riehl does not advocate recording all interactions, but she does recommend recordings be use until the nurse is able to respond effectively during on-the-spot interactions.
5. "It must be realized that it is not completely possible to take the role of the other, but genuine attempts to do so convey understanding of the other's position."
6. "Three additional elements must be included to meet the requirements of an effective conceptual model for nursing, namely, the source of difficulty, the intervention, and the consequences." Riehl equates the source of difficulty with the nursing diagnosis, and the intervention with the plan of care arrived at after role taking, interpretation, and process recordings.
7. The eclipse shown in her model (Fig. 28.1), "should never be complete, however, because maintaining a certain distance is essential for the preservation of the individuality of each person." As the nurse and patient gain knowledge and insight

from their interactions, the circles in the model move toward each other and form an ecliptical image. However, Riehl emphasizes that if the circles form a complete eclipse, objectivity and independence will be lost.

Riehl's theory uses deductive and inductive logic. It is deductive because Riehl draws relationships between nursing and the SI theory. Her statements are consistent with Mead's concepts of role raking and self-concept. Her theoretical assertions deduced from Rose's assumptions demonstrate further consistency. This allows for easy identification of the interrelationships between the theoretical components, and thus enhances the generation of hypotheses for empirical testing. It is inductive because Riehl utilizes SI as a foundation upon which to build and develop her concepts into a nursing theory.

Nursing Implications

Practice

Riehl's theory is becoming more widely accepted in the United States and is used fairly extensively in Canada, England, Japan, and the Middle East. It has been considered a middle range theory in nursing. Middle range constitutes a relatively broad scope of phenomena. However, Riehl's theory and model have been found applicable to all age groups and in a variety of clinical settings.

As Figure 28.1 illustrates, Riehl views the nurse therapist and the patient as actively exchanging information and gleaning knowledge. This is accomplished through mutual role taking in conjunction with the nurse selecting and using known theoretical approaches. The unshaded areas of the model indicate active process in the relationship, while the arrows represent the complex interdependencies of these elements, allowing for continual reassessment and evaluation.

Riehl's model provides a realistic approach for nursing practice in any situation where the focus in on role interaction in the nurse-patient relationship. Preisner demonstrates the applicability of Riehl's model in the psychiatric setting. The nurse selects from multiple theories, therapies, and allied health disciplines in planning and implementing effective nursing interventions.

Wood demonstrates the use of role taking in a patient's hospital admission. The nurse interprets the patient's response to the new environment and thereby helps the patient acquire the necessary perceptual changes or new role in the health care system.

The nursing implications are evident yet not restrictive to the interaction between the nurse and patient. The role interaction framework may also be effective in nurse-nurse relationships (nursing management, for example), nurse-physician dyads, nurse-patient-family triads, and other interactive situations. However, the model's emphasis is on the nurse-patient-family relationships.

Education

The SI theory has long gene prevalent among schools of sociology and psychology. The Riehl interaction model was introduced to the nursing discipline in 1980. The number of educational institutions that have incorporated it into their nursing curriculum is uncertain. The Riehl Interaction Model was considered as part of the organizing

372 Nursing Theories

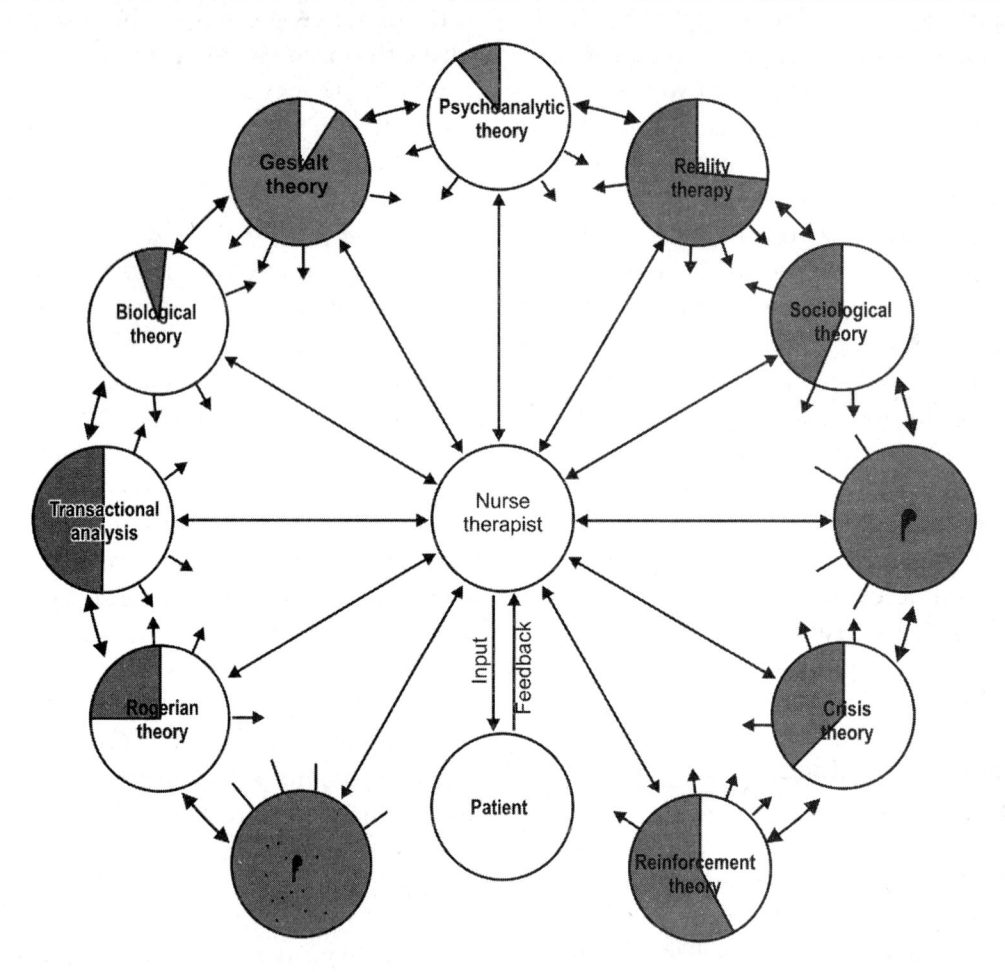

Figure 28.1: Riehl's model

framework of the curriculum at both Harrisburg Area Community College and Indiana University of Pennsylvania.

In addition, interaction models as a group are moderately employed in BSN programmes. Nursing is presently concerned with developing a distinct body of knowledge and delineating its professional role. Riehl's model, which focusses on the therapeutic processes in the nurse-patient and nurse-patient-family relationships, continues to contribute to these goals.

Research

The earliest research relevant to Riehl's theory can be found in her own doctoral dissertation. This study examines autistic children's ability to role take as compared with their "normal" siblings. It implicates a positive correlation between the level of development of self-concept and the ability to role take.

The generation of implications for further research is inherent in empirical studies. Riehl makes several suggestions for further testing dealing specifically with autistic children, such as investigating their perceptions of their patent's treatment of them and simply increasing the sample size to study more variables in this population. Examples of other recommendations include applying this study to other handicapped children and developing more tools for measuring self-conception.

Research on Riehl's theory and model supports their applicability to a wide variety of patients and clinical settings. These studies include use of the model with pregnant women, with adults in a medical clinic and the concept of personal space, with diabetic children and their self-esteem, with patients being transported by helicopter to acute care settings, and with a woman in postpartum psychosis. Continued research is needed for Riehl's theory to gain credibility, acceptance, and future application.

In operationalizing her model, Riehl has developed an assessment tool in the form of a matrix with the mnemonic FANCAP down the left side and the parameters physiological, psychological, sociological, cultural, and environmental across the top. With this approach, each factor intersects with each parameter and is therefore addressed (Table 28.1). After analyzing the collected data and making a diagnosis, a plan of care is made with the patient and/or family. The diagnosis and plan of care are prioritized (nurse with patient and/or family) and evaluated after implementation. This tool has been tested and Riehl indicates that it is valid and reliable.

Riehl has introduced an interesting and valuable model of SI to nursing. She has included further development of her theory in her third edition of *Conceptual Models for Nursing Practice*.

More explicit definitions of many concepts in the current model, including, *I, me, process recordings,* and *SI* itself are needed for in-depth descriptions in regard to the relationship statements between Blumer's concepts and nursing, and between Rose's assumptions and nursing. Furthermore, The theoretical assertions require refinement for lucidity and depth.

As a therapeutic nursing approach, Riehl's theory merits the involvement of the profession for progress in its development, understanding, and validation. Abundant potential for both nursing research and subsequent contributions to the theory seems to lie particularly in the psychiatric nurse setting. This testing may also generate new information. "Theory development is important to the growth of any discipline" and should be pursued.

Riehl is continuing to work with the theory and will be publishing papers in the future. A book, currently being written in England, compiles information from various sources about the use of the theory. Development of a consortium is being planned to add clarifications to the concepts as they apply to various nursing situations.

EVALUATION OF THEORY

- The Riehl interaction model contains several key concepts and theoretical relationships; thus, its complex. The future development of concepts and relationships will increase the level of complexity.
- Riehl's interaction model is generalizable to the broad scope of nursing. With a nonresponsive comatose patient, however, the model may be applied utilizing

Table 28.1: Riehl interaction model assessment tool

	Physiological	Psychological	Sociological	Cultural	Environmental
Fluids					
Aeration					
Nutrition					
Communication					
Activity					
Pain					

nonverbal form of communication. The exact interpretations may vary from patient to patient and nurse to nurse. A team approach is important and the help of family and friends is invaluable.

- The derived concepts from Blumer and Mead have been defined explicitly and grounded in observable reality within their parent discipline. Riehl does not clarify all her concepts with denotative definitions. "Peripheral nuances exist. Slight variations on the theme can be adjusted to the individual situation without changing the basic theory. The means for accurate testability and the degree of empirical precision will remain with the individual researcher.
- Riehl's interaction model uses the nursing process in implementing nursing care. Emphasis is on the nurse assessing and interpreting the patient's actions and then making predictions about the patient's behavior in order to plan interventions with the patient and his family. Furthermore, the evaluation phase in the theory, regarding potential patient problems, presents important nursing implications. The theory's usefulness is evident not only in the delivery of nursing care, but also in delineating the nurse's professional role

Riehl is continuing the development of her nursing theory, which is derived from SI. SI, as defined by Blumer, involves the interaction that transpires between people who "interpret or define each other's actions instead of just relating to them. Riehl uses Rose's genetic and analytic assumptions as her own. She identifies Blumer's concepts, the I and Me concepts of Mead, and the role reversal and sick role concepts in describing her model. Using these assumptions and concepts, Riehl relates nursing to the SI theory. She believes that the nurse must view the actions of the individual as he perceives them. By role playing, explicitly or implicitly the nurse is able to understand why the patient does what he does and is thus better able to identify the source of difficulty, or nursing diagnosis. Then, having interpreted the patient's action and studied the process recordings, the nurse is able to intervene with a plan of care. The plan of care involves helping the patient and/or family assume roles they have used in the past, or are currently using, to cope with the present illness. The evaluation process is then used to determine the success of this role taking. Riehl views this dynamic process as one that changes daily, requiring continuous assessment by both the nurse and the patient Although testing of Riehl's theory within the science of nursing has occurred only since 1985, its contribution to nursing is apparent.

Chapter 29

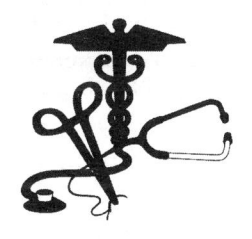

Barnard's Parent-child Interaction Model

Kathryn E. Barnard was born April 16, 1938, in Omaha, Nebraska. In 1956 she enrolled in a prenursing programme at the University of Nebraska and graduated with a Bachelor of Science in Nursing in June 1960. Upon graduation, she continued at the University of Nebraska in part-time graduate studies. That summer she accepted an acting head nurse position and in the fall became an assistant instructor in pediatric nursing. In 1961 Barnard moved to Boston, Massachusetts, where she enrolled in a Master's programme at Boston University. She also worked as a private duty nurse. After earning her Master's of Science in Nursing in June 1962 and a certificate of Advanced Graduate Specialization in Nursing Education, she accepted a position as an instructor in maternal and child nursing at the University of Washington in Seattle. In 1965 she was named Assistant Professor. She began consulting in the area of mental retardation, and coordinated training projects for nurses in child development and the care of children with mental retardation and handicaps. Barnard became the project director for a research study to develop a method for nursing child assessment in 1971. The following year she earned a Ph.D. in the Ecology of Early Childhood Development from the University of Washington.

In 1972 Barnard accepted a position at the University of Washington as a professor in parent-child nursing. From May 1985 to May 1986, Barnard was an adjunct professor of Psychology at the University of Washington. She was appointed Associate Dean for Academic Affairs at the University of Washington School of Nursing in 1987.

Since 1972 she has been the principal investigator of 18 research grants and co-investigator of two research grants. In addition to these research efforts, Barnard has provided consultation, presented lectures internationally, and served on multiple advisory boards. She has published articles in both nursing and non-nursing journals since 1966. Her books include a four-part series on child health assessment, two editions related to teaching the mentally retarded and developmentally delayed child and work focusing on families of vulnerable infants. Her most recent publications focus on the school-age follow-up of preterm infants' learning and social-emotional problems at the second-grade level.

Barnard is a member of the American Nurses' Association, where she has served on the Executive Committee for the Division on Maternal and Child Health Nursing. She is also an active member of ten other national organizations, including The Society for Research in Child Development, Sigma Theta Tau, the National League for Nursing, and the American Academy of Nursing. She has served on numerous advisory boards and committees of these professional organizations.

In 1969 Barnard was presented with the Lucille Perry Leone Award by the National League for Nursing for her outstanding contribution to nursing education. Since then she has been honored by several other associations, including the American Nurses' Association's Maternal and Child Health Nurse of the Year Award, which was presented at the 1984 convention. In 1987 Barnard was named Nurse Scientist of the Year by the Council of Nurse Researchers of the American Nurses' Association. She was the recipient of two research awards from Sigma Theta Tau in that same year. In May 1990, Barnard received an Honorary Doctor of Science Degree from the University of Nebraska Medical Center. In May 1992, The American Association for Care of Children's Health presented her with the T.B. Brazelton Lectureship Award.

Although Barnard cites various nursing theorists, such as Florence Nightingale, Virginia Henderson, and Martha Rogers, their direct influence on her research and theory development is uncertain.

Barnard refers to the Neal Nursing Construct, which has four expressions of health and illness: cognition, sensation, motion, and affiliation. Neal worked on a construct for practice and Barnard and her associates developed measures related to the period of infancy. Barnard later stated, "In reviewing both the Maryland construct and the Washington research, we were impressed with how the design and results of the Nursing Child Assessment Project (NCAP) fit into the [Neal] construct."

Barnard credits Florence Blake for the beliefs and values making up the foundation of current nursing practice. She describes Blake as:a great pediatric nursing clinician and educator who turned our minds towards an orientation on the patient rather than the procedure. Blake saw the principal function of parenthood and nursing to be the capacity to establish and maintain constructive and satisfying relationships with others. She amplified for nursing important acts such as mother-infant attachment, maternal care, and separation of child from parents. She helped nursing understand the importance of the family.

Many of Dr. Barnard's publications were co-authored by writers such as D. King and A.W. Pattullo, indicating a variety of influences. Barnard also published a book, entitled *Teaching the Mentally Retarded Child: A Family Care Approach*, with Marcene L. Powell. Four years later they developed a second edition, *Teaching Children with Developmental Problems: A Family Care Approach*. Of greater influence were the co-investigators and consultants of the Nursing Child Assessment Project, which includes Sandra Eyres, Charlene Snyder, and Helen Bee Douglas. Barnard et al state that they were influenced by child development theorists such as J. Piaget, J.S. Brunner, L. Sander, and T.B. Brazelton, in addition to nursing theorists.

EVOLUTION OF THEORY

Many researchers' findings were used as Barnard's work centering around the parent-child interaction evolved. Barnard used the work of T. Berry Brazelton and Bettye Caldwell. Once it was determined that the interaction/adaptation between parent and child was the area to focus on, Barnard used the research findings of many, such as H. Als, M.F. Waldrup and J.D. Goering, and L.M.S. Dubowitz. Their findings added to the growing body of usable knowledge that could be brought to bear on the task of developing tools to adequately assess that important interactional aspect of early child development.

In addition to tapping others' research, Barnard conducted her own. She began her research in 1968 by studying mentally and physically handicapped children and adults. In the early 1970s, she studied the activities of the well child and later expanded her study to include methods of evaluating growth and development of children. She also initiated a 10-year series of research projects to examine the effects of stimulation on sleep states in premature infants. The majority of these research studies were funded by grants from the US Department of Health, Education, and Welfare.

From 1976-1979, Barnard and colleagues from the University of Washington initiated work to determine how research results could be communicated to practicing nurses across the nation. This led to the evolution of the Nursing Child Assessment Satellite Training Project. In 1977 Barnard began researching methods for disseminating information about newborns and young children to parents. Projects have been funded by the National Foundation of the March of Dimes and Johnson and Johnson baby products. Barnard recently participated in a publication for parents entitled, "The Many Facets of Touch," which was also funded by Johnson and Johnson.

Today, Barnard continues to study the mother-infant relationship. Her research projects examine the nurse's role in relation to high-risk mothers and high-risk infants.

The Nursing Child Assessment Project (NCAP) formed the basis for Barnard's Child Health Assessment Interaction Theory. This was a longitudinal study "to identify poor [child development] outcomes before they occur and to examine the variability of the screening and assessment measures over time." The study population included 193 infants and their parents. Using various assessment scales and interviewing tools, the child and his or her parental relationships were assessed at six stages: prenatally, postnatally, at 1 month, 4 months, 8 months, and 1 year of age. Additional funds were obtained to continue the project by reassessing the child and parent at 2 years of age, and again when the children were in the second grade.

Researchers have used the Nursing Child Assessment Satellite Training (NCAST) instruments for diverse research purposes. Ruff used the tools to assess the interaction between unmarried teenage mothers and their infants. The NCAST instruments were used as an outcome measure to evaluate differences between mothers and high-risk infants who participated in a monitoring programme and those who did not. Farrel et al conducted a research study to examine the usefulness of the NCAST instruments for assessing the interaction between high-risk infants and their mothers to determine the need for intervention and the focus for such services. The findings suggest that the NCAST instruments may be useful in screening for dysfunctional interactions between high-risk infants and their mothers. As screening tools, the NCAST instruments appear to be valuable for directing more specialized intervention services in the high-risk infant population. Seideman *et al* conducted a research study using the NCAST instruments to assist in identifying issues and questions related to assessing urban American Indian parenting and the whole of the caretaker experience. This study evaluated the relationships of the findings from the three assessment instruments to the norms for those tools and to anecdotal data based on information from an interview with the caregiver. This study's findings indicate that NCAST tools reflect urban American Indian's cultural parenting practices and could be used to identify potentially problematic American Indian parenting situations.

Concepts Used by Barnard

A major focus of Barnard's work was the development of assessment tools to evaluate child health, growth, and development while viewing the parent and child as an interactive system. Barnard stated that the parent-infant system was influenced by individual characteristics of each member and that the individual characteristics were also modified to meet the needs of the system. She defines modification as adaptive behavior. The interaction between parent and child is diagrammed in the Barnard Model in Figure 29.1.

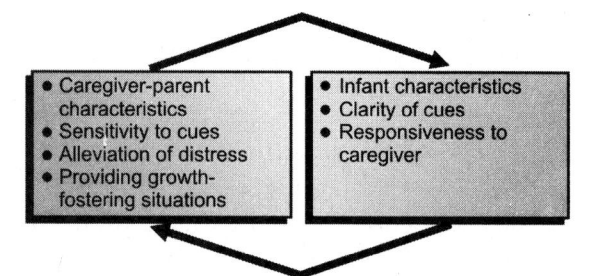

Figure 29.1: The Barnard model

Barnard has defined the terms in the diagram as follows:

Infant's clarity of cues: To participate in a synchronous relationship, the infant must send cues to his/her caregiver. The skill and clarity with which these cues are sent will make it either easy or difficult for the parent to "read" the cues and make the appropriate modification of his/her own behavior. Infants send cues of many kinds: sleepiness, fussiness, alertness, hunger and satiation, and changes in body activity, to name a few. Ambiguous or confusing cues sent by an infant can interrupt a caregiver's adaptive abilities.

Infant's responsiveness to the caregiver: Just as the infant must "send" cues so that the parent can modify his/her behavior, the infant must also "read" cues so that he/she can modify his/her behavior in return. Obviously, if the infant is unresponsive to the behavioral cues of his/her caregivers, adaptation is not possible.

Parent's sensitivity to the child's cues: Parents, like infants, must be able to accurately read the cues given by the infant if they are to appropriately modify their behavior. There are also other influences on the parents sensitivity. Parents who are greatly concerned about other aspects of their lives, such as occupational or financial problems, emotional problems, or marital stress, may be unable to be as sensitive as they would be otherwise. Only when these stresses are reduced are some parents able to "read" the cues of their young children.

Parents' ability to alleviate the infant's distress: Some cues sent by the infant signal that assistant from the parent is needed. The effectiveness of parents in alleviating the distress of their infants depends upon several factors. First, they must recognize that distress is occurring. Second, they must know (or figure out) the appropriate action which will alleviate distress. Finally, they must be available to put this knowledge to work.

Parent's social and emotional growth-fostering activities: The ability to initiate social and emotional growth-fostering activities depends upon more global parent adaptation. The parent needs to be able to play affectionately with the child, engage in social interactions such as those associated with eating, and to provide appropriate social reinforcement of desirable behaviors. To do these things the parent must be aware of the child's level of development and be able to adjust his/her behavior accordingly. This depends as much upon the parent's available energy as on his/her knowledge and skill.

Parent's cognitive growth fostering activities: It has been shown in a number of studies that cognitive growth is facilitated by providing stimulation which is just above the child's level of understanding. To do this, the parent must have a good grasp of the child's present level of understanding and the parent also have the energy available to use these skills.

As the NCAP continued, Barnard's model became the foundation for her Child Health Assessment Interaction Theory. Three major concepts form the basis of this theory.

- *Child:* In describing the child, Barnard used the characteristics of "newborn behavior, feeding and sleeping patterns, physical appearance, temperament and the child's ability to adapt to his/her caregiver and environment."
- *Mother:* Mother refers to the child's mother or caregiver and his or her important characteristics. The mother's characteristics include her "psychosocial assets, her concerns about her child, her own health, the amount of life change she experienced, her expectations for her child, and most important, her parenting style and her adaptional skills."
- *Environment:* The environment represents the environment of both child and mother. Characteristics of the environment include "aspects of the physical environment of the family, the father's involvement and the degree of parent mutuality in regard to child rearing."

Paradigm of Barnard Model

Nursing: Except for nursing, Barnard does not define her major assumptions. In 1966 she defined *nursing* as "a process by which the patient is assisted in maintenance and promotion of his independence. This process may be educational, therapeutic, or restorative: it involves facilitation of change, most probably a change in the environment." Five years later, in a 1981 keynote address to the first International Nursing Research

Conference, she defined nursing as "the diagnosis and treatment of human responses to health problems."

Person

When Barnard describes a person or human being, she speaks of the ability "to take in auditory, visual, and tactile stimuli but also to make meaningful associations from what he takes in." This term includes infants, children, and adults.

Health

Although Barnard does not define health, she describes the family "as the basic unit of health care." In the *Nursing Child Assessment Satellite Training Study Guide*, she states, "In health care, the ultimate goal is primary prevention." Barnard emphasizes the importance of striving to reach one's maximum potential. She believes "We must promote new values in American society, which up to now has valued not health, but the absence of disease." She wrote the definition for the scope of practice on maternal child health.

Environment

Environment is an essential aspect of Dr. Barnard's theory. In *Child Health Assessment, Part 2: The First Year of Life*, she states, "In essence, the environment includes all experiences encountered by the child: people, objects, places, sounds, visual and tactile sensations." She makes a distinction between the animate and inanimate environments. "The inanimate environment refers to the objects available to the child for exploration and manipulation. The animate environment includes the activities of the caretaker used in arousing and directing the young child to the external world."

Assertions of Barnard

Barnard's Child Health Assessment Interaction Theory is based on the following 10 theoretical assertions.

1. In child health assessment the *ultimate* goal is to identify problems at a point before they develop and when
2. Environmental factors, as typified by the process of parent-child interaction, are important for determining child health outcomes.
3. The caregiver-infant interaction provides information that reflects the nature of the child's ongoing environment.
4. The caregiver brings a basic style and level of skills that are enduring characteristics; the caregiver's adaptive capacity is more readily influenced by responses of the infant and her environmental support.
5. In the adaptive parent-child interaction, there is a process of mutual modification in that the parent's behavior influences the infant or child and in turn the child influences the parent so that both are changed.
6. The adaptive process is more modifiable than the mother's or infant's basic characteristics; therefore, in intervention the nurse should lend support to the mother's sensitivity and response to her infant's cues rather than trying to change her characteristics or styles.
7. An important quality of promoting the child's learning is in permitting child initiated behaviors and in reinforcing the child's attempt at a task.

8. A major issue for the nursing profession is support of the child's caregiver during the first year of life.
9. Interactive assessment is important in any comprehensive child health care model.
10. Assessment of the child's environment is important in any child health assessment model.

The Child Health Assessment Interaction Model was developed to illustrate Barnard's theory (Fig. 29.2). "The smallest circle represents the child and his/her important characteristics. The next largest circle represents the mother or caregiver and his/her important characteristics. The largest circle represents the environment of both the child and mother."

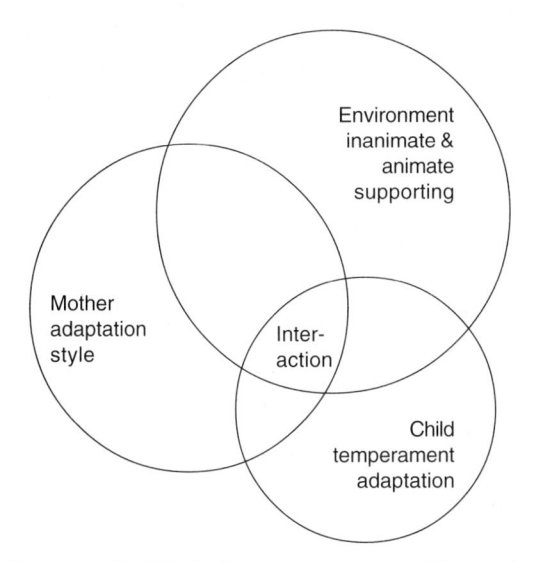

Figure 29.2: Child health assessment interaction model

Those portions of the model where two circles overlap represent interaction between the two concepts. The dark center area represents interaction among all three concepts. Barnard's theory focusses on this crucial mother-child-environment interactive process. The Nursing Child Assessment Project used this as the theoretical basis for the study of potential screening and assessment methods to be used with young children.

According to Chinn and Jacobs, "In inductive logic the reasoning method relies on observing particular instances and then combining those particulars into a larger whole." Inductive logic is the form Barnard used in developing her Child Health Assessment Interaction Theory. This theory was an outcome of the investigation and findings of the Nursing Child Assessment Project. Barnard concluded the most important aspect of child health assessment was the interaction and adaptation that occurs between parent and child.

Nursing Implications

Practice

The nursing satellite training project prepared about 4,000 nurses to use a series of standard assessment instruments. The exactness of the preparation in interrater reliability has increased observation skills applicable to other aspects of nursing. Now nurses use the assessment tools and their skills throughout the nation and in foreign countries.

Education

The nursing satellite training project initially used satellite communications and later videotaped classes to teach nurses how to use a series of standard assessment instruments. The concept of interrater reliability has encouraged nurses to share their knowledge and observations with co-workers. The explicitness of the observations has made the task of educating others easier.

Research

One of the outcomes of the contract to develop accurate assessment tools was the creation of a research project. The purpose of the satellite training programme was to quickly disseminate current research findings. Barnard is continuing to refine the assessment scales and continues to receive funds for research. She is well recognized for her work, having been cited in the Citation Indices at least 35 times between 1976 and 1984. She has received awards recognizing her work from several organizations, including the American Nurses' Association, the American Public Health Association, and the Nurses' Association of the American College of Obstetricians and Gynecologists.

Barnard stated she has a model of interaction. She does not believe that her model completes the criteria set forth for evaluation of a theory.

The greatest deficit of Barnard's theory is lack of clarity. Barnard does not explicitly define her major assumptions about nursing, person, health, and environment. Although the identification of major concepts is implied through the Nursing Child Health Assessment Interaction Model, Barnard fails to clearly define these concepts. This is an area requiring further development.

In the Child Health Assessment Interaction theory, the mother is identified as a major concept, and the father is included in the description of the environment. Although this classification may accurately describe the father's role in most families, a problem exists when the father assumes the role of primary caregiver. In these instances, Barnard's theory needs modification.

Barnard says her future endeavors will focus on further investigation of the child, his or her parents, and the environment. She plans to continue work in the area of teaching parents how to improve interaction skills with their children. From 1982 to 1988 she conducted research involving the high-risk infant. In 1987 she began a study to develop a nursing model for preterm infant follow-up. Although Barnard's theory is a micro theory, she does not intend to broaden her scope. Rather, she will be looking more closely at individual variables and how these affect a child's development.

EVALUATION OF THEORY

- Clarity in general refers to the lucidness and consistency of the theory. An extremely important aspect of semantic clarity is that of definition of concepts. Barnard does not identify or define her theoretical concepts. Rather, she describes and implies the definitions of these concepts. "In a theory with structural clarity, concepts are interconnected and organized into a coherent whole." By using Barnard's Child Health Assessment Interaction Model, it is relatively easy for the reader to understand the interrelationships of her theoretical concepts. Barnard is consistent in the use of an inductive form of logic.
- The Child Health Assessment Interaction Model is a simple way of communicating the main focus of Barnard's work as it relates to the parent-child interaction and the development of accurate assessment tools. However, there are several identified characteristics for both concepts

- and assertions, and consequently the complexity is great. It must also be noted that the research necessary to define and support the assertions is complex.
- Barnard's work with the interactive focus between parent and child is not generalizable to nursing. The original work involved interactions between parent and child during the child's first 12 months of life. Subsequent work lengthened the time period of the child assessment to 36 months. However, one can currently only generalize to parent-child interactions in the first 3 years of life. The parent-child interaction model approaches midrange theory as defined by Chinn and Jacobs. Despite the narrow scope, Barnard's theory is applicable, not only to nursing but also to other disciplines that deal with the parent-child relationship.
- Much research is included in Barnard's original work. She also used alternate research concurrently to validate test results obtained by one set of rates who made home visits with test results obtained by a set of testers from another discipline. Further development of the feeding and teaching assessment tools demonstrated test-retest reliability and validity of the original scales. Original videotapes were rescored using the revised scales.
- More than 4000 nurses have been trained to use the standardized assessment scales with 85% interrater reliability. Nurses across the nation and in other countries utilize the observational skills in daily practice.

Throughout her writings, Barnard emphasizes the need for strong links between nursing research, theory, and practice. She indicates, "There has been no more exciting time in nursing than now. We have the clinical, research, scholarship, administrative, and educational expertise so carefully developed over the past years." In discussing research, she states "We simply must attempt to be in closer alignment with practice from the beginning." In the Nursing Child Assessment Satellite Training Project, she identifies her goal as the dissemination of research findings and the application of these findings to practice. This goal is a prime example of Barnard's efforts to link research, theory, and practice.

Chapter 30

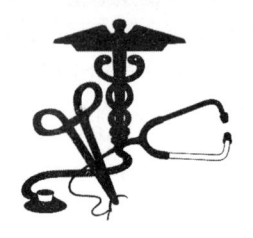

Pender's Health Promotion Model

Nola J. Pender made an early commitment to the profession of nursing when, at the age of 7 she observed the nursing care given to her hospitalized aunt. This desire to give care to others developed through experience and education to a belief that the goal of nursing was to help people care for themselves. Dr. Pender has made an impact on knowledge about the promotion of health through her research, teaching, presentations, and writings.

Pender was born in 1941 in Lansing, Michigan, as the only child of parents who were strong supporters of education for women. This family encouragement for her goal of becoming a Registered Nurse led her to attend the School of Nursing at West Suburban Hospital in Oak Park, Illinois. This school was chosen for its ties with Wheaton College and its strong Christian foundation. She received her nursing diploma in 1962 and began working on a medical surgical unit in a Michigan hospital.

In 1964 Pender completed her B.S.N. at Michigan State University in East Lansing. She credits Helen Penhale, the Assistant to the Dean, for helping to streamline her programm and foster her options for further education.

As was common in the 1960s, Pender changed her major from nursing as she pursued her graduate degrees. She earned her M.A. in Human Growth and Development from Michigan State University in 1965. Her Ph.D. in Psychology and Education was completed in 1969 at Northwestern University in Evanston, Illinois. Dr. Pender's dissertation investigated developmental changes in encoding processes of short-term memory in children.

At the time of earning her Ph.D., Pender notes a shift in her thinking toward defining the goal of nursing care as the optimal health of the individual. A series of conversations with Dr. Beverly McElmurry at Northern Illinois University and reading *High-level Wellness* inspired to her to look at health and nursing in a broader way. Her marriage to Albert Pender, an associate professor of business and economics who has collaborated with his wife in writing about the economics of health care, and the birth of a son and daughter provided personal influence in the desire to learn more about optimizing human health.

In 1975 Dr. Pender published "A conceptual model for preventive health behaviour," which was a basis for studying how individuals made decisions about their own health care in a nursing context. This article identified factors that were found to influence the decision-making and actions of individuals in preventing disease. In 1982 the first edition of the text *Health Promotion in Nursing Practice* was published with the concept of promoting optimal health superseding disease prevention. The health promotion model made its first appearance in the edition and appears in revision in the 1987 edition of the book.

A 6-year study was funded by the National Institutes of Health and conducted at Northern Illinois University in DeKalb by Pender's colleagues Susan Walker, Ed.D., Karen Sechrist, Ph.D., and Marilyn Frank-Stromborg, Ed.D. The study tested the validity of the health promotion model. An instrument, the Health Promoting Lifestyle Profile, was developed by the research team to study the health promoting behaviour of working adults, older adults, cardiac rehabilitation patients, and ambulatory cancer clients. Published results from these studies support the health promotion model, which Pender refers to as a model "in evolution."

Nola Pender has provided important leadership in the development of nursing research in the United Sates. Her work in support of the National Center for Nursing Research in the National Center for Nursing Research in the National Institutes of Health was instrumental to its formation in 1981. She has promoted scholarly activity in nursing through her involvement with Sigma Theta Tau, the Midwest Nursing Research Society, and the Council of Nurse Researchers of the American Nurses Association. Inducted as a Fellow of the American Academy of Nursing in 1981, she served as President of the Academy from 1991 until 1993. As director of the Center for Nursing Research at the University of Michigan School of Nursing since 1990, she is heavily involved in building nursing research. A child/adolescent health behaviour research center initiated in 1991 at the University of Michigan represents Dr. Pender's hopes to continue to study and influence the health promoting behaviours of individuals by understanding how these behaviours are first established in youth. Dr. Pender has published numerous articles on exercise, behaviour change, and relaxation training as aspects of health promotion. She is recognized as an expert and serves frequently as a speaker and consultant on these topics.

EVOLUTION OF THEORY

The health promotion model (Fig. 30.1) has its base in the social learning theory of Albert Bandura, which postulates the importance of cognitive processes in the changing of behaviour. Fishbein's theory of reasoned action, which asserts that behaviour is a function of personal attitudes and social norms is also important to the model's development. The health promotion model is similar in construction to the health belief model but is not limited to explaining disease prevention behaviour and expands to encompass behaviours for enhancing health. Dr. Pender's background in human development, experimental psychology, and education accounts for this foundation of social psychology and learning theory for her health promotion model.

The health promotion model, in its current form, identifies cognitive-perceptual factors in the individual that are modified by situational, personal, and interpersonal characteristics to result in the participation in

```
Cognitive-perceptual          Modifying              Participation in health-
       factors                 factors                promotion factors
```

- Importance of health
- Perceived control of health
- Perceived self-efficacy
- Definition of health
- Perceived health status
- Perceived benefits of behaviours
- Perceived barriers of health-promoting behaviours

Modifying factors:
- Demographic characteristics
- Biological characteristics
- Interpersonal influences
- Situational factors
- Behavioural factors

Participation in health-promotion factors:
- Likelihood of engaging in health-promoting behaviours
- Cues to action

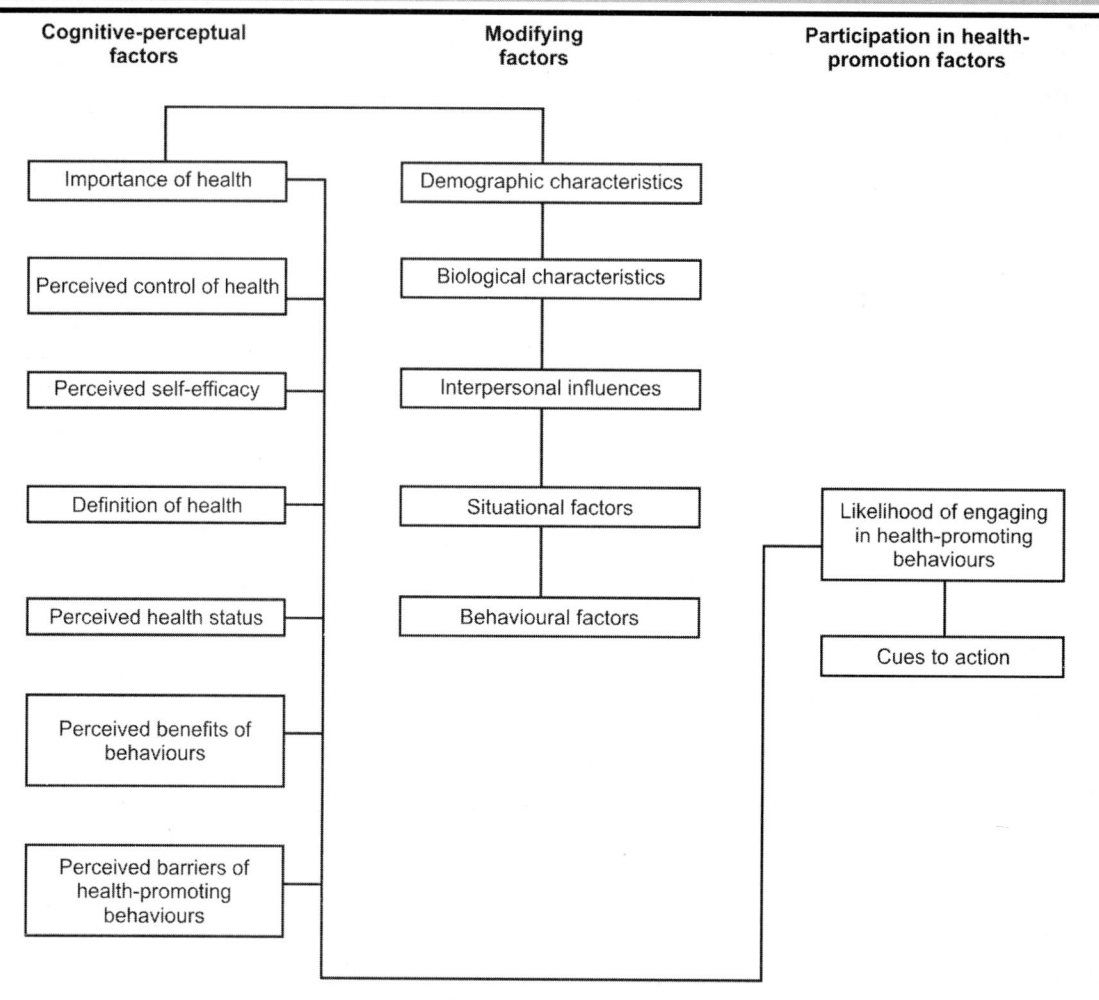

Figure 30.1: Health promotion model

health promoting behaviours in the presence of a cue to action. The identified proposed factors were determined by extensive review of health behaviour research. The health promotion model serves the function of identifying concepts relevant to health promoting behaviours and integrating research findings in such a way as to facilitate the generation of testable hypotheses.

Concepts Used by Pender

The following are cognitive-perceptual factors, defined as "primary motivational mechanisms" for the activities related to health promotion:

1. *Importance of health:* Individuals who value heath highly are more likely to seek it.
2. *Perceived control of health:* The individual's perception of his own ability to change his health can motivate his desire for health.
3. *Perceived self-efficacy:* The individual's strong belief that a behaviour is possible can influence the occurrence of that behaviour.
4. *Definition of health:* The individual's definition of what health means, ranging

from absence of disease to high-level well-being, can influence what behaviour changes will be attempted.
5. *Perceived health status:* The current state of feeling well or feeling ill can determine the likelihood that health-promoting behaviours will be initiated.
6. *Perceived benefits of behaviours:* Individuals may be more inclined to begin or continue health-promoting behaviours if the benefits to such behaviours are considered high.
7. *Perceived barriers to health-promoting behaviours:* The individual's belief that an activity or behaviour is difficult or unavailable may influence his intention to engage in it

Modifying factors such as age, gender, education, income, body weight, family patterns of health care behaviours, and expectations of significant others also play roles in the determination of health care behaviours. These modifying factors are seen as having indirect influence on behaviour, with the cognitive-perceptual factors bearing directly on behaviours.

Health is seen as a positive high-level state. The individual is assumed to have a drive towards health. The individual's definition of health for himself has more importance than a general denotative statement about health. Pender reviews major health views from medicine, nursing, psychology, and sociology.

The person is the individual and the focus of the model. Each person is uniquely expressed by his or her own pattern of cognitive-perceptual and modifying factors. Pender does not propose the model as explanatory for aggregates.

The model represents the interrelationships between cognitive-perceptual factors and modifying factors influencing the occurrence of health-promoting behaviours as this knowledge emerged from research findings. Specific theoretical assertions are not indicated by Pender.

The health promotion model has been formulated through induction by using existing research to form a pattern of knowledge. Middle range theories have commonly been built through this approach. The health promotion model is a conceptual model that was formulated with the goal of integrating what is known about health-promoting behaviour to generate questions for further testing. This model provides a framework for seeing more clearly how the results of previous research fit together and also how concepts can be manipulated for further study.

Nursing Implications

Practice

The concept of health promotion is a popular one in practice. Wellness as a nursing specialty has exploded in the past decade. Personal responsibility for health care is the cornerstone of every plan for health care reform in the United States. The financial, human, and environmental cost to society for individuals who do not engage in health prevention and promotion has been high. Understanding how consumers can be motivated to attain personal health has social relevance that will be of increasing importance to planners of health care delivery and those who provide the care. *Health Promotion in Nursing Practice* has proven to be a primary resource in the addition of health promotion to the practice of nursing.

Education

The use of the health promotion model has not been established in nursing education. Health promotion is a new emphasis that is currently placed behind illness care as clinical education is taking place in acute care settings.

Research

The health promotion model is primarily a tool for research. Dozens of research reports have been published that use the model and the Health Promoting Lifestyle Profile. The model has implications for application by emphasizing the importance of individual assessment of the factors believed to influence health behaviour changes.

The model continues to be refined and tested for its power to explain the relationships among the factors believed to influence health behaviour changes. Dr Pender plans further testing with populations across the life span, and aggregates, to determine the model's validity and expand the usefulness of the evolving model.

EVALUATION OF THEORY

- The health promotion model is simple to understand. Its language is clear and accessible to nurses. The relationships among the various factors in each set are linked, but the relationships require further clarification. The sets of factors, as being direct or indirect influences, are clearly set out in a visually simple diagram that shows their associations. Factors are seen as independent, but the sets have an interactive effect that results in action.
- The model is middle range in scope. It is highly generalizable to adult populations. The research used to derive the model was based on male, female, young, old, well, and ill samples. Applicability of the model to children ages 10 to 16 is currently being tested.
- The model has been supported through testing by Pender and others as a framework for explaining health promotion. The Health promoting Lifestyle Profile has emerged as an instrument to assess health-promoting behaviours.
- Dr. Pender has identified health promotion as a goal for the twenty-first century, just as disease prevention was a task of the twentieth century. The model can potentially influence the interaction between the nurse and the consumer. Pender has responded to the political, social, and personal environment of her time to clarify nursing's role in delivering health-promotion services to persons of all ages.

Chapter 31

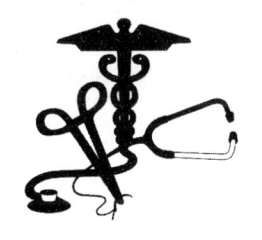

Other Theories

ET Patterson and ES Hale

A THEORY OF MENSTRUAL CARE ACTIVITIES OF DAILY LIVING

It is a Making Sure: Integrating menstrual care practices into activities of daily living (1985). This is derived from a grounded theory study to inductively develop a substantive theory about integrating menstrual care practices into daily activities. Making sure, the core concept of the theory, is defined as the process that enables menstruating women to continue their daily activities, knowing that their practices of menstrual care are effective and that the menstrual care demand can be met efficiently and effectively. Accidents are errors in making sure. Day of flow is a condition affecting making sure. Backup mechanisms are the strategies used to enhance making sure. Public and private are the contexts affecting making sure. Attending, calculating and juggling are the sub processes of making sure. Attending is the process of assessing the current menstrual demand. Calculating is a cognitive process of placing the menstrual care demand within the broader system of daily care demands that results in a decision about what to do with respect to menstrual self-care. Juggling is the process of assuring that time, space, and supplies coincide to meet menstrual self-care demands. The concepts of the theory are analogous to the concepts of Orem's general theory of self-care (1980).

Making sure is composed of the three sub-processes of attending, calculating, and juggling. The three sub-processes occur in stages that are sequential phases of the core process of making sure; they are analogous to Orem's estimative, transitional, and productive operation of self-care (1980). Making sure occurs in the context of accidents, day of flow, backup mechanisms, and public and private contexts. The context of the theory is that surrounding menstruating women and consists of cultural, social, and personal values regarding menstruation.

The theory was inductively generated with a grounded theory methodology. Interviews were conducted with 25 women who volunteered or were invited to participate because of theoretically relevant variables. In addition to the interviews, informal anecdotes and serendipitous sampling were used-stories volunteered by friends and colleagues or overheard conversations in public restrooms. The process of data analysis involved coding, memoing, and sorting; ongoing comparison of incidents and codes was done to collapse categories into higher-level categories.

The purpose for developing this theory was to provide insight into nursing care that can enhance a woman's self-care ability, particularly in the early experience with menstruation. The theory has implications for education related to self-care activities, particularly with anticipating menarche and in preventing toxic shock syndrome. Further development of the theory is advocated by systematically applying the theory in practice. The authors also note that the theory may have applicability in other circumstances involving involuntary eliminative processes, such as occurs with an ostomy, urinary incontinence, or lactation.

LR Phillips and VF Rempusheski

A THEORY OF QUALITY OF FAMILY CAREGIVING

It refers to a caring for the frail elderly at home: toward a theoretical explanation of the dynamics of poor quality family caregiving (1986). This is a grounded-theory approach to theory development to inductively describe dynamics of good-quality and poor quality family caregiving, explain the relationships among contextual and perceptual variables in caring for the elderly at home, and identify points at which interventions by nurses could be effective. Five major constructs were identified. Personal identity of the elder was defined as a mental image that the caregiver has of the elder being cared for. Image of caregiving was defined as the degree to which the caregiver's personal imperatives, standards, and values are realized by the caregiving situation. Caregiver's role beliefs were defined as the standards and values the caregiver held regarding the performance of the caregiver role; they include the caregiver's and the elder's expectations for role responsibilities. Caregiver behavioural strategies were defined as the behaviour the caregiver customarily uses in responding t the elder. Perception is defined as the caregiver's interpretation of the elder's response.

The five major concepts of the theory were structured as stages consistent with the framework of symbolic interactionsim. *Stage 1*, defining the process, consists of the personal identity of the elder and image of the caregiving. *Stage 2*, cognitive processes, consists of the caregiver's role beliefs. *Stage 3*, expressive processes, consists of the caregiver's behavioural strategies. *Stage 4*, evaluation processes, consists of perception.

The stage 1 construct of personal identity of the elder involves the associated concept of reconciliation of past with present, which in turn involves six distinct processes, each of which involves three separate steps of deriving a past image, deriving a present image, and reconciling past and present by using comparison. The reconcile image can be normalized or anormalized. Anormalized images can be either deified (viewing the elder as more adequate than is real) or stigmatised (viewing the elder as less adequate than is real).

The stage 1 construct of image of the caregiving involves the associated concept of reconciliation of reconciliation of proscriptions with the perceived reality of caregiving, or the degree to which the caregiver's observations and perceptions of the situation diverge from the caregiver's beliefs about propriety. Several interrelated categories of proscriptions are derived in the theory development process.

The stage 1 construct of image of the caregiving involves the associated concept of reconciliation of proscriptions with the perceived reality of caregiving, or the degree to which the caregiver's observations and perceptions of the situation diverge from the caregiver's beliefs about propriety. Several interrelated categories of proscriptions are derived in the theory development process.

The stage 1 constructs have a direct influence on the stage 2 construct of the caregiver's role beliefs, which has two associated concepts: role responsibilities of the caregiver and role responsibilities of the elder. The nature of the influence between the two stages is a major factor in determining the quality of caregiving.

The stage 3 construct, the caregiver's behavioural strategies, involves the concept of the caregiver's management strategies or the methods used to control the elder's behaviour and to resolve conflicts with the elder. Three types of management strategies were identified: positive, negative, and neutral.

The stage 4 construct of perception involves the concept of perception of the elder response, or the caregiver's interpretation of the elder's role support and role enactment. This process, over time, can positively or negatively modify state 1.

Details of the structure and context of the theory are presented in diagrams and clarified by definitions and examples from the data.

The theory was inductively generated with a grounded-theory methodology. In-depth interviews were conducted with 39 caregivers in tow geographic locations who responded to one of two newspaper advertisements. One advertisement solicited caregivers who had a good relationship with an elder for whom they cared, and the other solicited caregivers who had an abusive or neglectful relationship with the elder. Approximately 2000 large data bits comprised the beginning working sample, which was derived from the interviews. The data were subjected to constant comparative analysis, consisting of open and selective coding.

The authors state that therapeutic and cost-effective care for elders depends on the nurse's understanding of the dynamics of family caregiving and on knowing how to intervene to meet the needs of both the elder and the family members who are providing care. The hypotheses generated in this study provide the basis for further testing of the theory in practice, which can lead to the ability to predict caregivers who are at high risk for providing less than optimal care an to identify those points at which interventions by nurses will be most effective in high-risk caregiving situations.

MA Wewers and ER Lenz

A THEORY OF RELAPSE AMONG EX-SMOKERS

It refers to relapse among ex-smokers: An example of theory derivation (1987). This is a theory of relapse among ex-smokers derived from a theory of recovery from alcohol abuse; empiric testing of the derived theory with a prospective one-group-only design. Relapse is a central focus of the theory. The meaning of relapse among ex-smokers evolved from examining studies of the role of a specific factor in the relapse process and of alcohol relapse. Six factors that influence relapse were identified: Sociodemographic and pre-treatment smoking characteristics, nature of treatment received, and three posttreatment characteristics (stressors, coping responses, and family environment).

Relapse, the central concept of the theory, was postulated to be a function of three characteristics; patient-related characteristics, treatment-related characteristics, and posttreatment characteristics. Patient-related characteristics are the subfactors of sociodemographic factors and pre-treatment symptoms. There were no subfactors for treatment related characteristics. Subfactors under the concept of posttreatment characteristics were stressors, coping responses, and family environment.

Patient-related characteristics of sociodemographic factors, pretreatment symptoms, and the posttreatment characteristics of stressors, coping responses, and family environment were postulated to have a major explanatory role in the theory. Because of empiric evidence that countered any differential effect of various treatment techniques, treatment-related characteristics were assigned a minor explanatory role.

The context of ex-smokers was postulated to differ from the derived context of alcohol recovery in terms of the nature of stressful life event and physiologic factors arising from within the individual.

A study was conducted to examine the relationships between smoking relapse and five of the six major components of the theory with a one-group-only prospective design with 150 adults attending a smoking cessation clinic. Variables that operationalized the theory factors were measured prior to beginning the treatment and then 3 months later. The results of the study suggested that the role of posttreatment characteristics, stressors (particularly carving), and type of coping response may be useful in designing effective treatment to prevent relapse.

The purpose underlying the development of this theory was to assist nurse in designing effective treatments to help ex-smokers maintain long-term abstinence and prevent relapse. The results of this empiric test of the derived theory suggested two major areas of focus for application of the theory. First, symptoms of craving should be considered a high-risk predictor of relapse. Second, a focus on problem-versus emotion-focused coping responses may improve success rates.

MH Mishel

A THEORY OF UNCERTAINTY

It refers to a reconceptualization of the uncertainty in illness theory, (1990). This is a reconceptualization of uncertainty theory (Mishel, 1988) to include experiences of living with continual uncertainty processes. Reconceptualization is based on an examination of theory and prior empiric evidence, with particular attention to the outcome portion of the theory. The original version of the uncertainty theory includes the major concept of uncertainty, which is the inability to determine the meaning of illness because cues necessary to assigning value are insufficient. Therefore, outcome of illness events cannot be known.

Two subconcepts that identify processes for appraisal of illness events precipitating uncertainty are inference and illusion. Inference is the construction of meaning by reference to exemplary former situations. Illusion refers to construction of a generally positive belief system.

Two subconcepts defining outcomes of appraisal processes are identified: danger and opportunity. For the appraisal process outcome of dangers, two coping strategies are identified: mobilizing and affect-control strategies. For the appraisal process outcome of opportunity, the coping strategy of buffering is identified.

Adaptation, in the original version of the model, is identified as the outcome of all coping strategies, whether in response to uncertainty appraisal as danger or opportunity. Adaptation is a positive value and connotes stability and the return to equilibrium.

In the reformulated version of uncertainty theory, the concept of continual self-organization to increasing levels of complexity replaces adaptation as the outcome of uncertainty appraisal in situations of continuing and chronic uncertainty.

A structure of the outcome portion of an earlier version of the uncertainty theory (Mishel, 1988) is provided. A narrative also explains and adds structure to the visual of the earlier version, as well as the reformulated version of the theory. The structure is a time-ordered linear framework that begins with the situation of uncertainty in illness. Uncertainty is appraised by two processes: influenced by (i) the patient, (ii) the patient's social resources, and (iii) health care providers. Inference, or comparison of present situations with earlier situations, can result in appraisal of uncertainty as either danger or opportunity. Illusion, or the construction of a belief system that is positive, usually results in a view of uncertainty as opportunity. Whether appraised as danger or as opportunity, coping with uncertainty follows its appraisal. If appraised as danger, coping strategies seek to decrease uncertainty. If appraised as opportunity, coping maintains uncertainty. Two strategies to decrease uncertainty are structured: mobilizing or affect-control strategies. Strategies to maintain uncertainty are structured to include buffering strategies.

In the earlier version of the theory, which was developed in the context of acute illness with a generally downward course, adaptation was the outcome of coping. Adaptation was assumed to be a positive state in which uncertainty was successfully manipulated in the desired direction. Adaptation constituted the end point of the theory.

The original theory was structured to include cultural biases inherent in the Western worldview. Assumptions reflecting this bias were identified to include (i) a temporal invariability in the appraisal of uncertainty, (ii) uncertainty is generally aversive, and (iii) uncertainty is a stable state rather than a process. The author states that this bias is reflected in prior research findings and limits advancing the theory. The reformulation of the theory challenges these assumptions and utilizes theory derivation as described by Walker and Avant (1989).

The theory is reformulated for the context of long-term chronic uncertainty situations. In long-term illness situations the early acute disruptions that create uncertainty and a high level of instability provide the foundation for evolving a new sense of order within the human system. Chaos theory is the perspective borrowed for reformulation of the outcome portion of the uncertainty theory. New levels of self-organization become the end point or the continuing process in response to the uncertainty of chronic illness.

The reformulation also discards the concept of illusion as a way to appraise uncertainty and the possibility of appraising uncertainty as negative or as danger. Rather, the theory is structured so that uncertainty as opportunity is the view maintained by the environmental forces of support resources and health care providers. Four factors are identified that block re-revaluation of uncertainty and continual self-organization to higher levels of complexity. These blocks occur when (i) patient's supportive resources do not promote a probabilistic view of life, (ii) the patient caretakes others, (iii) the patient is isolated from social interactional contests, and (iv) providers focus on certainty and definite illness outcomes. Blocks to the continual reintegration of uncertainty to new levels of self-organization can result in posttraumatic stress syndrome.

The reconceptualization of uncertainty theory is grounded in assumptions inherent in Chaos theory that characterize far-from-equilibrium systems. The theory undergoing reconceptualization was the result of approximately 10 years of ongoing empiric research and theory formulation in a variety of health and illness contexts. The author suggests the need for empiric research for the newly reformulated theory. Also, practical use of the theory is suggested to promote a view of the uncertainty of life and the need to create unpredictable contingencies from seemingly unrelated situations.

The author does not specifically address research strategies for deliberative application aside from the suggested need for empiric research. Deliberative application might be accomplished through clinical application of the theory, with subsequent theory reformulation based on careful analysis of the experiences of clinicians.

AA Quinn

A THEORY OF PERIMENOPAUSAL PROCESS

It refers to a theoretical model of the perimenopasual process, (1991). This is a qualitative study to generate theory related to women's experience of perimenopausal processes. A core variable and four subprocesses emerged from date analysis. The core variable of integrating a changing me was the central concept. Four subprocesses were identified: (i) tuning in to me (my body and moods represented awareness of physical and emotional changes), (ii) facing a paradox of feeling included negative and positive feelings about the menopausal experience, (iii) contrasting impressions included processes of resolving conflicting information about the menopause, and (iv) making adjustments referred to changes and alterations made in response of life changes. Subprocesses were further defined by narrative discussion that included examples and delineation of additional subprocesses.

A theoretic structure of a pinwheel was provided. The core variable (integrating a changing me) was located at the center. The four subprocesses were integrated and linked with the core variable. The subprocesses were not depicted as sequential or linear. The subprocesses were further structured as follows: Tuning in to me included processes of changing control and uncertainty in relation to qualitative and quantitative changes surrounding the menstrual cycle, hot flashes, breast tenderness, weight fluctuation, skin character, energy levels, and moods. Facing a paradox of feelings included both negative and positive feelings around getting older, reproduction, physical vulnerability, and the uncertainty of the future. Contrasting impressions were structured to include processing conflicting information about menopause acquired from stories, communication with others, exposure to media, and self-beliefs. Making adjustments included self-care practices to maintain health, coping strategies to handle stress, and caring activities. Making adjustment processes were further structured into changing diets, exercising, taking vitamins and calcium, creating time for self, making life accommodations, seeking solitude, promoting change, recognizing physical limits, putting lives in perspective, and regaining control. Further structure was provided throughout by use of examples and quotes from participants.

The theory was contextualized for the perimenopausal process as experienced by women. The structuring assumed (i) menopause was a natural process, (ii) meaning attributed to the process was culturally based, (iii) women's health is not synonymous with reproductive health, and (iv) women's self-reports of their experience and validity.

The theory was generated with a grounded-theory methodology. Two main questions were asked: What is the process of menopause for perimenopausal women? What are the self-care practices used for? Perimenopause was defined as the cognitive, affective, and behavioural/physical responses of women aged 40 to 60. Self-care practices were defined as consistent with the self-care theory of Dorothea Orem (1980) to maintain life, health, and well being.

Twelve women who were not on hormone therapy and who had varied backgrounds of marital status, education, and parity participated in the study. Women were interviewed and kept daily logs for 2 months. Field notes also contributed data. Theoretic sampling was used throughout data generation and analysis. Data were coded, categorized, and sorted by ethnographs to produce the core variable and related subprocesses. The truth value was established by confirming study findings with the women experiencing the perimenopausal process.

The author suggests use of the theory to understand the perimenopausal process and facilitate women's integration of the process. Providing a forum for women to express their concerns, share their stories, and receive information about the experience is cited as a clinical application of the theory. The use of the clinician's experience in applying the theory to subsequently expand and refine it could represent deliberative application processes, although this is not suggested by the author. The author does suggest further research in a variety of cultural and socio-economic groups to broaden and expand the beginning theory.

PG Reed

A THEORY OF SELF-TRANSCENDENCE

Towards a nursing theory of self-transcendence: Deductive reformulation using development theories (1991). Here P.G. Reed using deductive reformulation as method for developing theory, the author reformulated life-span developmental theory from psychology, based on Rogers's general conceptual system of nursing. The definition of self-transcendence was based on reformulation that focused on areas of incongruence between life span development theory and Rogers's conceptual system for nursing. Self-transcendence was defined as expansion of self-boundaries multidimensionally-inwardly, outwardly, and temporally. Inward expansion involves introspective experience. Outward expansion involves reaching out to others. In temporal expansion past and future are integrated in the present. Self-transcendence is related conceptually to well-being, particularly in terms of mental health.

The structure and context of theory are expressed in two propositions that are set forth as central to the theory: (i) Self-transcendence is greater in persons facing end-of-own-life issues than in persons not confronted with such issues, and (ii) self-transcendence is positively related to indicators of well-being in persons facing end-of-own-life issues.

The propositions of the theory were tested in five studies by Reed (1986a, 1986b, 1987, 19889, 1991a) that examined spiritual and psychosocial self-transcendence. The people who participated in these studies were either terminally ill adults or middle-old and eldest-old adults. The author developed a Spiritual Perspective Scale to measure multidimensional personal boundary expansion and a self-transcendence scale to measure psychosocial expressions of self-transcendence in later life. In addition to the quantitative analyses, qualitative data were analysed by matrix analysis. The findings of all of the studies supported the initial propositions of the theory and provided a beginning empiric base for the theory.

The theory provides a rationale for nurses to attend to spiritual and psychosocial expressions of self-transcendence with clients who are experiencing end-of-own-life issues. The author notes that nursing therapies to help clients expand self-boundaries need to be tested in clinical practice. Potential approaches to nursing care that could be used in deliberative application include meditation, self-reflection, visualization, religious expression, peer counselling, journal keeping, and life-review processes.

KM Swanson

A THEORY OF CARING IN PERINATAL NURSING

It refers to a empirical development of a middle-range theory of caring (1991).This is an inductively developed theory of caring derived from three perinatal contexts. Caring is a central concept. Conceptual meaning was derived from empiric (phenomenologically based) study. The meaning of caring was expressed as five caring processes, each with four or five subprocesses. A discussion of each process further clarified meaning. An empirically based definition of caring was proposed. Conceptual meaning was validated by comparison with theoretic writings of Patricia Benner (1984), Nel Noddings (1984), and Jean Watson (1985).

Theory is structured in tabular form as five distinct but overlapping processes that define caring in the context of study. These five processes are (i) knowing, (ii) being with, (iii) doing for, (iv) enabling, and (v) maintaining belief. Subdimensions that further define each process are listed. The narrative discussion and the empirically derived definition of caring provide further structure for the dimensions of caring.

The context of derivation was perinatal nursing. Three subcontexts from which the theory was structured were (i) women who recently miscarried, (ii) caregivers in a newborn intensive care unit, and (iii) young mothers at social risk.

The theory was generated by successive phenomenologically based studies within separate but related contexts. Women who miscarried were interviewed, and the five dimensions of caring emerged. Successive studies confirmed and refined the dimensions of caring that had emerged from the initial study. The second study utilized participant observation of care providers, attendance at ethics grand rounds, and interviews with various care providers, including nurses, physicians, fathers, mothers, an ethicist, a nursing administrator and a social worker.

Deductive testing of the theory is in process. Woman who have miscarried are receiving counselling grounded in the theory of caring. Outcomes related to healing and the meaning of the human experience of health and illness will be assessed.

The generation and testing operations that gave rise to the theory constituted deliberately applying theory because the initial study formed the basis for second and third deliberative attempts to modify and strengthen the theory.

Cross-validation of the theory was provided by comparison of the emerging theory with work of Nel Noddings (1984), Patricia Benner (1984), and Jean Watson (1985).

Deliberative application is proposed for other contexts of caring to determine the generalizability of the theory. Findings that suggest congruence with nonnursing theories of caring support generalizability to nonnursing contexts.

JM Hitchcock and HS Wilson

A THEORY OF PERSONAL RISKING

This theory is related to personal risking: Lesbian self-disclosure of sexual orientation to professional health care providers (1992). This is an inductively developed theory of sexual identity disclosure processes of lesbians seeking traditional health care. The basic social process of personal risking is a central concept. Conceptual meaning was derived from in-depth interviews and from the assignment of meaning with grounded-theory methodology. The meaning of personal risking is ex-pressed through a series of complex conceptual networks of subconcepts representing processes and states related to personal risking.

Personal risking is conceptually divided into two phasic processes, which are both further defined by two subprocesses. Interactional stance is also an important concept and is defined by four subconcepts. Three additional concepts modify and determine the entire personal risking process: (i) personal attributes, (ii) health care context, and (iii) relevancy.

Conceptual meaning is provided by narrative description and examples from participants included in the report.

The concept of fear emerged as a basic social-psychologic problem that motivates the personal risking process.

The theoretic structure is derivable from the narrative. The basic social process of personal risking is a central concept. Personal risking is structured into two phases: (i) an anticipatory phase and (ii) an interactional phase. The anticipatory phase is structured into two subprocesses: imagining scenarios and cognitive strategizing. Cognitive strategizing is substructured as formalizing and scouting out. Imagining scenarios is not further structured by subprocesses. Interactional stance is substructured into four concepts: (i) passive disclosure, (ii) active disclosure, (iii) passive nondisclosure, and (iv) active nondisclosure. It also has two subprocesses: (a) scanning and (b) monitoring. Scanning occurs prior to contact with the provider. Monitoring occurs in the context of care provision.

Three additional concepts modify and determine the entire personal risking process: (i) personal attributes, (ii) health care context, and (iii) relevance. These concepts overlie the entire personal risking process. Personal attributes are structured to include the comfort level of the lesbian with sexual orientation, the relationship status of the lesbian, and the attitudes and beliefs about health care. Health care context includes provider characteristics (sexual orientation, gender, personal and professional attributes, the client's past experiences with providers), the health care environment, its location, and cues to its friendliness.

A linear structure for the major concepts is suggested in that the anticipatory phase is followed by the interactional phase. The concept of interactional stance is an outcome of the anticipatory phase, and interactional stance is an outcome of anticipatory phase, and interactional stance is implemented following the scanning process of the interactional phase. The interactional stance is continuously monitored during the implementation phase, with a feedback loop to interactional stance implied. The structure of the theory needs to consider stance modification (expect if the stance of active disclosure had been implemented), depending on personal attributes, health care context, and relevance of disclosure.

The concept of fear emerged as a basic social-phychologic problem that helped focus the structuring of the theory; fear is shared by all participants and becomes a focus for the basic social process. Thus the resolution or management of fear becomes a focal point for theoretic organization in that the basic social process of personal risking can be organized to show how it relates to the management of fear.

The theory was contextualized in relation to traditional health care environment processes and providers as experienced by lesbian women of broad ranges of age, income level, and years of formal education. The contextual variable of relationship status was also operating in that relationship status was not controlled.

The theory was inductively generated with a grounded-theory methodology. One-time in-depth interviews of participants were the source of data. A three-step coding process was used in data analysis. Level 1 codes were substantive codes that described experiences in the participant's own words. Level 2 codes were applied to initial clusters of level 1 data. Level 3 codes were those applied to the core concepts of the theory.

This is implied in suggestions for further development, which could accrue through deliberative application of the theory or focus on the theory-development process: generation and testing of theoretic relationships. Deliberative application in different contexts-for example, geographic location and ethnicity of respondents-would further define the context and provide information on generalizability of use findings. The authors suggest a theory-verifying approach for exploring conditions of personal attributes, health care context, and relevance (Particularly the effect each has on the personal risking process). Deliberative application also needs to focus on the reality of health care provider attitudes toward lesbian health issues and how they affect personal risking processes.

CL Winner and MJ Dodd

A THEORY OF ILLNESS TRAJECTORY

It is a coping amid uncertainty: An illness trajectory perspective (1993). This is a secondary analysis of qualitative data for congruity with an extant theoretic framework of illness trajectory; a test of the validity of this theoretic framework with cancer patients by interrelating concepts of illness trajectory, coping, and uncertainty. Illness trajectory is a central concept and names the theoretic framework to be validated. The meaning of illness trajectory evolved from studies of chronically ill people that began in the 1960s and continued through the late 1980s. Illness trajectory is defined loosely as the path of an illness course and is further defined by three major subconcepts. The course of the disease refers to an individual's life course of living with a chronic illness, which is additionally defined by three major concepts.

Other key concepts are cooping and uncertainty. The meaning of coping, as a correlate of stress, is consistent with the usage in Particia Benner's caring theory (1989). The dimensions of uncertainty evolved from extensive qualitative data analysis.

The illness trajectory theory is more specifically defined as work done over the total course of the disease. There are subconcepts or dimensions of work done: (i) the physical unfolding of the disease, (ii) the total organization of work done over the course of the disease, and (iii) the reciprocal consequences for family, health care professionals, and patients. The framework is undergirded by an assumption that work occurs in a social context. Subsequent research with the illness trajectory framework identified three interrelated elements around the course of disease as a life course: (i) conceptions of self and (ii) evolution of self over time that (iii) arise directly or indirectly from the body. The theoretic structure is consistent with the expectation that these three life course concepts work together to provide structure and continuity to living. The need for coping arises when illness, such as cancer, intrudes.

The theory developed from this base and reported in this research derived from the examination of the uncertainty data in relation to temporality, body, and identity-concepts directly related to the elements of subconcepts around the life course of disease. The major concepts evolved: uncertain temporality, uncertain body, and uncertain identity. The dimensions of uncertain temporality include (i) loss of temporal predictability (duration, pace, frequency of recurrence), (ii) sketching out and constriction of time, and (iii) time as limitless. These dimensions were correlates of patient concern about the efficacy of treatment, recurrence of illness, unreliability of symptoms, and risk inherent in treatment. The dimensions of the uncertain body included: (i) body failure (activity performance, appearance, physiologic function) and (ii) the body's response to treatment. These dimensions correlated with patient concerns with new bodily symptoms, with having the body's resistance in jeopardy, and with what was being done with the body. The uncertain identity arises through the body and the challenges to who the patient is.

These theoretic dimensions that evolved from interrelating uncertainty with one major facet of the illness trajectory (the life course of a disease) formed a basis for examining the second major concept of the illness (work done over this life course). This resulted in the structuring of four major concepts: illness-related work, everyday work, biographic work, and uncertainty-abatement work. Illness-related work included symptom management, following the management regimen, crisis prevention and management, and diagnostic-related work. Everyday work included house-keeping and repairing, occupational work, marital, child rearing, recreation and daily living activities. Biographic work included gathering and dispensing information, expressing concern, caring, anger; and diving tasks. Uncertainty-abatement work included pacing, becoming a professional patient, seeking reinforcing comparisons, engaging in reviews, setting goals, covering up, finding a safe place to let down, choosing a supportive network, and taking charge.

Uncertainty is both a response to and an outcome of work and life course processes within the illness trajectory. Coping is also a response to and outcome of uncertainty. Thus the concepts of coping, uncertainty, and illness trajectory are structurally interrelated to allow mutual, simultaneous interaction.

The theory derived from this research is contextualized for patients with an initial or ongoing cancer diagnosis who require chemotherapy and for their families.

Utilizing the borrowed theoretic framework of illness trajectory, uncertainty was examined in light of its three elements. Uncertainty data were part of a larger study of family coping and self-care during 6 months of a chemotherapy experience. The core variable of "tolerating the uncertainty that permeates the disease" emerged from qualitative data analysis. This research examined the work processes (that define the concept of illness trajectory) of coping in the face of uncertainty.

The uncertainty data examined were accrued from 100 interviews of a family member of a variety of patients with cancer. Each family member was interviewed 3 times during a 6-month period of chemotherapy, either initial or repeated. The authors acknowledge that the re-examination of existing data from the perspective of grounded-theory methodology departs from its original intent. The coding paradigm was adapted to retrospective data to elicit the dimensions of uncertainty and the management processes people use to deal with cancer and its consequences.

Deliberative application is suggested in relation to theoretic sampling under different cultural conditions or among patients with different chronic illness. Inherent in these suggestions is sampling with patients for whom uncertainty has varying significance.

That health care professionals use insights to provide care suggests the possibility for intervention studies to determine if nursing care deliberately structured to manage uncertainty and facilitate coping would have reciprocal positive effects on these experiences.

INDEX

A

Adaptation model 205
  adaptive modes 214
    interdependent mode 215
    physiological mode 214
    role function 215
    self-concept 215
  assumptions from
    adaptation level theory 210
    based on veritivity 211
    humanism 211
    philosophical assumptions 211
    scientific assumptions 211
    systems theory 210
  concepts used
    adaptation level 209
    adaptation problems 209
    adaptive (effector) modes 209
    adaptive responses 210
    cognator 209
    contextual stimuli 209
    focal stimulus 209
    interdependence 210
    physiological mode 210
    regulator 209
    residual stimuli 209
    role performance mode 210
    Roy adaptation model 210
    self-concept mode 210
    system 209
  elements of the Roy's adaptation model 212
    cognator subsystem 214
    coping mechanism 213
    output and feedback 213
    person theory 212
  evaluation of the theory 223
  evolution of theory 206
  metaparadigm and RAM 215
    environment 216
    health 216
    human being 215
    nursing 216
  nursing process and Roy's adaptation model 217
    assessment of stimuli 218
    behaviour assessment 217
    evaluation 219
    implementation 219
    nursing diagnosis 218
    planning 218
  Roy nursing process applied to nursing 219
  Sister Callista Roy 205
  work and the characteristics of a theory 220
Aesthetics 30, 32
Art of clinical nursing 130
  characteristics of theory and Wiedenbach's work 144
  concepts used 132
    art 135
    communication skills 134
    conferring 135
    consulting 135
    coordination 134
    deliberative action 136
    factual knowledge 133
    identification 134
    interpretation 135
    judgement 133
    knowledge 133
    ministration 134
    need for help 132
    nurse 132
    patients 132
    philosophy 133
    practical knowledge 133
    practice 133
    preconception 135
    procedural skills 134
    purpose 132
    rational action 135
    reactionary action 135
    reporting 135
    skills 134
    speculative knowledge 133
    stimulus 135
    validation 134
  Ernestine Wiedenbach's 130
  evaluation of theory 145
  evolution of theory 130
  framework of clinical nursing 136
  nursing practice and process 140
    identification 140
    ministration 140
    validation 140
  paradigm of Wiedenbach 143
    environment 144
    health 143
    human being 143
    nursing 144
  prescriptive theory 137
    central purpose 138
    prescription 138
  realities
    agent 139
    framework 140
    goal 139
    mean 139
    recipient 139

B

Behavioural system model 190
  behavioural system model 196
  concepts used 192
    achievement subsystem 193
    aggressive subsystems 194
    attachment-affiliative subsystem 193
    behaviour 192
    behavioural system 192
    biological subsystem 193
    dependency subsystem 193
    equilibrium 194
    sexual subsystem 193
    stressor 194
    subsystems 193
    system 192
    tension 194

development of model 194
Dorothy E Johnson 190
evaluation of theory 204
evolution of theory 190
nursing process and Johnson
    work assessment 200
    diagnosis 200
    evaluation 201
    implementation 201
    planning 201
paradigm
    environment 199
    health 199
    human being 199
    nursing 199
work and characteristics of a
    theory 201

C

Care and cure models 86
Caring in perinatal nursing 396
Concept 10, 19, 30
Conceptual models on nursing
    337
    concepts used 341
    conceptual models 22
        Johnson's behavioural
            systems model 22
        King's open system model
            23
        Levine's conservation
            model 23
        Neuman's health care
            systems model 23
        Orem's model of self-care
            24
        Roger's model of the
            unitary person 24
        Roy's adaptation model 24
    evaluation of theory 347
Evelyn Adam 337
evolution of theory 340
nursing implications 343
    consequences 346
    education 344
    intervention 346
    practice 343
    research 345
Conservation principles 242, 245
    concepts used 244
        conservation 245
        holism 245
        holistic 244
        integrity 245
conservation of social integrity
    250
evaluation of theory 256
evolution of theory 243
Myra Estrin Levine 242
nursing process and Levine's
    theory
    assessment 252
    evaluation 253
    implementation 253
    nursing diagnosis 252
    planning 253
paradigm of Levine theory
    250
    environment 251
    health 250
    human being 250
    nursing 251
theory of Levine
    adaptation 247
    conservation of energy 249
    conservation of personal
        integrity 249
    conservation of structural
        integrity 249
    integrity principles of
        conservation 248
    levels of behaviours 248
work and characteristics of a
    theory 253
Cultural care theory 257
assessment of nursing
    diagnosis 266
evaluation of theory 271
evolution of theory 258
    transcultural nursing 260
    cultural care theory 260
Madeleine M. Leininger 257
nursing process and
    Leininger's theory 266
orientational definitions 262
paradigm and Leininger's
    theory 264
    environment 265
    health 264
    human being 264
    nursing 266
    planning and implementation
        266
work and the characteristic of
    a theory 267

E

Empirics 28, 31
Environment model 40
    evolution of theory 41
    Florence Nightingale 40
    Nightingale and nursing
        process
        assessment 47
        evaluation 48
        implementation 48
        nursing diagnoses 47
        planning 48
Nightingale's theory on
    environment 42
    bed and bedding 44
    chattering hopes and
        advices 45
    health of houses 43
    light 43
    noise 43
    nutrition and taking food 45
    personal cleanliness 44
    social considerations 45
    variety 44
    ventilation and warning 43
paradigm of Nightingale's
    environment model 45
    environment 47
    health 47
    human being 47
    nursing 45
the characteristics of theory
    48
evaluation of theory 49
Typology or 21 problems 52, 54
    concepts used 55
    health 55
    nursing 55
    nursing problem 56
evaluation of theory 59
evolution of theory 53
Faye Glenn Abdellah 52
paradigm of Abdellah's
    typology 57
    environment 57
    health 57

human being 57
nursing 58
nursing process and Abdellah 58
work and characteristics of theory 58
Ethics 28, 31
Excellence and power 313
  assertions of theory 321
  concepts used
    advanced beginner 318
    competent 318
    expert 319
    novice 318
    proficient 318
  evaluation of theory 324
  evolution of theory 314
  nursing implications
    education 322
    practice 322
    research 323
  paradigm of Benners' theory 319
    health 320
    nursing 320
    person 320
    situation 321
  Patricia Benner 313

H

Health promotion model 384
  concepts used 386
  evaluation of theory 388
  evolution of theory 385
  Nola J. Pender 384
  nursing implications 387
Human-to-human relationships 304
  concepts used 305
    communication 306
    empathy 306
    hope 306
    hopelessness 306
    human being 305
    human-to-human relationship 306
    interaction 306
    nurse 305
    nurse-patient interaction 306
    nursing need 306
    pain 305
    patient 305
    rapport 306
    suffering 305
    sympathy 306
    therapeutic use of self 306
  evolution of theory 304
  Joyce Travelbee 304
  paradigm of theory
    assertions of theory 307
    human-to-human relationship 308
    nursing implications 309
    research 310

I

Illness trajectory theory 399
Interpersonal relations theory 109
  concepts used 111
  evaluation of theory 119
  evolution of theory 111
  Hildegard E. Peplau 109
  interpersonal process and nursing process 116
    assessment 117
    nursing diagnosis 117
    nursing roles 114
      counselling role 115
      leadership role 115
      role of resource person 114
      role of the stranger 114
      surrogate role 115
      teaching role 115
  paradigm of Peplau's theory 115
    environment 116
    health 115
    human being 115
    nursing 116
  phases of interpersonal relationship 112
    exploitation 113
    identification 113
    orientation 112
    resolution 114
  work and characteristics of theory 117

M

Man-living-health theory 348
  evolution of theory 349
    environment 351
    health 350
    man 350
    nursing 350
  assertions of theory 352
  assumptions of theory 355
    becoming assumptions 356
    human assumptions 355
  concepts used 351
  evaluation of theory 364
  nursing implications 362
    education 362
    practice 362
    research 363
  paradigm and Parse theory 358
    health 358
    human being 358
    nursing 358
  Parse's work and characteristics of theory 359
  principles 356
  Rosemarie Rizzo Parse's 348
  structures 357
Maternal role attainment 327
  assertions of theory/model 332
  concepts used 330
  evaluation of theory 335
  evolution of theory 328
  nursing implications 334
  paradigm of Mercebs theory 332
    environment 332
    health 332
    nursing 332
    person 332
  Ramona T. Mercer 327
Menstrual care activities of daily living 389

N

Nursing process theory 121
  characteristics of theory and Orlando's work 127
  concepts used 123
    nurse's action 125
    nurse's reaction 124
    patient behaviour 124

professional function 123
evaluation of theory 128
evolution of theory 122
Ia Jean Orlando 121
nursing process and Orlando process discipline 126
    assessment phase 127
    nursing diagnosis 127
paradigm of Orlando
    health 126
    human being 126
    nursing 126

P

Parent-child interaction model 375
    assertions of Barnard 380
    concepts used 378
    evaluation of theory 382
    evolution of theory 377
    Kathryn E. Barnard 375
    nursing implications 381
    paradigm of Barnard model 379
Pattern of knowing 33
Perimenopausal process 394
Personal risking 397
Philosophy and science on caring 96
    characteristic of theory and Watson's work 106
    curative factors 102
        allowance for existential-phenomenological factors 104
        assistance with the gratification of human needs 104
        cultivation of sensitivity of self and others 102
        helping-trust relationships 102
        humanistic-altruistic system of values 102
        instillation of faith-hope 102
        promotion and acceptance of the expression of feelings 103
        promotion of interpersonal teaching learning 103
        provision of suitable conducive environment 104
        use of scientific problem-solving for decision-making 103
    evaluation of theory 107
    evolution of theory 98
    (Margaret) Jean Harman Watson 96
    nursing process and Watson 106
    paradigm of Watson theory 105
        environment 105
        health 105
        human being 105
        nursing 105
    theory of caring 100

Q

Quality of family caregiving 390

R

Relapse among ex-smokers 391
Rhythm model 298
    concepts used 299
    evaluation of theory 302
    evolution of theory 299
    Joyce J. Fitzpatrick 298
    logical form 300
    nursing implications 302

S

Science of unitary human beings 273
    characteristics of theory and research work 281
    evaluation of theory 284
    evolution of theory 274
    Martha E. Rogers 273
    nursing process and Rogers' homeodynamics 281
    paradigm of Rogers' theory
        environment 280
        health 280
        nursing 280
    principles of homeodynamics 278
        helicy 279
        integrality 279
        resonancy 279
    Rogers' basic assumptions 276
Self-care theory 72
    concepts used by Orem 75
        developmental self-care requisites 76
        self-care requisition 75
        theory of self-care 75
        universal self-care requisites 75
    Dorothea Elizabeth Orem 72
    evolution of theory 73
    general theory of nursing 75
    Orem's on nursing process
        designing for regulatory operation 82
        nursing diagnosis and prescription 82
        production and managing nursing system 82
    paradigm of Orem's theory 80
        environment 81
        health 81
        human being 80
        nursing 81
        nursing technologies 81
    theory of nursing system 77
        partly compensatory nursing system 79
        supportive-educative nursing system 80
        wholly compensatory nursing system 78
    theory of self-care deficit 76
    work and characteristics of theory 92
Self-transcendence 395
Symbolic interactionism 366
    assertions of theory/model 370
    assumptions 368
        analytic 369
        genetic 369
    concepts used 367
    evaluation of theory 373
    evolution of theory 367
    Joan Riehl 366
    nursing implications 371
        education 371
        practice 371

Index

Systems model 225
  Betty Neuman 225
  evaluation of theory 239
  evolution of theory 226
  Neuman system model 228
    degree of reaction 233
    environment 229
    normal line of defenses 232
    open system 229
    prevention of intervention 233
    reconstitution 234
    stressors 232
    wholistic client approach 229
  paradigm of Neuman's model 234
    environment 235
    health 235
    human being 234
    nursing 235
  propositions of the Neuman systems model 235
  systems model and the characteristics of a theory 237
  systems model and the nursing process 236

T

Theory 1, 25
  analysis and evaluation 7
  categories 26
  characteristics 6
  classification 14
  definitions 1-3
  developing nursing's patterns of knowing 37
  level of theory 25
  nursing theory and knowledge 26
    concepts of knowing and knowledge 26
    pattern of knowing in nursing 27
  nature 5
  patterns gone wild 36
  purpose of theory in a nursing research 16
    purpose as a declarative statement 19

purpose as a hypothesis 19
purpose as a question 19
research frameworks 17
selection of theory in research 18
statement of the purpose of the study 18
purposes 3
steps of theory development 9
  criticism of fault finding 9
  statement of the problem 9
testing theory 11
theory and nursing research 12
theory construction 10
theory of structure and development 8
types of theory to be tested 25
validation of theory 11
Theory of goal attainment 147
  evaluation of theory 166
  evolution of theory 148
  Imogene King 147
  interpersonal system 153
    communication 154
    interaction 154
    role 154
    stress 155
    transactions 154
  open system framework 151
  paradigm of King's theory 159
    environment 160
    health 160
    human being 159
    nursing 161
  personal systems 152
    body image 153
    growth and development 153
    learning 153
    perceptions 152
    self 152
    space 153
    time 153
  social system 155
    authority 156
    control 157
    decision-making 157
    organization 156
    power 156

status 156
theory of goal attainment 157
  interaction 157
  perception 158
theory of goal attainment and the nursing process 161
work and the characteristics of a theory 163
Theory of health 286
  concepts used 289
    consciousness 289
    health 289
    movement 290
    pattern 289
    time and space 290
  evaluation of theroy 296
  evolution of theroy 287
  Margaret A. Newman 286
  Newman model of health 290
  nursing process and theory of health 293
  paradigm and theory of health 291
    environment 292
    health 292
    human being 292
    nursing 293
  work and the characteristics of a theory 294
Theory of humanistic nursing 169
  elements of humanistic nursing 173
  evolution of theory 170
  Josephine G Paterson and Lorett T Zderad 169
  nursing as dialogue 173
    call and response 174
    community 174
    phenomenologic nursology 174
    presence 174
    relating 173
  nursing process and phenomenologic nursology 175
    assessments 176
    evaluation 176
    nursing diagnosis 176
    planning and implementation 176

paradigm and theory on
    humanistic nursing 172
  health 172
  nursing 172
  Paterson and Zderad's work 177
Theory of modelling and role
    modelling 179
  adaptive potential 182
  affiliated-individuation 182
  aims of intervention 180
  APAM model 182
  evaluation of modelling 184
  modelling 179
  paradigm of theory 182
    environment 183
    health 183
    human beings 182
    nursing 183
  role modelling 180
Theory of nursing as caring 186
  Anne Boykin and Savina
    Schoenhofer 186
  conception of nursing as a
    discipline and profession 187

nursing as caring and
    paradigm 189
nursing as caring and the
    nursing process 189
perception of persons as
    caring 186
theory of nursing as caring 187
Theory of uncertainty 392

U

Unique function of nurses 61
  concepts used 64
    needs 64
  concepts used by Hall 88
  evaluation of theory 70
  evaluation of theory 94
  evolution of definition of
    nursing 63
  evolution of theory 62
  evolution of theory 86
  Henderson on nursing
    process 68
  nursing assessment 68
  nursing diagnosis 68

nursing evaluation 69
nursing implementation 69
nursing plan 69
Henderson's 14 basic needs 65
metaparadigm of Henderson
    theory 66
  environment 67
  health 67
  human 66
  nursing 67
nursing process and Hall 91
paradigm of Hall 90
  environment 91
  health 91
  human being 90
  nursing 91
presentation of theory 89
  care 89
  core 90
  cure 90

W

Work and characteristics of
    theory 83
  evaluation of theory 84